NATIONAL ACADEMIES

Scie
Eng
Me

T0221662

Essential Health Care Services Addressing Intimate Partner Violence

Susan J. Curry, and Crystal J. Bell,
Editors

Committee on Sustaining Essential
Health Care Services Related to
Intimate Partner Violence During
Public Health Emergencies

Board on Health Care Services

Board on Health Sciences Policy

Board on Population Health and Public
Health Practice

Health and Medicine Division

Consensus Study Report

NATIONAL ACADEMIES PRESS 500 Fifth Street, NW Washington, DC 20001

This activity was supported by a contract between the National Academy of Sciences and the Health Resources and Services Administration of the U.S. Department of Health and Human Services. Any opinions, findings, conclusions, or recommendations expressed in this publication do not necessarily reflect the views of any organization or agency that provided support for the project.

International Standard Book Number-13: 978-0-309-71389-4
International Standard Book Number-10: 0-309-71389-7
Digital Object Identifier: https://doi.org/10.17226/27425
Library of Congress Control Number: 2024937618

This publication is available from the National Academies Press, 500 Fifth Street, NW, Keck 360, Washington, DC 20001; (800) 624-6242 or (202) 334-3313; http://www.nap.edu.

Printed in the United States of America.

Suggested citation: National Academies of Sciences, Engineering, and Medicine. 2024. *Essential health care services addressing intimate partner violence.* Washington, DC: The National Academies Press. https://doi.org/10.17226/27425.

The **National Academy of Sciences** was established in 1863 by an Act of Congress, signed by President Lincoln, as a private, nongovernmental institution to advise the nation on issues related to science and technology. Members are elected by their peers for outstanding contributions to research. Dr. Marcia McNutt is president.

The **National Academy of Engineering** was established in 1964 under the charter of the National Academy of Sciences to bring the practices of engineering to advising the nation. Members are elected by their peers for extraordinary contributions to engineering. Dr. John L. Anderson is president.

The **National Academy of Medicine** (formerly the Institute of Medicine) was established in 1970 under the charter of the National Academy of Sciences to advise the nation on medical and health issues. Members are elected by their peers for distinguished contributions to medicine and health. Dr. Victor J. Dzau is president.

The three Academies work together as the **National Academies of Sciences, Engineering, and Medicine** to provide independent, objective analysis and advice to the nation and conduct other activities to solve complex problems and inform public policy decisions. The National Academies also encourage education and research, recognize outstanding contributions to knowledge, and increase public understanding in matters of science, engineering, and medicine.

Learn more about the National Academies of Sciences, Engineering, and Medicine at **www.nationalacademies.org**.

Reviewers

This Consensus Study Report was reviewed in draft form by individuals chosen for their diverse perspectives and technical expertise. The purpose of this independent review is to provide candid and critical comments that will assist the National Academies of Sciences, Engineering, and Medicine in making each published report as sound as possible and to ensure that it meets the institutional standards for quality, objectivity, evidence, and responsiveness to the study charge. The review comments and draft manuscript remain confidential to protect the integrity of the deliberative process.

We thank the following individuals for their review of this report:

DAVID M. ABRAMSON, New York University
ANDREIA ALEXANDER, Indiana University School of Medicine
KAMILA A. ALEXANDER, Johns Hopkins University School of
  Nursing
CATHERINE CERULLI, University of Rochester
MELISSA L. GILLIAM, Ohio State University
TONDA L. HUGHES, Columbia University School of Nursing
KATHERINE M. IVERSON, Boston University
DEAN G. KILPARTRICK, Medical University of South Carolina
ALEXANDER KRIST, Virginia Commonwealth University
ANNIE LEWIS-O'CONNOR, Brigham and Women's Hospital
CLINT OSBORN, DC Homeland Security and Emergency Management
  Agency
SARAH M. PEITZMEIER, University of Michigan School of Nursing

JENNIFER L. PIATT, Arizona State University
JESSICA R. WILLIAMS, University of North Carolina at Chapel Hill

Although the reviewers listed above provided many constructive comments and suggestions, they were not asked to endorse the conclusions or recommendations of this report, nor did they see the final draft before its release. The review of this report was overseen by **BETTY R. FERRELL,** City of Hope National Medical Center, and **MARSHALL H. CHIN,** University of Chicago. They were responsible for making certain that an independent examination of this report was carried out in accordance with the standards of the National Academies and that all review comments were carefully considered. Responsibility for the final content rests entirely with the authoring committee and the National Academies.

Acknowledgments

The committee extends its sincere thanks to the many individuals who shared their time and expertise to support its work and inform its deliberations. The study was sponsored by the Health Resources and Services Administration's (HRSA's) Office of Women's Health. The committee extends its thanks to HRSA for initiating this effort to identify the essential health care services related to intimate partner violence and hopes that the report will positively affect HRSA's programming in this field. In particular, the committee thanks Timothy Corrigan, Stephen Hayes, Ellen Hendrix, and Helen Wesley for their guidance and support. The committee benefited greatly from discussions with the individuals who presented at the committee's open sessions: Maria Balata, Gregory J. Della Roca, Marianne Gausche-Hill, Lorena Halwood, Hirsch Handmaker, Lisa D. Martin, Nancy Mautone-Smith, Ivon Mesa, Sarah Peitzmeier, Anita Ravi, Athena Sherman, Melissa Simon, and Rob Stephenson. Agendas for the public meetings are located in Appendix C.

Our appreciation goes to the reviewers for their invaluable feedback on an earlier draft of the report and to the monitor and coordinator who oversaw the report review. The committee acknowledges the many staff within the Health and Medicine Division who provided support in various ways to this project, including Crystal J. Bell (study director), Taylor King (associate program officer), Lyle Carrera (research associate), Marjani Cephus (research associate), Anesia Wilks (senior program assistant), Karen Helsing (senior program officer), Scott Wollek (senior program officer), Rose Marie Martinez (senior director, Board on Population Health and Public Health Practice), Arzoo Tayyeb (finance business partner), and

Julie Wiltshire (senior finance business partner). The committee extends great thanks and appreciation to Sharyl Nass, senior director, Board on Health Care Services, who oversaw the project. The committee also appreciates Anne Marie Houppert's (senior librarian) research assistance. The report review, production, and communications staff all provided valuable guidance to ensure the success of the final product. Catherine McKinley and Lisa Fedina drafted papers for the committee, which were valuable contributions to the narrative.

Finally, the committee thanks Allie Boman of Briere Associates for drafting technical writing and editorial assistance in preparing the report and Robert Pool, copyeditor for the final report.

Contents

Boxes, Figures, and Tables

TABLES

Acronyms and Abbreviations

ACA	Patient Protection and Affordable Care Act
ACS	alternate care site
AI/AN	American Indian and Alaska Native
ART	antiretroviral therapy
ASPR	Administration for Strategic Preparedness and Response
CCR	Coordinated Community Response
CDC	U.S. Centers for Disease Control and Prevention
CFPI	Colorado Family Planning Initiative
CMS	Centers for Medicare & Medicaid Services
CSC	crisis standards of care
DCM	disaster case management or manager
DHS	U.S. Department of Homeland Security
DMAT	Disaster Medical Assistance Team
DOVE	Domestic Violence Enhanced Home Visitation Program
DV	domestic violence
ED	emergency department
EMAC	Emergency Management Assistance Compact
EMTALA	Emergency Medicine Treatment and Active Labor Act
ESF	Emergency Support Function
ESP	Essential Services Package
EUA	Emergency Use Authorization

FDA	U.S. Food and Drug Administration
FEMA	Federal Emergency Management Agency
FMS	federal medical station
FQHC	Federally Qualified Health Center

HCC	Health Care Coalition
HHS	U.S. Department of Health and Human Services
HIPAA	Health Insurance Portability and Accountability Act
HIV	Human Immunodeficiency Virus
HRSA	Health Resources and Services Administration

IFRC	International Federation of the Red Cross and Red Crescent
IHS	Indian Health Service
IPV	intimate partner violence
IPVAP	Intimate Partner Violence Assistance Program

LARC	long-acting reversible contraceptive
LBTQ	lesbian, bisexual, transgender, and queer
LGBTQ	lesbian, gay, bisexual, transgender, and queer
LEP	limited English proficiency

MISP	Minimum Initial Services Package

NDMS	National Disaster Medical System
NDRF	National Disaster Recovery Framework
NEA	National Emergencies Act
NEISS–AIP	National Electronic Injury Surveillance System–All Injury Program
NISVS	National Intimate Partner and Sexual Violence Survey
NRF	National Response Framework
NVDRS	National Violent Death Reporting System

OB-GYN	obstetrician/gynecologist
OPA	Office of Population Affairs
OWH	Office of Women's Health (at HRSA)

PHE	public health emergency
PHS	Public Health Service
PHSA	Public Health Service Act
PPE	personal protective equipment
PREP	Pandemic Readiness and Emergency Preparedness Act
PRAMS	Pregnancy Risk Assessment Monitoring System
PROMiSE	Promoting Safety in Emergencies

PTSD   post-traumatic stress disorder
PurpLE   Purpose, Listen and Engage (health foundation)

RISE   Recovering from Intimate Partner Violence through Strengths
            and Empowerment
RSF   Recovery Support Functions

SANE   sexual assault nurse examiner
SCBHC   school- and college-based health center
SLTT   state, local, tribal, and territorial
STI   sexually transmitted infection
SUD   substance use disorder

TBI   traumatic brain injury

UNFPA   United Nations Population Fund
USPHS   U.S. Public Health Service
USPSTF   U.S. Preventive Services Task Force

VAWA   Violence Against Women Act
VHA   Veterans Health Administration
VOAD   volunteer organization active in disasters

WHO   World Health Organization
WPSI   Women's Preventive Services Initiative

Preface

Intimate partner violence (IPV) is deeply troubling and complex. A comprehensive approach that focuses both on providing a broad range of services and on ultimately eliminating IPV would extend far beyond the health care delivery system. Moreover, the committee recognized that even in steady state conditions our current health care system does not equitably deliver essential health care services. While the committee desired to address a broader scope of how to eliminate IPV and improve our overall health care system, the committee operated within the scope of our statement of task and with the body of research available. This committee's task and this consensus report focus specifically on the essential health care services for IPV, first during steady state conditions, then in the context of public health emergencies (PHEs).

The committee members brought diverse thought and multidisciplinary expertise to the statement of work put forth by HRSA. It became apparent early in our committee discussions and public sessions that IPV care providers and those responsible for planning and carrying out PHE response can benefit from learning more about each other's respective fields. Thus, our report includes both basic information about IPV and PHE response to facilitate future cooperation in PHE preparation, planning, and response. Through hard work, deliberation, and careful review of the evidence, the committee achieved consensus on the 11 recommendations highlighted in this report. The recommendations are pragmatic, actionable, and address key gaps in responding to IPV during PHEs that were identified over the course of this study.

Given the complexities of both IPV and PHEs, there are multiple sectors involved in the response (clinicians, disaster responders, emergency planners, etc.). Due to the various ways these response systems are structured across municipalities, the committee did not name specific local and state organizations that might lead the efforts in standing up the essential services during PHEs. The committee dedicated time and deep consideration to recommendations that call out specific national entities, ensuring that those entities were the most appropriate to take charge in those specific recommendations. I am convinced that implementation of these recommendations will be transformative for providing health care services to those experiencing IPV in steady state and PHE conditions.

Susan J. Curry, Ph.D.
Committee Chair

Summary[1]

Intimate partner violence (IPV) refers to abuse or aggression committed by a current or former intimate partner. IPV includes, but is not limited to, physical violence, sexual violence, stalking, psychological aggression, and reproductive coercion. While estimates of IPV prevalence vary, primarily due to under-reporting and terminology inconsistencies, the data generally indicate that it is common in the United States. The most commonly used source to estimate the population-level prevalence of IPV in the United States is the Centers for Disease Control and Prevention's (CDC's) National Intimate Partner and Sexual Violence Survey (NISVS). The most recent survey, conducted in 2016 through 2017, estimated that nearly half of women in the United States had experienced IPV in some form during their lifetime.

A substantial body of literature has documented adverse health outcomes associated with experiencing IPV. Women with a documented history of experiencing IPV had 4.5 times more emergency department (ED) visits than those without according to an analysis of insurance claims from across the United States. Some of the most common and most serious injuries include injuries to the head, face, and neck; traumatic brain injury; injuries due to strangulation; and musculoskeletal injuries. Escalating injury severity is often a precursor to homicide at the hands of an intimate partner. Additionally, the effects of IPV on gynecologic and reproductive health can be severe. IPV is associated with numerous adverse reproductive health

---

[1] This summary is intended to provide a high-level overview of the report itself. This summary does not include references. Evidence and citations to support the text and recommendations herein are provided in the body of the report.

1

outcomes, including abnormal vaginal bleeding, unintended and rapid repeat pregnancies, sexually transmitted infections, and HIV infection. During pregnancy, IPV increases the risk of preterm delivery, low-birthweight infants, preeclampsia, other obstetric complications, and fetal and neonatal death. Experiencing IPV is also associated with substantial adverse mental health outcomes, including post-traumatic stress disorder, anxiety, depression, substance misuse, and suicidality.

Women's[2] health and well-being are disproportionately adversely affected by public health emergencies (PHEs).[3] Women are at greater risk for experiencing violence, including IPV, during PHEs. Multiple studies conducted in the United States after Hurricane Katrina, after the Deepwater Horizon oil spill, and throughout the COVID-19 pandemic have found increases in the prevalence and severity of IPV against women in the aftermath of these events. Women who experience IPV during a disaster or PHE are exposed to physical and psychological trauma due to IPV and from the PHE. In light of this, the Health Resources and Services Administration's (HRSA's) Office of Women's Health (OWH) identified a need to identify the essential health care services related to IPV for women and how to plan for and sustain access to essential health care services related to IPV during PHEs.

COMMITTEE'S CHARGE

HRSA's OWH contracted with the National Academies of Sciences, Engineering, and Medicine to convene a multidisciplinary panel of experts to address the statement of task (Box S-1) and produce recommendations for delivering essential health care services for women related to IPV.

Study Scope

This study focuses on women aged 13 and older that directly experience IPV, based on guidance from the study sponsor. The committee acknowledges that the experience of IPV is not limited to women. There is a growing body of research into the effects of experiencing IPV on men, including transgender men. However, health care interventions specifically for men experiencing IPV are beyond the scope of this study. Additionally,

---

[2] The committee used an inclusive approach to define woman/women as used throughout this report. For the purpose of this report, woman/women encompass cisgender women, transgender women, and people whose gender identity is not male, who are non-binary or otherwise gender expansive.

[3] The committee applied the following definition for public health emergency throughout the report: a situation with health consequences whose scale, timing, or unpredictability threatens to overwhelm the routine capabilities of the affected geographic area.

BOX S-1
Statement of Task and Charge to the Committee

An ad hoc committee of the National Academies of Sciences, Engineering, and Medicine shall develop a conceptual framework for delivering essential preventive and primary health care services related to Intimate Partner Violence (IPV) during public health emergencies (PHEs), using an all-hazards approach.[a] The committee's framework shall:

- Identify essential health care services related to IPV in non-PHEs (steady state) based on currently available evidence;
- Define essential health care services related to IPV in PHEs based on currently available evidence;
- Identify ways to prepare for and prioritize the provision of essential health care services related to IPV before PHEs;
- Describe health disparities related to IPV in PHEs;
- Identify innovations and best practices to prepare for and operationalize the equitable delivery of essential health care services related to IPV during PHEs;
- Identify promising practices in the prevention of IPV; and
- Develop strategies to overcome barriers faced by HRSA-supported and safety-net care settings in providing essential health care services related to IPV during PHEs, particularly for underserved populations.

---

[a] An all-hazards approach is an integrated approach to emergency preparedness planning that focuses on capacities and capabilities that are critical to prepare for, respond to, and recover from the full spectrum of emergencies or disasters, whether human-made or natural. The committee notes that their application of an all-hazards approach acknowledges that not all disasters and emergencies are identical, nor are their effects on different populations and communities.

---

while the committee identifies several promising prevention strategies, consideration of health care services for individuals who engage in IPV is outside of the scope of the committee's charge. While child abuse is a serious issue that can intersect with IPV and witnessing IPV can have adverse effects on a child, addressing these issues also falls outside of the parameters of the statement of task.

The committee acknowledges that the complex nature of addressing IPV may necessitate a broad array of supports and strategies to address the many effects of IPV as well as its root causes. However, the scope of this study is limited to health care services.[4] As such, when considering essential health care services for IPV, the committee limited its consideration to IPV care that is delivered in or referrable from a health care setting. The committee did consider a specific group of support services that are directed at protecting the immediate health and safety of women experiencing IPV and that often serve as an initial point of contact for women to access IPV-related care, including health care.

The Committee's Approach

The statement of task emphasized the value of having an overarching conceptual framework to guide the committee's process for identifying essential health care services related to IPV. The committee selected the Social Ecological Model as the conceptual framework to guide its understanding of the health care needs of women experiencing IPV and to identify the essential health care services related to IPV (Figure S-1).[5] Health care services related to IPV are delivered in multiple settings within the health care system as well as in community-based settings outside of a defined health care system. Examples of these community-based settings include shelters for women experiencing IPV and community centers that provide support groups or advocacy services for women. In some cases, people experiencing IPV may be referred to community-based care from the traditional health care setting. In other cases, these community-based settings may be the first site of care. As noted in the Care Coordination Model, high-quality referrals and transitions to resources outside of the traditional health care system are a key component of effective health care delivery. Therefore, the committee felt that it was important to acknowledge the role of community-based organizations in IPV-related care and emphasize the importance of warm referrals to that care, recognizing the value and interdependence of connections between the health care system and community-based care settings.[6]

The committee recognizes that some of the essential health care services identified may be unavailable due to state-level restrictions placed on reproductive health care services or federal restrictions that may apply to the use of federal funding for such services. However, significant scientific evidence of increased risk for serious adverse maternal and fetal health outcomes,

---

[4] The committee defines *health care services* as care delivered in or referrable from a health care setting.

[5] An explanation of the Social Ecological Model can be found at https://www.cdc.gov/violenceprevention/about/social-ecologicalmodel.html (accessed October 20, 2023).

[6] *Warm referrals*, or warm handoffs, are transfers of care between members of a health care team that occur with the patient's permission, often with an in-person introduction. This approach can also be used when referring a patient to community-based services.

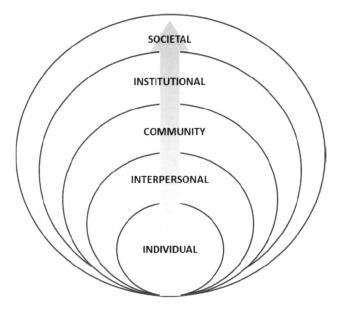

FIGURE S-1 Social Ecological Model.
SOURCE: Concept from McLeroy et al., 1988. Figure adapted from NASEM report *Getting to Zero Alcohol-Impaired Driving Fatalities: A Comprehensive Approach to a Persistent Problem* (2018).

including death, as well as elevated risk for increased severity or frequency of IPV and intimate partner homicide in the perinatal period support the inclusion of these services.

Health Care Services

Health care services related to IPV are delivered in multiple settings across health care systems, including primary and specialty care, such as practices specific to women's health (e.g., reproductive health care clinics), perinatal-specific care settings, and orthopedic clinics; emergency departments; and behavioral health care settings. Women experiencing IPV report at least 20 percent more health care utilization than those who have not reported experiencing IPV, a difference that continues after the abuse has ended.

Several federal programs have been established to deliver health care to people residing in under-resourced communities, including women from populations that are disproportionately affected by IPV. These include HRSA-supported Federally Qualified Health Centers and clinics supported by provisions of Title X, the federal program that supports the delivery of family planning and related reproductive health care services to individuals with lower incomes.[7]

Essential Health Care Services Related to Intimate Partner Violence

The committee's process for identifying essential health care services related to IPV during steady state conditions was informed by an extensive review of evidence from literature searches; recommendations from the U.S. Preventive Services Task Force (USPSTF), the IIRSA-funded Women's Preventive Services Initiative (WPSI), and the World Health Organization (WHO); and insight gleaned from a commissioned paper and presentations to the committee by experts in IPV-related care.

The committee identified the following criteria for identifying essential health care services related to IPV:

- evidence-based health care services that address the most common and most serious health outcomes related to experiencing IPV;
- preventive services recommended by USPSTF and WPSI; and
- specific support services required to meet the basic safety and housing needs of people experiencing IPV.

This analysis identified several serious and high-prevalence adverse health effects related to experiencing IPV. These health issues can be grouped into the general categories of acute physical injuries, gynecologic and reproductive health issues, perinatal and obstetric health issues, behavioral health issues (including mental health and substance use), and other chronic health issues that are either exacerbated by acute IPV or related to experiencing long-term IPV. The committee also prioritized health care services that facilitate disclosure and protect the safety of those experiencing IPV and their children, if needed. After reviewing the evidence with the above criteria in mind, the committee identified a list of essential health care services related to IPV.

> **Recommendation 1: The committee recommends that the Health Resources and Services Administration and all U.S. health care systems classify the following as essential health care services related to intimate partner violence (IPV):**
> - **Universal IPV screening and inquiry**
> - **Universal IPV education**
> - **Safety planning**

---

[7] *Title X of the Public Health Service Act* 42 USC § 300 to 300a-6.

- Forensic medical examinations
- Emergency medical care
- Treatment of physical injuries
- Reproductive health care, including all forms of Food and Drug Administration–approved contraception and pregnancy termination
- Screening and treatment of sexually transmitted infections and HIV
- Treatment for substance use disorders and addiction care
- Pharmacy and medication management
- Obstetric care, including perinatal home visits
- Primary and specialty care
- Mental health care
- Support services, including shelter, nutritional assistance, and child care
- Dental care

Universal IPV screening and education often serve as the point of entry for accessing IPV-related health care services. Pairing education with screening can help women understand the health effects of IPV and increase their awareness of the resources available to them. It can also provide an opportunity for women who may not be ready to disclose to a clinician that they are experiencing IPV to become aware of their options and available resources. Universal education involves offering information about healthy relationships, the intersections of IPV and health, and relevant supports and services during all clinical encounters. It can be delivered through prominently displayed posters and brochures as well as patient education discussions during the clinical encounter. Universal screening for IPV is an established standard of routine preventive health care for women in the United States. It involves inquiring about IPV with all women, regardless of the presence of signs, symptoms, or health conditions. The USPSTF and WPSI recommendations for IPV screening also recommend that those who screen positive should be provided with or referred to care and support services. Connecting women who screen positive for IPV with person-centered support and interventions that reduce exposure to IPV and improve health outcomes is critical. Safety planning is one of those crucial interventions. This is the process of collaborating with the woman experiencing IPV to empower her to develop strategies that increase safety by enhancing situational awareness of IPV-related risks in a manner that is consistent with her identified concerns and priorities. It is also an urgently important harm reduction strategy for women who do not feel they can leave an abusive relationship. Notably, when a woman leaves a partner who is engaging in IPV, this can be a period of increased risk for her, including escalating violence that can lead to her being killed by her partner.

Recommendation 2: Health care providers should consistently pair intimate partner violence (IPV) screening with universal IPV education and, for women who disclose IPV, provide warm referrals for health care and support services during both steady state conditions and public health emergencies.

Health Inequities and Barriers to Care

Health inequities and other barriers can make accessing essential health care services related to IPV even more challenging. Data indicate that many populations experiencing health inequities also report higher prevalence of IPV. These populations include non-Hispanic Black women; American Indian and Alaska Native women; Hispanic women; multiracial women; lesbians, bisexual, and transgender women; women from immigrant populations; and women with disabilities. When women experiencing health inequities also experience IPV, poor health outcomes are more likely.

Women face a variety of barriers to disclosing that they are experiencing IPV and to accessing needed care. For example, some women may face pressure from family members or their community to stay silent so as not to bring shame to the community by making what is considered a private problem public. Women from minoritized populations that have historically experienced discrimination and abuse when they sought medical care may distrust the health care system and be reluctant to disclose that they are experiencing IPV or seek care. Women who are immigrants often face additional hurdles when trying to access IPV-related health care services due to language barriers.

Maldistribution of health care and mental health providers, in which the distribution of providers does not match the health care needs of a geographic area, has led to health care deserts across the United States. These health care deserts have created additional barriers for women experiencing IPV to access the care that they need.

Health care systems have a responsibility to reduce barriers to IPV care by taking steps informed by the communities that they serve to reduce health inequities.

Recommendation 3: In order to reduce health inequities related to intimate partner violence (IPV), health care systems should:
- **Ensure that individuals from historically marginalized communities and other communities adversely affected by health inequities are included in IPV care program development and planning.**
- **Provide culturally and linguistically specific resources for IPV care.**
- **Evaluate and monitor the reach of their IPV care programs' efforts to ensure equitable access to those programs.**

Prevention

Primary prevention of IPV is crucial for reducing IPV, its consequences across the lifespan, and for promoting healthy families and communities. A key component of primary prevention is promoting healthy, respectful, and nonviolent relationships. Services for supporting survivors to increase their safety and reduce harm are key components of secondary prevention of IPV. Tertiary prevention strategies seek to address the long-term effects of experiencing IPV. Comprehensive approaches for IPV prevention combine these three components.

CDC developed guidance that highlights evidence-based prevention strategies to address known risk and protective factors for IPV. These include specific prevention strategies for adolescents that can disrupt the developmental pathways toward IPV. Sadly, IPV is not uncommon among adolescents, and many adults report that they first experienced IPV when they were younger than 25. The CDC guidance highlights strategies for adolescents that teach safe and healthy relationship skills and engage influential adults and peers in IPV education and prevention programs. Prevention strategies that are evidence based, easily implemented, and scalable are important tools for preventing IPV in this age group.

Recommendation 4: The Health Resources and Services Administration should disseminate best practices for ensuring that multi-sector, confidential services are available for adolescents experiencing intimate partner violence, including prevention services.

INTIMATE PARTNER VIOLENCE AND PUBLIC HEALTH EMERGENCIES

PHEs include infectious disease outbreaks; extreme weather events such as hurricanes, heat waves, and wildfires; earthquakes; and technological disasters such as mass power outages or oil spills. PHEs disrupt and stress communities and individuals, adversely affecting health and well-being at all levels of society. As previously noted, PHEs are associated with increased severity and frequency of IPV. The committee concluded that essential health care services are determined by the health care needs of the affected populations and not the ability to provide them. Therefore, essential health care services retain their designation of essential, regardless of whether a PHE has occurred. In light of this, as well as the serious adverse health effects associated with experiencing IPV, the committee determined that the essential health care services related to IPV during steady state conditions remained essential during PHEs.

The committee sought to address the balance between essential services and the substantial service obstacles created by a PHE. This led them

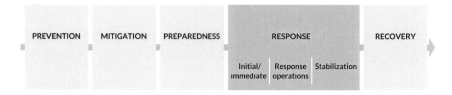

FIGURE S-2 Emergency management phases with divided response phase.

to draw on the Federal Emergency Management Agency's Community Lifelines approach as an organizing framework for sustaining essential health care services for IPV during a PHE. This approach prioritizes ensuring the delivery of services that are critical to protecting life safety, followed by those services that are essential but less time sensitive given the resource constraints during various points of the PHE.

The committee recognizes that not all essential health care services related to IPV can be restored simultaneously in the immediate wake of a disaster or during a PHE. Therefore, it recommends a phased approach to restoration of services. The committee defined three phases within the response phase of emergency management for the purpose of this report, described below, and delineated which essential services to reestablish during each phase of PHE response (Figure S-2).[8]

The *initial* or *immediate response phase* occurs while the situation is unstable and before supplementary resources can be deployed to the affected area or resources within the community can be redirected. During this phase, disaster health responders' efforts are focused on saving and sustaining life using limited resources.[9] The *response operations phase* occurs once the health care system and associated jurisdictional authorities have assessed the incident and have stood up relevant incident coordination structures. During this phase, disaster health responders have begun to receive additional resources, such as supplies and staff to support temporary care delivery sites. At this point, while health care delivery capacity has increased beyond life-saving and -sustaining activities, resources are not adequate to support the full delivery of all essential health care services related to IPV for all individuals. The *stabilization phase* occurs when basic lifeline services have been provided to PHE survivors, either by rapid reestablishment of lifeline services or through the employment of a contingency response solution. At this point all essential health care services related to IPV are available for all individuals.

---

[8] Emergency management generally involves five phases, prevention, mitigation, preparedness, response, and recovery. The committee divided the response phase into three parts to organize its phased approach to restoration of essential health care services related to IPV during PHEs.

[9] For the purposes of this report, *disaster health responders* are the leaders and staff with expertise in public health and health care who are working and providing care in those settings during response to a PHE.

Recommendation 5: Essential health care services related to intimate partner violence (IPV) during steady state conditions remain essential during public health emergencies (PHEs), but health care systems should restore them in phases that consider the obstacles to delivering this care during different phases of PHE response. (See Table S-1.)

TABLE S-1 Essential Health Care Services for IPV During Public Health Emergencies—A Phased Return to Steady State

Essential Health Care Service	PHASE WHEN SERVICE SHOULD BE RESTORED		
	Initial	Response operations	Stabilization
Universal IPV screening/inquiry and education			
Safety planning			
Forensic medical exams			
Emergency medical care			
Treatment of physical injury			
Gynecologic and reproductive health care including pregnancy termination	Urgent	Non-urgent	
Obstetric care	Urgent	Non-urgent	
Perinatal home visits			
Contraception and emergency contraception	Contraceptives not requiring procedures or immediate follow-up	All types of contraceptives	
Screening and treatment of sexually transmitted infections and HIV	Treatment and rapid testing	Treatment and all screening	
Substance abuse treatment	Withdrawal mitigation	All treatment	
Pharmacy/medication management			
Primary and specialty care			
Mental health care	Urgent/Crisis	Non-urgent	
Dental care	Urgent treatment for acute injuries	Urgent treatment for acute injuries	
Support services including shelter, nutritional assistance, child care			

Restore services for all patients

Selectively restore services for acute needs or restore targeted services

Do not restore services during this phase

The committee prioritized the delivery of essential health care services related to IPV that are most integral to protecting life safety during the initial phase of PHE response. In some cases, specific components of an essential health care service are essential for protecting life due to the severity and time-sensitive nature of certain IPV-related health conditions. In other cases, these components are critical for women from groups that have an elevated risk for serious or life-threatening outcomes, such as pregnant women. Those components should be available during the initial phase of PHE response with delivery efforts focused on those presenting with an immediate need. Then, as health care staff and supplies become more available, the full essential health care service can be delivered more broadly. For example, unintended pregnancy, as well as IPV during pregnancy, are associated with serious adverse health outcomes, including fetal death and intimate partner homicide. Thus, women who have experienced IPV-related rape or IPV-related unintended pregnancy that need to prevent or terminate a pregnancy have a time-sensitive need to access care.

Health Inequities, Public Health Emergencies, and Intimate Partner Violence

Historically and structurally marginalized populations experience worse outcomes than many other populations during PHEs. There is a substantial overlap between populations that are likely to experience worse outcomes during PHEs and populations that are more likely to experience health inequities. The interaction of weather- and climate-related disasters with the built environment causes damage to critical infrastructure that is essential for the health of communities, such as access to food, water, shelter, health care, transportation, and electrical power. Widening social inequalities, increasing urbanization, and rapid population growth—particularly in coastal areas—predispose certain groups to disaster-related disparities. Women who experience IPV in this context are more vulnerable to serious adverse health outcomes, particularly if the disaster health responders who they encounter are not adequately prepared to care for them.

Planning and Operationalization of Intimate Partner Violence Care During Public Health Emergencies

Immediately following a disaster, emergency health care may be delivered by federal and state, local, tribal, and territorial (SLTT) response teams or volunteer organizations active in disasters. These teams have diverse health care backgrounds, so IPV training may not be a requirement of their usual role. Additionally, local health care providers, emergency medical services staff, police officers, and community health workers could all be considered disaster health responders during a PHE. Given the increased severity and prevalence of IPV associated with PHEs, disaster health responders need to be able to recognize the signs and symptoms of IPV and feel confident in addressing IPV. This requires education, training, and protocols for IPV care during PHEs.

Scant evidence exists among federal disaster response entities and national volunteer organizations regarding training, protocols, or guidance for IPV care during PHEs. The committee found that most public-facing federal PHE preparedness and response guidance did not address protocols related to IPV. Some guidance mentioned IPV as part of domestic violence, but that guidance framed violence in the context of families with children, which can lead planners and disaster health responders to overlook the possibility of IPV in families that do not have children, couples that do not live together, or former intimate partners. The public-facing federal preparedness and response guidance that did address IPV did not offer specific guidance for development of IPV care protocols, but rather mostly encouraged planners and responders to have domestic violence hotline numbers available and to know the hours and contact information for local domestic violence shelters.

Education and training focused on IPV recognition and care is important for developing the capacity for disaster health responders to care for people experiencing IPV during PHEs. Despite preparedness planning, disaster health responders may need more preparation for the setting and type of care needs of the affected community. This is often addressed through just-in-time training. Just-in-time training is an opportunity to reinforce prior disaster knowledge and convey other vital information about the PHE. This training represents a unique opportunity to provide IPV-specific education and training.

The *2023–2025 HRSA Strategy to Address Intimate Partner Violence* recommends integrating training for IPV care into existing programs and providing training and technical assistance specific to IPV for the health care workforce. One of HRSA's National Training and Technical Assistance Programs, Health Partners on IPV and Exploitation, provides training about trauma-informed services during steady state conditions, education and tools for building partnerships, policy development, and integration of processes to promote prevention and increase referrals to services for individuals at risk for and experiencing IPV. The Administration for Strategic Preparedness and Response (ASPR) collaborates with SLTT governments, hospitals, community members, and other members of the private sector to improve their medical and public health PHE readiness and response capabilities. ASPR has developed a collection of technical resources, including guidance on training and protocol development for PHE preparedness and response. The committee concluded that ASPR and HRSA were well suited to developing and disseminating training and guidance for IPV care during PHEs.

International guidance, such as that developed by WHO and the United Nations Population Fund (UNFPA) can also be used to inform development of domestic protocols. Additionally, collaboration with IPV care providers outside of health care institutions to develop plans before PHEs occur is important to ensuring safety, security, and community acceptance.

> **Recommendation 6: The Health Resources and Services Administration should partner with the Administration for Strategic Preparedness and Response to add an open access training hub on intimate partner violence (IPV) for disaster health responders and other personnel in health care and community settings that includes education about:**
> - **Recognizing the signs and symptoms of IPV during public health emergencies;**
> - **Appropriate use of supplies and care protocols unique to IPV-related health care services, including those related to reproductive health and forensic medical examinations; and**
> - **Best practices for providing care and connections to support services for individuals experiencing IPV.**

> **Recommendation 7: The Health Resources and Services Administration should partner with the Administration for Strategic Preparedness and Response to develop and disseminate standardized guidance for developing protocols for intimate partner violence care for disaster health responders as well as the essential supplies required for delivering that care.**

> **Recommendation 8: Federal and state, local, tribal, and territorial government emergency response leaders should ensure that coordinated planning and response protocols for sustaining essential health care services related to intimate partner violence (IPV) during public health emergencies (PHEs) are in place before PHEs occur. Key steps in the planning process include:**
> - **At the federal level, the Department of Health and Human Services should ensure that protocols for IPV care are integrated into the planning and execution of all of the core competencies of the Emergency Support Function 8 Public Health and Medical Services Annex.**
> - **At the state, local, tribal, and territorial government level, IPV care planning and coordination should be assigned to a specific office or division that is part of the emergency planning or emergency management team.**

- At all levels, jurisdictional emergency planning teams should include representation from social service providers and IPV-related community-based organizations to ensure that strong partnerships exist between disaster health responders and the organizations providing care for IPV survivors.

Supplies for Intimate Partner Violence Care in Emergencies

Emergency medical supply caches are a key component of PHE preparedness and response. Several federal systems exist to supply disaster health responders during emergencies, including the Strategic National Stockpile, supplies deployed with Disaster Medical Assistance Teams, and resources included as part of a Federal Medical Station's deployment kit. While these caches are typically supplemented by supplies maintained by private and SLTT actors, kits meant for acute deployment are pre-packaged and standardized. Many of the essential health care services related to IPV during PHEs are the same as those for individuals not experiencing IPV, but there are some unique supply considerations, particularly related to caring for a woman who has experienced IPV-related sexual assault or rape. However, standard protocols to guide the allocation of resources, such as supplies and medications, when providing IPV care in austere settings or in disrupted health care environments during PHEs are not currently widely available in the United States. UNFPA maintains guidelines, the Inter-Agency Emergency Reproductive Health Kits for Use in Humanitarian Settings, which describe necessary supplies and their use across a variety of women's health needs. Emergency reproductive health kits are designed for use in conditions similar to those of the initial response phase of a PHE and are tailored to the knowledge, competencies, and qualifications required to use each of the supplies in the kit. Different kits exist for different types of care. Examples include a post-rape treatment kit, oral and injectable contraception kit, and sexually transmitted infection kit. The committee acknowledges that those located in certain geographic areas in the United States may encounter challenges procuring specific and vital supplies for IPV care, such as emergency contraception. However, it emphasizes that caches should include the necessary supplies to support delivery of all essential health care services related to IPV regardless of location.

Recommendation 9: Federal, state, local, tribal, and territorial governments' planning should take the following actions to ensure the availability of necessary supplies to deliver essential health care services for intimate partner violence (IPV) during public health emergencies:
- Conduct an annual review of disaster response caches to ensure that appropriate supplies related to IPV are included.

- Establish logistics and procurement plans for needed supplies for all entities that will be responsible for delivering that care, including disaster health responders, emergency shelter staff, and community-based support service providers engaged in IPV care.

Intimate Partner Violence Research

As previously noted, the committee engaged in an extensive review of the literature to inform its work. However, it encountered difficulties when attempting to compare data and findings across studies. Most studies and surveys, including different years of the NISVS, differed in terms of the terminology used related to IPV, demographic categories, and approaches to data collection. These inconsistencies were also noted in IPV research that used clinic-based data, such as that extracted from electronic health records. This included variations in the definitions and descriptions used for the different forms of IPV (physical violence, sexual violence, stalking, psychological aggression, and reproductive coercion). Most systematic reviews of IPV-related research identified inconsistencies in terminology among studies as a substantial limitation to drawing strong conclusions.

Without comparable data sets, it is difficult to develop accurate estimates of IPV prevalence and identify temporal trends, particularly among different populations and geographic areas that may be under-represented in a single study's data collection. Furthermore, demographic data collection and analysis approaches are often inconsistent. Thus, data specific to some smaller populations in a data set may not be represented accurately or at all. Inconsistencies in terminology and data also make it difficult to compare effectiveness of different IPV interventions across studies. These data inconsistencies undoubtedly have slowed the process of identifying effective, scalable interventions for IPV and led to an incomplete understanding of its prevalence. CDC developed its *Intimate Partner Violence Surveillance: Uniform Definitions and Recommended Data Elements* to reduce these inconsistencies, but it has not been widely adopted.

> **Recommendation 10: In order to improve consistency in intimate partner violence (IPV)-related terminology used in both the research and clinical setting, the Health Resources and Services Administration (HRSA) and all U.S. health care systems should adopt the IPV-related terminology defined in the Centers for Disease Control and Prevention *Intimate Partner Violence Surveillance: Uniform Definitions and Recommended Data Elements*. HRSA and other federally funded health care agencies can further support better alignment of clinical and survey data in IPV research by requiring use of the recommended data elements in their funded projects.**

The committee recognized several challenges in conducting high-quality studies involving women experiencing IPV. These women navigate complex and evolving circumstances related to their safety when they disclose IPV and seek care. Often these circumstances are beyond their control. For example, a study participant may experience a change in her safety during the study, requiring services that differ from the intervention to which she was randomized. Failure to modify the intervention would pose an unethical risk to the participant's safety. Moreover, people experiencing IPV may need to relocate for their safety, which disrupts the administration of the intervention, long-term follow-up, and outcome measurement. These challenges likely contribute to the relatively small study populations of many IPV-related studies and many of the gaps in IPV-related research specific to this study's statement of task. The committee concluded that HRSA is well-positioned to support efforts to address these gaps and build a more robust evidence base.

> **Recommendation 11: The Health Resources and Services Administration should fund research efforts that address:**
> - Best practices for identifying and managing intimate partner violence (IPV) in routine clinical practice and during public health emergencies (PHEs);
> - The effectiveness of IPV interventions in improving physical and mental health outcomes in steady state conditions and PHEs;
> - The potential harms of IPV identification and management in steady state and PHE and strategies to prevent or reduce those harms;
> - The prevalence and characteristics of IPV among specific populations, particularly those populations experiencing adverse effects of health disparities; and
> - The effect of PHEs on IPV frequency and severity.

CONCLUDING THOUGHTS

Women who experience IPV have complex and substantial health care needs. Women experiencing IPV and their clinicians face barriers to accessing and delivering evidence-based IPV-related care. When IPV occurs in the context of a PHE, the challenges encountered by both the women experiencing IPV and the disaster health responders who must care for them become more complex. The recommendations put forth by this committee outline critical measures that, if acted on, will increase access to essential health care services related to IPV and ultimately save lives.

1

Introduction

BACKGROUND

Women's well-being and safety are often disproportionately negatively affected during disasters and public health emergencies (PHEs) (Thurston et al., 2021). International and domestic studies have reported that violence against women increases in the context of PHEs and disasters (Thurston et al., 2021). Multiple studies conducted in the United States after Hurricane Katrina, after the Deepwater Horizon oil spill, and throughout the COVID-19 pandemic have found increases in the prevalence and severity of intimate partner violence (IPV) against women in the aftermath of these events (First et al., 2017; Lauve-Moon and Ferreira, 2016; Viero et al., 2021). Women who experience IPV during a disaster or PHE are exposed to physical and psychological trauma due to IPV in addition to traumas from the PHE. With this in mind, the Health Resources and Services Administration's (HRSA's) Office of Women's Health (OWH) identified a need to identify, highlight, and describe essential health care services related to IPV that should be prioritized and made available during PHEs. Thus, HRSA's OWH contracted with the National Academies of Sciences, Engineering, and Medicine's Health and Medicine Division to convene an expert multidisciplinary panel of 14 members to address the statement of work (see Box 1-1) and produce a report with recommendations and conclusions within an 18-month timeframe. The committee on Sustaining Essential Health Care Services Related to Intimate Partner Violence During Public Health Emergencies was formed and convened four in-person meetings and four virtual meetings in response to HRSA's request.

BOX 1-1
Statement of Task and Charge to the Committee

An ad hoc committee of the National Academies of Sciences, Engineering, and Medicine shall develop a conceptual framework for delivering essential preventive and primary health care services related to Intimate Partner Violence (IPV) during public health emergencies (PHEs), using an all-hazards approach. The committee's framework shall:

- Identify essential health care services related to IPV in non-PHEs (steady state) based on currently available evidence;
- Define essential health care services related to IPV in PHEs based on currently available evidence;
- Identify ways to prepare for and prioritize the provision of essential health care services related to IPV before PHEs;
- Describe health disparities related to IPV in PHEs;
- Identify innovations and best practices to prepare for and operationalize the equitable delivery of essential health care services related to IPV during PHEs;
- Identify promising practices in the prevention of IPV; and
- Develop strategies to overcome barriers faced by HRSA-supported and safety-net care settings in providing essential health care services related to IPV during PHEs, particularly for underserved populations.

STUDY APPROACH AND SCOPE

Defining Intimate Partner Violence

The committee adopted the Centers for Disease Control and Prevention's (CDC's) definition of *intimate partner violence* as abuse or aggression committed by a current or former intimate partner (Breiding et al., 2015). An intimate partner is a person with whom one has a close romantic and consensual physically intimate relationship and is characterized by regular interaction. IPV can include, but is not limited to, physical violence, sexual violence, stalking, psychological aggression, and reproductive coercion (ACOG, 2012; CDC, 2022). *Physical violence* or *physical IPV* refers to the intentional use of physical force to inflict injury (Breiding et al., 2015). Examples include but are not limited to pushing, grabbing, choking, hair pulling, the use of a weapon, the use of restraints, or coercing others to commit such acts (Breiding et al., 2015). *Sexual violence* or *sexual IPV* refers to forcing a partner to take part in a sexual act without his or her consent or when the partner is not able to freely give consent and includes drug- or alcohol-facilitated acts and non-physical acts (Breiding et al., 2015). Some examples are forced sexual touching, rape, sexual coercion, sexting, or forcing sexual contact with a third party. *Stalking* is a pattern of repeated behavior that involves unsought attention and contact by a current or former intimate partner that creates a sense of fear for one's safety or that of someone with a close relationship to the victim (Breiding et al., 2015). Some examples are following or repetitive phone calls or text messages. *Psychological aggression* or *psychological IPV* refers to using verbal and non-verbal communication to intentionally harm a partner mentally or emotionally or to wield control over a partner (ACOG, 2012; Breiding et al., 2015; CDC, 2022). Some examples include name-calling, isolation, degradation, reproductive coercion, or intentional deprivation of resources such as food, medication, health care, or economic resources. *Psychological IPV* often co-occurs with other forms of IPV. *Reproductive coercion* refers to actions that exert control over a partner's reproductive health and can occur in the absence of physical or sexual violence (ACOG, 2012). Some examples include contraception sabotage, refusal to practice safe sex, forced pregnancy, forced pregnancy termination (either through forced abortion or infliction of injury with the intent to cause a miscarriage), and controlling access to reproductive health services (ACOG, 2012).

IPV is different from domestic violence (DV). DV is a broader category that refers to abuse or aggression committed by a family member or member of a household against another family member or member of a household (Merriam-Webster, 2023). DV may include IPV, but it also includes child abuse, elder abuse, and abuse or aggression between other family members or household members. Some organizations, researchers, reporting bodies, and legal jurisdictions use IPV and DV interchangeably, which can create challenges in interpreting data and research findings. The committee considered research and data specific to IPV. It only included references and data that referred to DV for consideration if the source's definition of DV was limited to abuse and aggression between current or former intimate partners.

IPV should not be confused with interpersonal violence. Interpersonal violence is the intentional use of violence or aggression by an individual or small group of individuals against another individual or small group (Mercy et al., 2017).

Study Scope

The experience of IPV is not limited to women. However, to remain consistent with the guidance from the study sponsor, the committee limited its focus to women (see next section for the committee's definition of women) over the age of 13 who directly experience IPV. Additionally, consideration of health care services for individuals who engage in IPV, beyond those specifically addressed in prevention strategies, is beyond the scope of this study. The committee acknowledges that IPV is also directed at men, including transgender men, and there is a growing body of research into the effects of experiencing IPV on men. However, health care interventions specifically for men experiencing IPV are also beyond the scope of the study. Additionally, while elder abuse and child abuse are significant issues that can intersect with IPV, these issues also fall outside of the parameters of the statement of task. Undoubtedly, the pediatric health care setting represents a point of contact with the health care system for parents or adolescents to disclose that they are experiencing IPV (Randell and Ragavan, 2020). However, services for children witnessing IPV are beyond the scope of the statement of task. Of note, several studies have identified a parent's concern about the safety of their children or losing custody of their children as a frequently reported barrier to IPV disclosure (Heron and Eisma, 2021). The committee considers essential health care services for the parent or caregiver experiencing IPV that reduce barriers to disclosure and IPV care by supporting the safety of their child or children. The committee also considers IPV in relationships among adolescents as detailed in the chapters that follow.

The committee acknowledges that the complex nature of addressing IPV may necessitate a broad array of supports and strategies to address the many effects of IPV as well as its root causes. However, the scope of this study is limited to health care services, which are defined later in this chapter. As such, when considering essential health care services for IPV, the committee limited its consideration to IPV care that is delivered in or referrable from a health care setting. The committee did consider a specific group of support services that are directed at protecting the immediate health and safety of women experiencing IPV and that often serve as an initial point of contact for women to access IPV-related care, including health care.

Women

The committee used an inclusive approach to define woman/women as the population of interest in this report. For the purpose of this report, woman/women encompass cisgender women, transgender women, and people whose gender identity is not exclusively male who are non-binary or otherwise gender expansive. This is a modified version of the approach used by the HRSA-funded Women's Preventive Services Initiative (WPSI) (WPSI, 2022). The committee emphasizes that inclusion of people who are gender non-binary or otherwise gender expansive as part of the population they refer to when using the word woman throughout this report is done with the intent of being inclusive of individuals whose gender identity is not exclusively male and not with the intent of disregarding the gender identity of those who are gender non-binary or otherwise gender expansive. Unfortunately, there is very little research in the literature about IPV in the gender non-binary or otherwise gender expansive population. This limited the frequency with which this population could be discussed specifically when discussing the research evidence throughout the report.

The Committee's Approach

The committee conducted an extensive review of the literature pertaining to IPV and PHEs. This review included websites maintained by such organizations as the World Health Organization (WHO), United Nations, Futures Without Violence, National Resource Center on Domestic Violence, and multiple pertinent state and federal agencies. Committee members and project staff identified additional salient literature and information using traditional academic research methods and online searches throughout the course of the study. The committee also drew on information gleaned from presentations given by experts in the health effects of IPV; IPV in lesbian, gay, bisexual, transgender, and queer populations; IPV care delivery in American Indian and Alaska Native populations; individuals with lived experience of IPV; and individuals with lived experience providing IPV care during PHEs.

Conceptual Framework

The statement of task identified the value of an overarching conceptual framework to guide the committee's process for identifying essential health care services related to intimate partner violence. The committee selected the Social Ecological Model (SEM) as the conceptual framework to guide their understanding of the health care needs of women experiencing IPV and to identify the essential health care services related to IPV (see Figure 1-1) (Bronfenbrenner, 1977; McLeroy et al., 1988). The model has been widely applied to public health and clinical health care services challenges, including IPV and public health disaster response (Bell et al., 2021; Di Napoli et al., 2019; Nyambe et al., 2016). The committee considered the effect of factors consistent with the scope of the study at each level of the SEM on the health care needs of women experiencing IPV and the essential health care services to address those needs.

Health care services are delivered in multiple settings within the health care system as well as in community settings outside of a defined health care system (Aday and Andersen, 1974). In some cases, people experiencing IPV may be referred to community-based care from the traditional health care

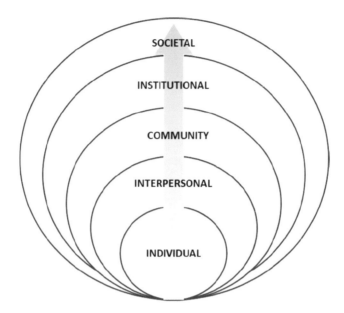

FIGURE 1-1 Social Ecological Model.
SOURCE: Concept from McLeroy et al., 1988. Figure adapted from NASEM report *Getting to Zero Alcohol-Impaired Driving Fatalities: A Comprehensive Approach to a Persistent Problem* (2018).

setting. In other cases, these community-based settings may be the initial site of care. The committee appreciates the value and interdependence of connections between the health care system and community-based care settings. The importance of these connections is further developed in the Care Coordination Model, which emphasizes high-quality referrals and transitions to outside resources for clinicians and patients (Wagner et al., 2014). Therefore, while this report is focused on health care services, the committee felt that it was important to acknowledge the role of community-based organizations in IPV-related care and emphasize the importance of warm referrals to that care.[1]

---

[1] *Warm referrals*, or warm handoffs, are transfers of care between members of a health care team that occur with the patient's permission, often with an in-person introduction. This approach can also be used when referring a patient to community-based services.

Determination Criteria for Essential Health Care Services for Intimate Partner Violence

The committee's process for identifying essential health care services related to IPV was informed by an extensive review of evidence from several literature searches; recommendations from the U.S. Preventive Services Task Force (USPSTF), WPSI, and WHO; and insight gleaned from presentations to the committee by experts in IPV-related care. The committee notes that not all essential health care services related to IPV are delivered within the health care system or by clinicians. The committee identified the following criteria for essential health care services related to IPV:

- Evidence-based health care services that address the most common and most serious health outcomes related to experiencing IPV;
- Preventive services recommended by USPSTF and WPSI; and
- Specific support services required to meet the basic safety and housing needs of people experiencing IPV.

The committee recognizes that some of the essential health care services identified may currently be unavailable due to state-level restrictions placed on reproductive health care services and federal restrictions that may apply to the use of federal funding for such services. However, significant scientific evidence of increased risk for negative maternal and fetal health outcomes, including death, as well as elevated risk for increased severity or frequency of IPV and intimate partner homicide in the perinatal period support their inclusion (Black, 2011; D'Angelo et al., 2022; Dillon et al., 2013; Liu et al., 2016; Nelson et al., 2022; Roberts et al., 2014; Smith et al., 2023; Stubbs and Szoeke, 2022; Vicard-Olagne et al., 2022). These risks are discussed in further detail in Chapter 4 of the report.

Research Considerations

Evaluating studies of the effectiveness of IPV interventions requires understanding the complexities of conducting this type of research. In biomedical science and health care research, evidence is typically evaluated using hierarchical levels based on the inherent biases of specific study designs (Burns et al., 2011). While multiple classification systems exist, they consistently rank randomized controlled trials (RCTs) and systematic reviews of RCTs as the highest level of evidence and expert opinion and case series as the lowest (Burns et al., 2011). The quality (internal validity or risk of bias) of intervention studies is evaluated using criteria based on the study design components of RCTs, such as randomization, blinding, selection of appropriate measurements, control of confounding variables, and loss to follow-up (Balshem et al., 2011; Higgins et al., 2023). These criteria apply primarily to interventions conducted in controlled settings where an intervention has low variance, such as drug trials. These criteria are not relevant to interventions that are ethically or operationally inappropriate for randomization, blinding, and other conditions of drug trials (Walshe, 2007). Most interventions for IPV fit into this latter group.

The committee understood several important challenges in conducting high-quality studies of IPV interventions. This research has been characterized as methodologically limited due to inconsistent randomization, inadequate control groups, no blinding, lack of long-term follow-up, or insufficient outcome measures (Zink and Putnam, 2005). Several issues specific to IPV research underlie these limitations.

First, the experience of IPV incorporates multiple confounding variables that can obscure the treatment effect of an IPV intervention (O'Campo et al., 2011). The most recent National Intimate Partner and Sexual Violence Survey results estimate that 63.3 percent of women had concerns for their safety during their lifetime because of IPV (Leemis et al., 2022). These issues differ for each individual and are often unanticipated and beyond their control. People experiencing IPV navigate complex and evolving circumstances related to their safety when they disclose IPV and seek care (Zink and Putnam, 2005). A study participant may experience a change in her or his safety during the study, requiring services that differ from the intervention to which the participant was randomized. Failure to modify the intervention would pose an unethical risk to the participant's safety (Zink and Putnam, 2005). Moreover, people experiencing IPV may need to relocate for their safety, which disrupts the administration of the intervention, long-term follow-up, and outcome measurement.

IPV intervention studies rely on self-reported, unverified predictors (disclosure) and outcome variables that lack standardization (Zink and Putnam, 2005). Since many individuals experiencing IPV do not disclose when first asked, the IPV status of study participants may be inaccurate (Korab-Chandler et al., 2022). Study outcomes may also be inaccurate, particularly when participants are concerned about the legal or social repercussions of ongoing or escalating IPV. Additional attempts to verify IPV status and outcome data could violate confidentiality and cause harm (Zink and Putnam, 2005).

In most IPV intervention studies, the control group is provided with usual or alternate care for ethical reasons. However, these non-interventions could increase participants' awareness of IPV, affect their use of services, and influence trial outcomes by creating a Hawthorne effect (i.e., the phenomenon that study participants change their behavior because of being involved in the study; see Franke and Kaul, 1978) (Nelson et al., 2012). As a result, differences between intervention and control groups may be diminished, and the effectiveness of the intervention may be underestimated.

The committee kept these challenges in mind throughout their consideration of the research evidence. Much of the research into effectiveness of different interventions for IPV had mixed results that were confounded by the variables discussed above. This limited the number of interventions that the committee could describe as effective based on the research evidence. However, the committee was able to identify several care models that it considered promising based on the committee's expert opinion and their review of the evidence. Those are discussed in Chapters 5 and 7 of this report.

Guiding Principles

Person-First Language

The committee acknowledges that stigma creates barriers to care, and language contributes to stigma. The Veterans Health Administration's Intimate Partner Violence Assistance Program uses person-first language as part of its approach to reducing the stigma associated with IPV (VA, 2021). Throughout this report, the terms *woman* or *women* or *person* or *people experiencing IPV* will be used instead of *victim* or *battered spouse*, and the term *person* or *people engaging in IPV* will be used instead of *batterer* or *perpetrator*.

Health Equity, Health Disparities, and Resilience

The committee sought to center health equity in developing a framework for delivering essential health care services related to IPV during PHEs. In the article "Systems of Power, Axes of Inequity: Parallels, Intersections, Braiding the Strands," Camara P. Jones offers this description of health equity: "Health equity is assurance of the conditions for optimal health for all people. Achieving health equity requires valuing all individuals and populations equally, recognizing and rectifying historical injustices, and providing resources according to need. Health disparities will be eliminated when health equity is achieved" (Jones, 2014, p. S74). Populations adversely affected by health disparities include racially and ethnically minoritized populations, people with low incomes, populations residing in underserved rural areas, and sexual and gender minoritized populations (NIMHD, 2023).[2] Some of these populations have been historically marginalized through discriminatory policies and systems that have led to intergenerational trauma, which may exacerbate health disparities. Many underserved communities lack access to quality health care services,

---

[2] The term *minoritized* refers to the active marginalization of certain groups into minority status, as well as what that status has historically entailed.

including perinatal health care, perpetuating health disparities (Brigance, 2022). The committee acknowledges that the health care services identified as essential during steady state and PHE conditions are substantially less accessible or inaccessible in underserved communities (Frakt, 2019). These underserved communities often experience a lack of access to health care services during steady state conditions which resembles the lack of access encountered by wealthier, better resourced communities during disasters (Topchik et al., 2021).

Inadequate access to health care services is one of many factors that affect community resilience, or its ability to maintain its essential functions despite shocks or stressors, such as PHEs (Clark-Ginsberg et al., 2020). In public health, the evaluation of community resilience is frequently focused on using defined neighborhood characteristics to describe factors such as vulnerability or social capital, with improving resilience being defined as a positive outcome. However, these evaluations can overlook the adverse effects of the interdependence of neighborhoods that occur during disasters. The COVID-19 pandemic provided an example of the negative effect of this interdependence. During the pandemic, essential workers continued to work, frequently outside of their neighborhoods, providing services for those who could work from home in more affluent neighborhoods (Hong et al., 2021). Essential workers and the less affluent neighborhoods where they lived bore a heavier contagion rate than those more affluent neighborhoods (Hong et al., 2021; Maroko, 2020). The resilience of more affluent neighborhoods is often bolstered by the labor of those residing in other, less affluent neighborhoods during disasters. Committee members kept this in mind throughout their work. They sought to develop a framework for delivering essential primary care and preventive health care services related to IPV during PHEs that did not reinforce pre-existing health care disparities or improve access for one community at the expense of another.

PHEs, by their nature of overwhelming system capacities, lay bare inadequate resilience among communities and systems, as well as disparities between them. The COVID-19 pandemic highlighted the degree to which longstanding health disparities and economic inequality had undermined the resilience of many communities. It also revealed that many government and community institutions were not adequately equipped to meet the compounding needs of those under-resourced communities in the face of a global pandemic (OASH, 2022). This revelation was the impetus for development of the Federal Plan for Equitable Long-Term Recovery and Resilience.[3] The interagency workgroup that developed the plan noted that, in light of the significant disparities that existed prior to the onset of the

---

[3] See https://health.gov/our-work/national-health-initiatives/equitable-long-term-recovery-and-resilience (accessed August 25, 2023).

COVID-19 pandemic, recovery efforts should not seek to restore systems and communities to pre-pandemic conditions (OASH, 2022). Instead, they aimed to develop a long-term recovery plan that would improve community and national resilience, which included improving health and well-being. The committee notes that while recovery planning is beyond the scope of this project, the factors that undermine resilience and contribute to adverse outcomes in PHEs, such as health disparities, exacerbate the adverse outcomes of IPV (this is discussed in greater detail in Chapter 3).

Key Terminology

Public Health Emergency

In 2020, the National Academies consensus study report *Evidence-Based Practice for Public Health Emergency Preparedness and Response* defined the term *public health emergency* as "a situation with health consequences whose scale, timing, or unpredictability threatens to overwhelm routine capabilities" (NASEM, 2020, p. 43). This committee acknowledges that routine capabilities vary broadly across communities. Therefore, the committee modifies the definition of a PHE as follows: a situation with health consequences whose scale, timing, or unpredictability threatens to overwhelm the routine capabilities of the affected geographic area. The committee applies this definition to the term *public health emergency* throughout this report. The committee notes that this is different from a declared PHE. The committee acknowledges that the declaration of a disaster or PHE typically involves one or more statutes or other legal authorities, which vary from jurisdiction to jurisdiction. Within the confines of this report, the committee defines a declared PHE as a formal emergency or disaster declaration or determination made by federal, state, local, tribal, or territorial authorities in response to an actual or potential PHE, as defined above to account for those many varied statutes and legal authorities. This report will note specific statutory declarations when the specifics of those legal authorities are central to the committee's findings, conclusions, or recommendations.

Steady State

In the context of this report, *steady state* refers to periods when a community's routine capabilities have not been disrupted due to a PHE. It represents the period when health care systems, businesses, schools, support services, and community-based organizations are operating without impediment from a PHE or its aftermath. Infrastructure, homes, and other buildings are intact and functioning without damage from a PHE.

Health Care Services

The committee defines *health care services* as care delivered in or referrable from a health care setting. This is a modification of the description of primary care services that is used by the USPSTF Topic Prioritization Workgroup: care that can be delivered in or referred from the primary care setting (Barry et al., 2023). *Referrable services* are those targeted at addressing the immediate social risk factors and social needs of a person experiencing IPV in order to protect that person's health and safety. *Social risk factors* are specific negative social conditions that have a negative effect on health at the individual level, such as housing instability (Alderwick and Gottlieb, 2019). *Social needs* reflect the social contributors to health, such as housing stability or access to food, that an individual has identified as a priority (Alderwick and Gottlieb, 2019). The committee acknowledges that the complex nature of addressing IPV may necessitate a broad array of supports and strategies to address the many effects of IPV as well as its root causes. However, the scope of this study is limited to health care services. As such, when considering essential health care services for IPV, the committee limited its consideration to IPV care that is delivered in or referrable from a health care setting.

Health Care System

The health care system is referred to throughout the report. For the purposes of this report, the health care system refers to the care delivery component, including individuals and institutions, clinicians, ancillary and support personnel, hospitals, and other health care facilities. The committee acknowledges that the U.S. health system is complex and involves an expansive variety of entities that are responsible for different aspects of health care, including financing, care delivery, regulation, and research. This report covers topics and makes recommendations that affect many elements and actors within the system. Throughout the report, entities of the U.S. health care system not included in the delivery component described above are referred to as different specified entities.

Prevention

The committee was asked to identify promising practices for the prevention of IPV. HRSA described three categories of public health prevention strategies applicable to IPV in its *2023–2025 HRSA Strategy to Address Intimate Partner Violence*.[4] Those three are:

---

[4] See https://www.hrsa.gov/office-womens-health/addressing-intimate-partner-violence (accessed August 28, 2023).

- Primary prevention, defined as preventing IPV before it occurs;
- Secondary prevention, defined as immediately responding to occurrences of IPV; and
- Tertiary prevention, defined as responding to the long-term effects of IPV (HRSA, 2023).

All-Hazards Approach

The statement of task asks the committee to use an all-hazards approach to develop its conceptual framework. An *all-hazards approach* is an integrated approach to emergency preparedness planning that focuses on capacities and capabilities that are critical to prepare for, respond to, and recover from the full spectrum of emergencies or disasters, whether human-made or natural (CMS, 2017). The committee notes that their application of an all-hazards approach acknowledges that not all disasters and emergencies are identical, nor are their effects on different populations and communities (Benevolenza and DeRigne, 2018; Mendenhall et al., 2023).

Disaster Health Responders

For the purposes of this report, *disaster health responders* are the leaders and staff with expertise in public health and health care who are working and providing care in those settings during response to a PHE.

Emergency Personnel

For the purposes of this report, the term *emergency personnel* refers to general leads and staff within emergency management infrastructures deployed throughout the emergency environment, including social services and other entities supporting the emergency response.

IPV Care Providers

For the purposes of this report, *IPV care providers* refer to staff and administrators whose expertise and role are focused on providing care for people experiencing IPV in the health care, social services, and support services settings.

Social Services and Support Services

For the purposes of this report, the committee defines *social services* as services provided by government agencies that are targeted at addressing the needs and promoting the well-being of individuals, families, and communities. Examples include programs operated by government agencies such as food and nutrition support programs, adult and child day care programs, and unemployment assistance programs. For the purposes of this report, the committee defines *support services* as services provided outside of the clinical health care setting by community-based organizations that are targeted at addressing the social needs and promoting the well-being of individuals and families.

Warm Referral

Warm referrals, or warm handoffs, as defined by the Agency for Healthcare Research and Quality, are transfers of care between members of a health care team that occur with the patient's permission, often with an in-person introduction (AHRQ, 2017). Warm referrals have been used in many domains of patient care in a wide variety of settings, including for behavioral health treatment and in successful social needs screening and referral programs.

ORGANIZATION OF THE REPORT

Chapter 1 of this report explains the committee's charge and approach to meeting that charge and defines key terminology and language used throughout the report. Chapter 2 describes IPV in the United States during steady state conditions, including prevalence, population-specific considerations, and factors affecting access to IPV-related care. Chapter 3 is organized into two parts. It begins with a high-level overview of core components of PHE response planning, including key related U.S. laws and regulations, existing federal frameworks and response resources, and a discussion of the interaction between PHEs and health disparities. The second part of Chapter 3 addresses the intersection of IPV with PHEs and discusses effects of PHEs on the prevalence and severity of IPV, the double-survivorship experience of those who have experienced both IPV and a PHE, barriers to accessing IPV-related care during PHEs, and existing guidance for providing health care related to IPV during PHEs. Chapter 4 discusses the most common and most serious health conditions related to experiencing IPV. Chapter 5 identifies the essential health care services related to IPV, the settings where care is typically delivered during steady state conditions, and promising models for IPV care during steady state conditions. Chapter 6 discusses the essential health care services related to IPV during PHEs and sustaining access to those services during PHEs, including a discussion of insights gleaned from international guidance and crisis standards of care, as well as approaches for addressing challenges in sustaining access. Chapter 7 discusses the planning and delivery of essential health care services related to IPV during PHEs, including opportunities to integrate IPV care into existing systems and settings, promising models for IPV care during PHEs, key supply considerations, training for disaster health responders, and existing guidance related to sheltering. Chapter 8 presents all of the committee's recommendations.

REFERENCES

ACOG. (American College of Obstetricians and Gynecologists). 2012. ACOG committee opinion no. 518: Intimate partner violence. *Obstet Gynecol* 119(2 Pt 1):412-417.

Aday, L. A., and R. Andersen. 1974. A framework for the study of access to medical care. *Health Serv Res* 9(3):208-220.

AHRQ (Agency for Healthcare Research and Quality). 2017. *Warm handoff: Intervention.* https://www.ahrq.gov/patient-safety/reports/engage/interventions/warmhandoff.html (accessed August 25, 2023).

Alderwick, H., and L. M. Gottlieb. 2019. Meanings and misunderstandings: A social determinants of health lexicon for health care systems. *Milbank Q* 97(2):407-419.

Balshem, H., M. Helfand, H. J. Schunemann, A. D. Oxman, R. Kunz, J. Brozek, G. E. Vist, Y. Falck-Ytter, J. Meerpohl, S. Norris, and G. H. Guyatt. 2011. Grade guidelines: 3. Rating the quality of evidence. *J Clin Epidemiol* 64(4):401-406.

Barry, M. J., T. A. Wolff, L. Pbert, K. W. Davidson, T. M. Fan, A. H. Krist, J. S. Lin, I. R. Mabry-Hernandez, C. M. Mangione, J. Mills, D. K. Owens, and W. K. Nicholson. 2023. Putting evidence into practice: An update on the U.S. Preventive Services Task Force methods for developing recommendations for preventive services. *Ann Fam Med* 21(2):165-171.

Bell, S. A., L. K. Krienke, S. Dickey, and R. G. De Vries. 2021. "Helping fill that gap": A qualitative study of aging in place after disaster through the lens of home-based care providers. *BMC Geriatr* 21(1):235.

Benevolenza, M. A., and L. DeRigne. 2018. The impact of climate change and natural disasters on vulnerable populations: A systematic review of literature. *Journal of Human Behavior in the Social Environment* 29(2):266-281.

Black, M. C. 2011. Intimate partner violence and adverse health consequences. *American Journal of Lifestyle Medicine* 5(5):428-439.

Breiding, M. J., K. C. Basile, S. G. Smith, M. C. Black, and R. R. Mahendra. 2015. *Intimate partner violence surveillance: Uniform definitions and recommended data elements. Version 2.0.* Edited by Centers for Disease Control and Prevention. Atlanta, GA: National Center for Injury Prevention and Control.

Brigance, C., R. Lucas, E. Jones, A. Davis, M. Oinuma, K. Mishkin, and Z. Henderson. 2022. *Nowhere to go: Maternity care deserts across the U.S. 2022 report.* March of Dimes.

Bronfenbrenner, U. 1977. Toward an experimental ecology of human development. *American Psychologist* 514-531.

Burns, P. B., R. J. Rohrich, and K. C. Chung. 2011. The levels of evidence and their role in evidence-based medicine. *Plast Reconstr Surg* 128(1):305-310.

CDC (Centers for Disease Control and Prevention). 2022. *Fast facts: Preventing intimate partner violence.* https://www.cdc.gov/violenceprevention/intimatepartnerviolence/fastfact.html (accessed October 5, 2022).

Clark-Ginsberg, A., B. McCaul, I. Bremaud, G. Caceres, D. Mpanje, S. S. Patel, and R. B. Patel. 2020. Practitioner approaches to measuring community resilience: The analysis of the resilience of communities to disasters toolkit. *Int J Disaster Risk Reduct* 50.

CMS (Centers for Medicare and Medicaid Services). 2017. *Frequently asked questions emergency preparedness regulation: Clarifications on definitions.* CMS.

D'Angelo, D. V., J. M. Bombard, R. D. Lee, K. Kortsmit, M. Kapaya, and A. Fasula. 2022. Prevalence of experiencing physical, emotional, and sexual violence by a current intimate partner during pregnancy: Population-based estimates from the pregnancy risk assessment monitoring system. *J Fam Violence* 38(1):117-126.

Di Napoli, I., F. Procentese, S. Carnevale, C. Esposito, and C. Arcidiacono. 2019. Ending intimate partner violence (IPV) and locating men at stake: An ecological approach. *Int J Environ Res Public Health* 16(9).

Dillon, G., R. Hussain, D. Loxton, and S. Rahman. 2013. Mental and physical health and intimate partner violence against women: A review of the literature. *Int J Family Med* 2013:313909.

First, J. M., N. L. First, and J. B. Houston. 2017. Intimate partner violence and disasters. *Affilia* 32(3):390-403.

Frakt, A. B. 2019. The rural hospital problem. *JAMA* 321(23):2271-2272.

Franke, R. H., and J. D. Kaul. 1978. The Hawthorne experiments: First statistical interpretation. *American Sociological Review* 43(5):623-643.

Heron, R. L., and M. C. Eisma. 2021. Barriers and facilitators of disclosing domestic violence to the healthcare service: A systematic review of qualitative research. *Health Soc Care Community* 29(3):612-630.

Higgins, J. P. T., J. Thomas, J. Chandler, M. Cumpston, T. Li, M. J. Page, and V. A. Welch, eds. 2023. *Cochrane handbook for systematic reviews of interventions,* version 6.4. Cochrane. www.training.cochrane.org/handbook.

Hong, B., B. J. Bonczak, A. Gupta, L. E. Thorpe, and C. E. Kontokosta. 2021. Exposure density and neighborhood disparities in COVID-19 infection risk. *Proc Natl Acad Sci U S A* 118(13):e2021258118.

HRSA (Health Resources and Services Administration). 2023. *2023-2025 HRSA strategy to addressing intimate partner violence.* Rockville, MD: HRSA.

Jones, C. P. 2014. Systems of power, axes of inequity: Parallels, intersections, braiding the strands. *Med Care* 52(10 Suppl 3):S71-S75.

Korab-Chandler, E., M. Kyei-Onanjiri, J. Cameron, K. Hegarty, and L. Tarzia. 2022. Women's experiences and expectations of intimate partner abuse identification in healthcare settings: A qualitative evidence synthesis. *BMJ Open* 12(7):e058582.

Lauve-Moon, K., and R. J. Ferreira. 2016. An exploratory investigation: Post-disaster predictors of intimate partner violence. *Clinical Social Work Journal* 45(2):124-135.

Leemis, R. W., N. Friar, S. Khatiwada, M. S. Chen, M.-j. Kresnow, S. G. Smith, S. Caslin, and K. C. Basile. 2022. *The national intimate partner and sexual violence survey: 2016/2017 report on intimate partner violence.* Atlanta, GA: Centers for Disease Control and Prevention.

Liu, F., J. McFarlane, J. A. Maddoux, S. Cesario, H. Gilroy, and A. Nava. 2016. Perceived fertility control and pregnancy outcomes among abused women. *J Obstet Gynecol Neonatal Nurs* 45(4):592-600.

Maroko, A. R., D. Nash, and B. T. Pavilonis. 2020. COVID-19 and inequity: A comparative spatial analysis of New York City and Chicago hot spots. *J Urban Health* 97(4):461-470.

McLeroy, K. R., D. Bibeau, A. Steckler, and K. Glanz. 1988. An ecological perspective on health promotion programs. *Health Educ Q* 15(4):351-377.

Mendenhall, R., J. C. Shin, F. Adibu, M. M. Yago, R. Vandewalle, A. Greenlee, and D. S. Grigsby-Toussaint. 2023. Lessons (not) learned: Chicago death inequities during the 1918 influenza and COVID-19 pandemics. *Int J Environ Res Public Health* 20(7).

Mercy, J. A., S. D. Hillis, A. Butchart, M. A. Bellis, C. L. Ward, X. Fang, and M. L. Rosenberg. 2017. Interpersonal violence: Global impact and paths to prevention. In *Disease control priorities, third edition (volume 7): Injury prevention and environmental health*. Pp. 71-96.

Merriam-Webster. 2023. Domestic violence. In *Merriam-Webster Dictionary*. https://www. merriam-webster.com/dictionary/domestic%20violence (accessed April 20, 2023).

NASEM (National Academies of Sciences, Engineering, and Medicine). 2018. *Getting to zero alcohol-impaired driving fatalities: A comprehensive approach to a persistent problem*. Edited by S. M. Teutsch, A. Geller and Y. Negussie. Washington, DC: The National Academies Press.

NASEM. 2020. *Evidence-based practice for public health emergency preparedness and response*. Edited by N. Calonge, L. Brown and A. Downey. Washington, DC: The National Academies Press.

Nelson, H. D., C. Bougatsos, and I. Blazina. 2012. Screening women for intimate partner violence: A systematic review to update the U.S. Preventive services task force recommendation. *Ann Intern Med* 156(11):796-808, W-279, W-280, W-281, W-282.

Nelson, H. D., B. G. Darney, K. Ahrens, A. Burgess, R. M. Jungbauer, A. Cantor, C. Atchison, K. B. Eden, R. Goueth, and R. Fu. 2022. Associations of unintended pregnancy with maternal and infant health outcomes: A systematic review and meta-analysis. *JAMA* 328(17):1714-1729.

NIMHD (National Institute on Minority Health and Health Disparities). 2023. *HD pulse: An ecosystem of health disparities and minority health resources*. https://hdpulse.nimhd.nih. gov/#def3 (accessed June 5, 2023).

Nyambe, A., G. Van Hal, and J. K. Kampen. 2016. Screening and vaccination as determined by the social ecological model and the theory of triadic influence: A systematic review. *BMC Public Health* 16(1):1166.

O'Campo, P., M. Kirst, C. Tsamis, C. Chambers, and F. Ahmad. 2011. Implementing successful intimate partner violence screening programs in health care settings: Evidence generated from a realist-informed systematic review. *Soc Sci Med* 72(6):855-866.

OASH (Office of the Assistant Secretary for Health). 2022. *Equitable long-term recovery and resilience*. https://health.gov/our-work/national-health-initiatives/equitable-long-term-recovery-and-resilience (accessed August 25, 2023).

Randell, K. A., and M. I. Ragavan. 2020. Intimate partner violence: Identification and response in pediatric health care settings. *Clin Pediatr (Phila)* 59(2):109-115.

Roberts, S. C., M. A. Biggs, K. S. Chibber, H. Gould, C. H. Rocca, and D. G. Foster. 2014. Risk of violence from the man involved in the pregnancy after receiving or being denied an abortion. *BMC Med* 12(1):144.

Smith, E. J., B. A. Bailey, and A. Cascio. 2023. Sexual coercion, intimate partner violence, and homicide: A scoping literature review. *Trauma, Violence, & Abuse* 25(1):341-353. https:// doi.org/10.1177/15248380221150474.

Stubbs, A., and C. Szoeke. 2022. The effect of intimate partner violence on the physical health and health-related behaviors of women: A systematic review of the literature. *Trauma, Violence, & Abuse* 23(4):1157-1172.

Thurston, A. M., H. Stockl, and M. Ranganathan. 2021. Natural hazards, disasters and violence against women and girls: A global mixed-methods systematic review. *BMJ Glob Health* 6(4).

Topchick, M., T. Brown, M. Pinette, B. Balfour, and H. Kein. 2021. *Rural communities at risk: Widening health disparities present new challenges in aftermath of pandemic*. The Chartis Group.

VA (U.S. Department of Veterans Affairs). 2021. *Intimate partner violence assistance program*. https://www.socialwork.va.gov/IPV/About.asp (accessed May 1, 2023).

Vicard-Olagne, M., B. Pereira, L. Rouge, A. Cabaillot, P. Vorilhon, G. Lazimi, and C. Laporte. 2022. Signs and symptoms of intimate partner violence in women attending primary care in Europe, North America and Australia: A systematic review and meta-analysis. *Fam Pract* 39(1):190-199.

Viero, A., G. Barbara, M. Montisci, K. Kustermann, and C. Cattaneo. 2021. Violence against women in the COVID-19 pandemic: A review of the literature and a call for shared strategies to tackle health and social emergencies. *Forensic Sci Int* 319:110650.

Wagner, E. H., N. Sandhu, K. Coleman, K. E. Phillips, and J. R. Sugarman. 2014. Improving care coordination in primary care. *Med Care* 52(11 Suppl 4):S33-S38.

Walshe, K. 2007. Understanding what works–and why–in quality improvement: The need for theory-driven evaluation. *Int J Qual Health Care* 19(2):57-59.

WPSI (Women's Preventive Services Initiative). 2022. *Women's preventive services initiative*. https://www.womenspreventivehealth.org/wpsi-statements/ (accessed August 18, 2023).

Zink, T., and F. Putnam. 2005. Intimate partner violence research in the health care setting: What are appropriate and feasible methodological standards? *J Interpers Violence* 20(4):365-372.

2

Intimate Partner Violence in Steady State Conditions

PREVALENCE OF INTIMATE PARTNER VIOLENCE

Intimate partner violence (IPV) is common among women in the United States. It affects women of all races and ethnicities, all levels of income, and all sexualities and gender identities, regardless of whether they live in rural, suburban, or urban areas. The Centers for Disease Control and Prevention (CDC) National Intimate Partner and Sexual Violence Survey (NISVS) is the most commonly used tool in the field of IPV research for estimating the prevalence of IPV in the United States. NISVS is a nationally representative random-digit-dial telephone survey. Data are collected from non-institutionalized English- and Spanish-speaking adult women who completed the survey. The most recent NISVS, conducted in 2016–2017 (N=15,152 women), estimated that 47.3 percent of women have experienced IPV in the form of contact sexual violence, physical violence, or stalking; and 49.4 percent have experienced psychological aggression by an intimate partner in their lifetimes (see Table 2-1) (Leemis, 2022). The past 12 months prevalence was 7.3 percent for experiencing any form of IPV, with 3.2 percent of women experiencing contact sexual violence, 4.5 percent experiencing any physical violence, 2.5 percent experiencing stalking, and 6.7 percent experiencing psychological abuse. A higher percentage of Black (12.3 percent), Hispanic (7.2 percent), and multiracial women (17.4 percent) women respondents reported a past-year experience of IPV, compared with only 6 percent of White women (Leemis, 2022). Prevalence rates of IPV are useful for identifying populations and characteristics associated with higher levels of IPV and related

TABLE 2-1 Lifetime Prevalence by Victimization Type for U.S. Women from the National Intimate Partner and Sexual Violence Survey: 2016–2017 Report[a]

Victimization Type[b]	Lifetime Prevalence Percentage[c]
Total N[d]	15,152
Any contact sexual violence, physical violence, and/or stalking	47.3
Psychological aggression	49.4
Physical violence	42.0
Contact sexual violence	19.6
Stalking	13.5

[a] Definitions used in the survey: Physical violence includes a range of behaviors from slapping, pushing, or shoving to severe acts that include being hit with a fist, kicked, hurt by pulling hair, slammed against something, choked, beaten, burned on purpose, or use of a weapon. Contact sexual violence includes rape, being made to penetrate someone else, sexual coercion, and unwanted sexual contact. Stalking refers to a pattern of harassing or threatening tactics used by people engaging in IPV that is both unwanted and causes fear or safety concerns in the woman experiencing abuse. Psychological aggression includes expressive aggression (e.g., name-calling, insulting, or humiliating an intimate partner) and coercive control (e.g., monitoring, controlling, or threatening an intimate partner).
[b] The summation of the percentage of respondents for each victimization type is different from the total percentages of respondents because respondents may have experienced multiple victimization types.
[c] All percentages are weighted to the U.S. non-institutionalized English- or Spanish-speaking adult population.
[d] N=number of respondents.
SOURCE: Leemis et al. (2022).

health conditions, guiding appropriate screening and interventions, and designing effective prevention efforts.

Lifetime prevalence rates of IPV are also high for all women, with the highest rates in American Indian or Alaska Native (AI/AN; 57.7 percent), non-Hispanic Black (53.6 percent), and multiracial groups (63.8 percent) (see Table 2-2) (Leemis, 2022). In addition to population-based survey data, such as those reported in NISVS, police-reported IPV rates are two to three times higher among Black and Hispanic women than among White women (Lipsky et al., 2009).

Prevalence estimates from NISVS survey results are the most referenced, but they are not the only source of information about IPV prevalence. Clinic and other site-based surveys have examined the prevalence of different forms of IPV in various demographic and geographic groups. However, the research methodology differs across studies, which limits comparisons. Many surveys, including different years of the NISVS, differ in terms of the

TABLE 2-2 Lifetime Prevalence by Race and Ethnicity for U.S. Women from the National Intimate Partner and Sexual Violence Survey: 2016–2017 Report

Lifetime Prevalence	Total	Hispanic	Non-Hispanic, Black	Non-Hispanic, White	Asian or Pacific Islander	American Indian or Alaska Native	Multiracial
N[a]	15,152	2,197	1,864	9,879	849	91	257
Any contact sexual violence, physical violence, and/or stalking percentage[b]	47.3	42.1	53.6	48.4	27.2	57.7	63.8

[a] N=number of respondents
[b] All percentages are weighted to the U.S. non-institutionalized English- or Spanish-speaking adult population.
SOURCE: Leemis et al. (2022).

terminology used related to IPV, demographic categories, and approaches to data collection. This makes it difficult to compare data and findings across studies. CDC released the first version of its *Intimate Partner Violence Surveillance: Uniform Definitions and Recommended Data Elements* in 1999 with the goal of improving consistency in IPV surveillance research (Breiding et al., 2015a; Saltzman et al., 1999). CDC released its second version of *Intimate Partner Violence Surveillance: Uniform Definitions and Recommended Data Elements* in 2015 with updated and added terminology, again with the intention of improving data gathering for IPV surveillance. This tool provides recommended uniform definitions, guidance about data elements for record-based and survey surveillance, and recommended data elements (RDEs). The uniform definitions can be used both in the clinic for documentation or data collection and in research, including survey data collection. The RDEs included in the guidelines address four types of violence: physical, sexual, stalking, and psychological. Each RDE has a corresponding definition or description, type of surveillance for which it is recommended, and coding instructions. The majority of the RDEs focus on collecting data about the most recent incidence of IPV as well as the very first experience of IPV but could be used to gather further information (Breiding et al., 2015a). While the CDC document is not all-encompassing, broader application of its guidance would greatly improve the usefulness of data collected in clinical and research settings, including surveys.

POPULATION-SPECIFIC CONSIDERATIONS

As noted earlier in this chapter, some populations are disproportionately affected by IPV. The committee found that many of those populations are under-represented in the IPV research literature, including those discussed in this section. The populations and considerations included in this section are those for which the committee identified adequate evidence to support an informed discussion. Additionally, the committee prioritized considerations that were most relevant to the study's statement of task.

American Indian and Alaska Native Women

There are currently 574 federally recognized American Indian and Alaska Native (AI/AN) tribes in the United States (BIA, 2022). The committee recognized that these tribes are distinct entities with unique languages, traditions, and structures and sought to avoid treating them as a monolith. This report refers to specific tribes when information is available. Unfortunately, tribal affiliation is rarely reported in studies relevant to IPV.

Data Collection

Much of the epidemiologic data and analysis about AI/AN populations, including IPV-related data, are subject to important methodological limitations. These include racial misclassification, in which individuals are incorrectly classified as a different race or ethnicity instead of AI/AN (Petrosky et al., 2021; Yellow Horse and Huyser, 2021). The demographic information section of forms in many states and in surveys often does not allow for the selection of multiple races or does not include a category for AI/AN (Yellow Horse and Huyser, 2021). This limits the response option to *other* and aggregates that data with the data of the rest of the respondents that are placed in the *other* category (Huyser et al., 2021). Also, in statistical analysis, data from a very small group are frequently combined with data from another group that, while smaller than other groups, is much larger than the very small group; such as the case with aggregating data from Asian American and Pacific Islander populations (Korngiebel et al., 2015). In this case, data from the smaller group, Native Hawaiians and other Pacific Island populations, can be obscured by data from the much larger group, Asian Americans (Korngiebel et al., 2015). These limitations result in inaccurate findings.

Violent crimes against AI/AN women are under-reported, which adds additional opacity to an understanding of the prevalence of violence inflicted by current and former intimate partners (BIA, n.d.). This is highlighted by the epidemic of missing and murdered Indigenous women and girls. An examination of reports of missing AI/AN women and girls found that in 2016 there were 5,712 reports of missing AI/AN women and girls in the U.S. Department of Justice federal missing persons database (BIA, n.d.). However, only 116 of those cases were logged in the National Missing and Unidentified Persons System, which serves as the national information clearinghouse for missing, unidentified, and unclaimed person cases (BIA, n.d.).

Prevalence of Intimate Partner Violence Among American Indian/Alaska Native Women

AI/AN women are a population that experiences exceptionally high rates of IPV. The 2016–2017 analysis of the NISVS found that 57.7 percent of non-Hispanic AI/AN women in the survey had experienced IPV in the form of physical violence, contact sexual violence, or stalking in their lifetime (Leemis et al., 2022). Among 230 undergraduate students self-identifying as AI/AN attending 20 medium- and large-sized universities across the United States, 28.9 percent reported having experienced any violence from a current or past intimate partner in the previous 6 months (Edwards et al., 2023). A study funded by the National Institute of Justice found that 66.4 percent of AI/AN women (N=2,473, n=1,642) had experienced psychological aggression from an intimate partner during their lifetime (Rosay, 2016). This study also found that AI/AN women experiencing IPV were 1.5 times more likely than non-Hispanic White women to be physically injured due to IPV and 2.3 times more likely to need medical care. AI/AN women were also 2.5 times more likely to lack access to needed IPV services (Rosay, 2016). Among AI/AN women, IPV is associated with poorer physical and mental health (Fedina et al., 2022; Stockman et al., 2015). Economic inequalities among these women are a salient predictor of IPV health outcomes, which demographic and geographic contexts may compound (Fedina et al., 2022). A CDC National Violent Death Reporting System analysis of AI/AN homicides in 34 states and the District of Columbia from 2003 to 2018 found that the suspect in murders of AI/AN women was most likely to be a current or former intimate partner in 38.4 percent of reported cases (Petrosky et al., 2021).

Sociological Factors

In the literature, the substantially higher rates of IPV in AI/AN populations have been attributed to historical violence, including forced relocation, traumas inflicted through residential schools, retraction of tribal sovereignty and associated economic rights leading to economic deprivation, and jurisdictional uncertainty, which contributes to a lack of legal consequences for people engaging in IPV (Fedina et al., 2022; Wahab and Olson, 2004). Studies have noted that exposure to intergenerational violence contributes to the normalization of IPV (Jock et al., 2022). AI/AN women have reported that contextual factors contributing to IPV include controlling relationships, losing a sense of priorities, using children as manipulation tools, socioeconomic stress, family pressures, and restricting relationships (McKinley and Liddell, 2022). Additional challenges include living in remote, rural areas that limit access to support or the ability to leave a dangerous relationship, or living in areas that isolate AI/AN women from their extended family, community ties, and culture (Gauthier et al., 2021; Raponi et al., 2023). Language barriers, fear of losing custody of children, lack of culturally congruent services, inconvenient location of services, and economic stress and its consequences also limit help seeking for AI/AN women experiencing IPV (Fedina et al., 2022; Wahab and Olson, 2004).

Pregnant and Postpartum Women

Prevalence of Intimate Partner Violence in the Perinatal Period

Studies comparing IPV prevalence before and during pregnancy have had mixed findings, with some reporting a decline during pregnancy and others reporting an increase, particularly under conditions of an unwanted pregnancy or paternal uncertainty (Cizmeli, 2018; Saltzman et al., 2003). A study using Pregnancy Risk Assessment Monitoring System (PRAMS) data from 16 states from 1996 to 1998 found a prevalence rate of 5.3 percent (N=64,994, n=3,444) for physical abuse during pregnancy (Saltzman et al., 2003). Studies using clinic-based data for IPV in the perinatal period usually consider more than one type of IPV and have found higher prevalence rates (Hahn et al., 2018). Perinatal IPV rates were 16.4 percent (N=104) for physical IPV and 73 percent (N=104) for psychological IPV in a review of studies using clinic-based data (Flanagan et al., 2015; Hahn et al., 2018). A large global systematic review found that for reported IPV prevalence during pregnancy in North America, physical violence occurred at a rate of 9 percent (11 studies, N=11,204), psychological abuse occurred at a rate of 28.6 percent (eight studies, N=9,680), and sexual IPV occurred at a rate of 8.9 percent (five studies, N=942) (Román-Gálvez et al., 2021). An analysis of PRAMS data from six states in 2016–2018 found that women younger than age 25 experienced both psychological and physical IPV at a higher rate than those in an older age range during pregnancy (D'Angelo et al., 2022). The analysis found that AI/AN, mixed race, and Black women experienced emotional violence at a higher rate than White women throughout the perinatal period (D'Angelo et al., 2022). This analysis also found that AI/AN and Black women experienced physical violence during pregnancy at higher rates than White women (D'Angelo et al., 2022). Few U.S.-based studies reported rates of sexual IPV during the perinatal period. However, a study of 104 southern Appalachian women found that 20.2 percent experienced sexual abuse at the hands of a current or former intimate partner during the perinatal period (Bailey and Daugherty, 2007).

An analysis of PRAMS data for 43,811 persons who had a live birth between 2018 and 2020 highlighted the role of sociodemographic factors and disability status of those experiencing IPV during the perinatal period (Alhusen et al., 2023). The analysis found that the odds of experiencing IPV during the perinatal period were higher for those who had less than a college education, had a household income less than 200 percent of the federal poverty level, or identified as White (Alhusen et al., 2023). The study also found that the odds of experiencing perinatal IPV were twice as high for women with at least one disability as compared to those without a disability (Alhusen et al., 2023).

Intimate Partner Violence Screening in the Perinatal Period

While the nature of perinatal care, which involves multiple visits with a clinician during that period, provides greater opportunity for IPV detection, screening rates are generally inconsistent and suboptimal (IPV screening is discussed further in Chapter 5) (ACOG, 2012). Data related to physical IPV from the 2016 to 2019 PRAMS (N=158,338) indicated that 65.7 percent of respondents reported not being screened for IPV before pregnancy, 29.7 percent reported not being screened during pregnancy, and 48 percent reported not being screened for IPV during the postpartum period (Kozhimannil et al., 2023). Of the 3.5 percent of women in the dataset reporting physical IPV in the perinatal period, 58.7 percent reported not being screened for IPV before pregnancy, 26.9 percent reported not being screened during pregnancy, and 48.3 percent reported not being screened after pregnancy (Kozhimannil et al., 2023). The American College of Obstetricians and Gynecologists and the American Academy of Pediatrics Bright Futures Guidelines recommend that clinicians discuss IPV during perinatal appointments (Hagan et al., 2017).

Perinatal Intimate Partner Homicide

The most severe outcome of abuse from a current or former intimate partner during the perinatal period is death. In an analysis of data from 2003 to 2007 from the National Violent Death Reporting System (NVDRS), 42.4 percent (N=139, n=59) of pregnancy-related homicides were found to have been carried out by an intimate partner (Campbell et al., 2021). A systematic review of research investigating intimate partner homicide during pregnancy or postpartum also concluded that current or former intimate partners were most frequently the perpetrator of the murder (Noursi et al., 2020). Additionally, in a case-control study, severe physical IPV during pregnancy (described in the study as women being "beaten") was a risk factor for intimate partner homicide, while less severe IPV was not (Campbell, 2003). Another analysis of NVDRS data found that suicide, although less frequent than homicide, was also a common cause of maternal mortality highly associated with IPV (Palladino et al., 2011).

Adolescent Girls

Teen dating violence (also referred to as adolescent dating abuse or dating abuse) includes emotional, physical, sexual, or economic abuse by an intimate or sexual partner, which can occur in person, via social media, or texting (McCauley et al., 2014). Examples of adolescent relationship abuse are similar to those for IPV in adults and include monitoring a partner's cell phone, telling partners what they can wear, limiting social interactions, refusing to use condoms, preventing contraceptive use, coercing sexual behaviors (including insisting on receiving nude or seminude photos from a partner), coercing a partner to use substances, and other controlling behaviors (Scott et al., 2023).

Reports on teen dating violence in the adolescent girl population demonstrate that violence and abuse are not uncommon in adolescent relationships. Among teens (ages 12–18) who have dated, 69 percent (N=1,804) report ever having experienced physical, psychological, or sexual relationship abuse (Taylor and Mumford, 2016). Many adults report that they first experienced IPV before age 25 (Breiding et al., 2014; Leemis et al., 2022). Several studies, including CDC's Youth Risk Behavior Surveillance System, document that female respondents reported significantly higher prevalence of either physical or sexual dating violence than male respondents (20.9 vs. 10.4 percent; N=9,900) (Vagi et al., 2015).

Youth who experience marginalization and social disadvantage have had a higher reported prevalence of IPV in the literature. An evaluation of differences in the prevalence of relationship abuse among youth suggests higher prevalence among Black/African American and Hispanic youth, including experiences of reproductive coercion (Miller et al., 2014).

Black Women

Non-Hispanic Black women experience some of the highest rates of IPV when compared to other racial and ethnic groups. Most recent data from the NISVS reported non-Hispanic Black women have a lifetime prevalence of IPV of 53.6 percent (Leemis, 2022). An analysis of 2003–2017 data from the National Violent Death Reporting System found that pregnancy-related intimate partner homicide (IPH) rates were three times higher for Black woman than White or Hispanic women (Kivisto et al., 2022). Despite this, published research specifically addressing IPV and Black women is limited. Studies investigating rates of reproductive coercion have reported that Black women are subjected to this form of abuse at higher rates than White, Hispanic, and Asian women (Alexander et al., 2021). Studies investigating severe IPV and IPH in Black women have identified some common themes. These researchers have noted that Black women may delay contacting law enforcement due to concerns related to historically prejudicial treatment during interactions with law enforcement or fear of unjust treatment of their partner during or after arrest (Harper, 2022; Vil et al., 2022). Researchers have also highlighted that while studies have suggested that Black women may underutilize formal IPV services, many also lack access to these services in their community (Vil et al., 2022)

LBTQ Populations

The prevalence data for IPV experienced by the lesbian, bisexual, transgender, and queer (LBTQ) population varies, but is generally higher than that for the general population. A systematic review of 14 studies that investigated the prevalence and correlates of IPV in same-sex relationships of self-identified lesbians found that IPV prevalence ranged from 9.6 to 51.5 percent (Badenes-Ribera, 2016). A majority of the included studies found that reported lifetime physical IPV for these women ranged from 40 to 50 percent and psychological IPV ranged from 18 percent to 84 percent (Badenes-Ribera, 2016). A systematic review of 85 articles found that compared with cisgender individuals, transgender individuals were 1.7 times more likely to experience any IPV, 2.2 times more likely to experience physical IPV, and 2.5 times more likely to experience sexual IPV (Peitzmeier et al., 2020). A systematic review including nine studies looking specifically at bisexuality and IPV found that in three of those studies, women who identified as bisexual had an increased risk of experiencing IPV (Corey et al., 2023).

IPV in sexual minority women is associated with poorer physical health and mental health outcomes, including stress, depression, anxiety, alcohol abuse, and emotional regulation difficulties (Porsch et al., 2022). IPV also increases overall health care costs for LBTQ people experiencing abuse (Porsch et al., 2022). There are several minority stressors that affect those in the LBTQ community, including stigma, facing prejudice and discrimination, internalized homophobia, and concealment of sexual identity, which can contribute to poor mental health outcomes (Porsch et al., 2022). Providing trauma-informed care for LBTQ IPV survivors can increase their empowerment to begin working toward safety and recovery (Scheer and Poteat, 2021).

Rural Populations

Women who experience IPV and reside in rural areas face unique challenges related to geographic isolation. Research investigating geographic differences in the prevalence of IPV has had mixed findings. However, comparison of findings is limited by variations in the types of data collection methods, inconsistent distinctions between definitions of different regions, and different types of regional mapping.

A systematic review of 32 studies comparing frequency of IPV by locale found that the prevalence of IPV was similar regardless of urban or rural location (Edwards, 2015). The authors noted that the five studies included that used National Crime Victimization Survey data reported prevalence rates that were similar or greater for urban women compared with rural and suburban women (Edwards, 2015). A study of more specific geographic regions (urban core, suburban, exurban, small town, and dispersed rural)—found that those residing in small towns, defined as "the urbanized portions of nonmetropolitan counties," were at higher risk of IPV (DuBois, 2022).

Women experiencing IPV in rural and remote communities are more likely to have worse mental and physical health outcomes, including intimate partner homicide (AbiNader, 2020; Edwards, 2015). They are likely to stay longer with a partner engaging in IPV, more likely to experience torture, and more likely to be shot by a partner engaging in IPV than women living in urban areas (Hart and Klein, 2013). Women living in rural areas are at a disadvantage regarding accessing IPV-related resources. A cross-sectional clinic-based survey of 1,478 women in Iowa found that the average distance to the nearest IPV resource for rural women was substantially greater than the distance for urban women (29.4 to 29.6 miles versus 6.5 miles) (Peek-Asa et al., 2011). Researchers have suggested that women experiencing IPV who live in rural areas may have worse physical and mental health outcomes due to inadequate availability, accessibility, and quality of IPV resources in their area (Edwards, 2015; Peek-Asa et al., 2011; Reckdenwald et al., 2017). Faith-based organizations are often the most likely place for women experiencing IPV in rural communities to find services (Hart and Klein, 2013).

ADDITIONAL CONSIDERATIONS

Disability

A secondary analysis of data from the 2010 NISVS found that women with a disability (N= 9,086, n=2,162) were substantially more likely than women without a disability (N= 9,086, n=6,924) to report each type of IPV measured, including rape (1.7 vs. 0.4 percent), sexual violence other than rape (4.5 vs. 1.8 percent), physical violence (7.1 vs. 3.3 percent), stalking (6.5 vs. 2.1 percent), psychological aggression (21.0 vs. 12.2 percent), and control of reproductive or sexual health (2.4 vs. 1.4 percent) (Breiding and Armour, 2015b). There is a limited body of research about IPV and women with disabilities. An analysis of PRAMS data from 2018 to 2020 found that women with disabilities experienced much higher prevalence of abuse from a current or former intimate partner (N=3,024) than those with no disabilities (N=70,813) both before (9.5 versus 2.4 percent) and during pregnancy (5.8 versus 1.7 percent) (Alhusen et al., 2023). An analysis of data from the 2001–2005 National Epidemiologic Survey of Alcohol and Related Conditions found that both physical and mental disabilities were significantly associated with experiencing IPV (Hahn et al., 2014).

Women living with disabilities experience higher levels of poverty and social isolation, and may be more likely to stay with a partner engaging in IPV if that person is providing their physical or financial care (Breiding and Armour, 2015). There are added barriers for women with disabilities related to disclosing and seeking care for IPV because the partner engaging in IPV may be providing transportation or communication assistance, which hinders one's ability to reach out for help when experiencing IPV (Breiding and Armour, 2015).

Immigration Status

Disparities related to immigration status can adversely affect the physical and mental health outcomes of IPV, particularly for racial and ethnic minority women (Stockman et al., 2015). Hispanic and Asian immigrant women experiencing IPV face significant social, cultural, structural, and political barriers to communication with IPV care providers which affect their help-seeking behaviors related to IPV (Stockman et al., 2015). Acculturative stress, the stress of adapting to a new context in the United States, has been demonstrated to be among the strongest predictors of experiencing IPV among Hispanic women who are immigrants (Cao et al., 2023; González-Guarda et al., 2012).

Immigrant populations, especially those arriving through irregular or extra-legal immigration routes, are particularly at risk for experiencing IPV (Salgado and Gurm, 2020). These women face unique barriers to reporting IPV related to the perceived threat that law enforcement involvement may lead to deportation and concerns about public charge status that may affect permanent legal status determination (Ballard et al., 2019).

Housing and Food Insecurity

IPV contributes to homelessness and housing insecurity for women and their children (Adams et al., 2021; Fraga Rizo et al., 2022). Women who reported recent housing or food insecurity were significantly more likely to experience all forms of IPV than women without housing or food insecurity (Breiding et al., 2017). Additionally, lack of access to safe and affordable housing is a barrier for women experiencing IPV to leave a partner engaging in abuse (Decker et al., 2022; Pavao et al., 2007). An analysis of data from the 2003 California Women's Health Survey (N=3,619), found that women who had experienced IPV in the previous year were almost four times more likely to have reported housing instability than women who had not experienced IPV (adjusted OR=3.98, 95% CI: 2.94–5.39) (Pavao et al., 2007). Higher rates of housing, food, and health care insecurity have been observed among women who identified as Black/African American, Hispanic, AI/AN, and other racial and ethnic minority groups (Fedina et al., 2022).

Reducing housing insecurity may help prevent IPV revictimization. A quasi-experimental evaluation of on-site transitional housing and community-based rehousing was conducted to meet the safety and stability needs of individuals made homeless because of IPV. Both IPV revictimization and housing instability had significantly improved by the 6-month follow-up point (p<0.001) (Decker et al., 2022).

Substance Use

Women using illicit drugs may be at greater risk of experiencing IPV (Testa et al., 2003). Among 414 women enrolled in methadone maintenance treatment programs in New York City, 88 percent reported having experienced physical and sexual IPV during their lifetime (El-Bassel et al., 2004). Nearly 50 percent reported having experienced physical or sexual IPV in the previous 6 months, and slightly more than 20 percent indicated that the physical or sexual IPV experienced in the past 6 months was severe (El-Bassel et al., 2004). Lifetime prevalence estimates of IPV among women with opioid use disorders range from 36 (N=114, n=41) to 94 percent (N=406, n=381) (Stone and Rothman, 2019). Women who used heroin were twice as likely to experience IPV and 2.7 times more likely to report IPV-related injury than those who did not report using heroin (El-Bassel et al., 2005).

The evidence related to the relationship between alcohol use in women and experiencing IPV is mixed and shows no clear causal relationship. Some studies have shown an association between alcohol use and experiencing IPV (Temple and Freeman, 2011; Testa et al., 2003; White and Chen, 2002). However, after reviewing the literature, Capaldi et al. (2012) suggested that the relationship may not be strong because substance use tends to co-occur with other risk factors for experiencing IPV. Moreover, the temporal direction of this association has not been consistently demonstrated (Dardis et al., 2021; Devries et al., 2014; Keller et al., 2009). Some studies have found that there is no significant association between alcohol use in women and experiencing IPV (Sabina et al., 2017; Thompson and Kingree, 2006).

HIV Infection

Women living with HIV infection are more likely than the general population to experience IPV, and women in IPV relationships are more likely to acquire HIV and other sexually transmitted infections (Campbell et al., 2008; Marshall et al., 2018). State-level IPV prevalence is positively associated with higher rates of state-level HIV diagnosis among women (Willie et al., 2018). Researchers have suggested that increased rates of HIV infection among women who experience IPV may be due to these women being sexually assaulted by a male partner with an HIV infection, directly affecting their HIV susceptibility (Dunkle and Decker, 2013; Li et al., 2014; Maman et al., 2000; Stockman et al., 2013). Additionally, women in relationships with controlling partners may not be able to negotiate safer sex practices. Finally, the chronic stress and trauma related to experiencing IPV may negatively affect the immune system (Campbell et al., 2008). While the literature has not shown a direct mechanical association, this may make these women more susceptible to acquiring sexually transmitted infections (Campbell et al., 2008). In an examination of data from the National Epidemiologic Survey on Alcohol and Related Conditions, among 13,928 women in a relationship in the last year, 11.8 percent of cases of HIV infection among women were attributable to past-year IPV (Sareen et al., 2009).

Involvement in Sex Work

Women involved in sex work may face increased vulnerability to IPV and barriers to reporting IPV and accessing health care. In a convenience sample of 346 HIV-negative, drug-involved women in relationships recruited in New York City, women reporting sex trading were three times as likely to report recent severe physical or sexual IPV than women who did not report sex trading, after accounting for sociodemographic factors (Jiwatram-Negrón and El-Bassel, 2019).

A couples-based study of 214 women engaged in sex work explored the context in which IPV occurred (Ulibarri et al., 2019). In this study, couples reported that conflict arose over the financial need for women to engage in sex work, men's inability to provide for female partners, men feeling uncomfortable that their female partners had sex with other men as part of work, and relationship power dynamics (women being considered head of the household due to higher income than a partner). They also reported conflict while under the influence of drugs or while going through drug withdrawal (Ulibarri et al., 2019).

RISK FACTORS FOR PEOPLE ENGAGING IN INTIMATE PARTNER VIOLENCE

While this report focuses on women experiencing IPV, research on factors associated with IPV risk has concentrated on characteristics associated with people engaging in IPV. Understanding risk and protective factors for people engaging in IPV is fundamental to IPV prevention. In addition, recognizing these factors can guide responses to public health emergencies by focusing on risk factors that are likely to worsen during and in the wake of an emergency.

Multiple factors are associated with an increased likelihood for engaging in IPV and have been classified by CDC as occurring at the individual, relationship, community, and society levels (see Figure 2-1) (Capaldi et al., 2012; CDC, 2021). These risk and protective factors may be contributing

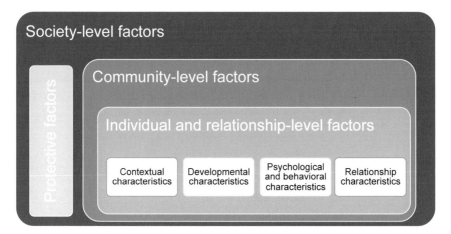

FIGURE 2-1 Risk and protective factors contributing to people engaging in IPV. NOTE: Multiple factors are associated with IPV. These include individual, relationship, community, and societal factors. Factors that increase the likelihood of IPV may be contributing factors and not direct causes.

factors to—not direct causes of—IPV, and they commonly include combinations of factors operating at different levels (e.g., coexisting individual- and community-level factors).

Individual- and relationship-level risk factors identified in observational studies relevant to the general U.S. population are listed in Table 2-3. Individual-level factors include contextual characteristics, such as low education or income, young age, and economic stress (e.g., unemployment). Developmental characteristics include a history of demonstrating previous physically abusive behavior, experiencing or witnessing physical or emotional abuse or violence in childhood, experiencing poor parenting, and having parents with less than a high school education (Capaldi et al., 2012; CDC, 2021). Psychological and behavioral characteristics include low self-esteem, aggressive or delinquent behavior, depression, suicide attempts, antisocial or borderline personality, and heavy alcohol and drug use. Also included in this category are beliefs in strict gender roles and hostility toward women (Capaldi et al., 2012).

Community-level risk factors include high poverty rates, unemployment, violence, and crime (Table 2-4). Communities with easy access to drugs and alcohol, limited educational and economic opportunities, low community involvement among residents, and a lack of sanctions against IPV are also at higher risk. Society-level risk factors include cultural norms that support traditional gender roles, gender inequality, and aggression toward others. Income inequality and weak policies or laws related to

TABLE 2-3 Individual- and Relationship-Level Risk Factors for Engaging in IPV

Contextual characteristics	Low education or income Young age Economic stress, such as unemployment
Developmental characteristics	History of being physically abusive History of physical or emotional abuse in childhood History of experiencing physical discipline as a child History of experiencing poor parenting as a child Parents with less than a high school education Witnessing violence between parents as a child
Psychological and behavioral characteristics	Low self-esteem Aggressive or delinquent behavior Depression and suicide attempts Anger and hostility Heavy alcohol and drug use Lack of nonviolent social problem-solving skills Antisocial personality traits and conduct problems Poor behavioral control and impulsiveness Traits associated with borderline personality disorder Emotional dependence and insecurity Belief in strict gender roles, such as male dominance and aggression in relationships Having few friends and being isolated from other people Hostility toward women Attitudes accepting or justifying violence and aggression
Relationship characteristics	Relationship conflicts, including jealousy, possessiveness, tension, divorce, or separation Dominance and control of the relationship by one partner over the other Families experiencing economic stress Unhealthy family relationships and interactions Association with antisocial and aggressive peers

SOURCES: Modified from Capaldi et al. (2012); CDC (2021).

health, educational, economic, and social needs also contribute to risk for people engaging in IPV.

The absence of risk factors is associated with a lower likelihood of people engaging in IPV. Protective factors specifically identified in studies include strong social support networks; neighborhood collective efficacy; coordination of resources and services among community agencies; and access to housing, medical care, and economic and financial help (CDC, 2021).

TABLE 2-4 Community- and Society-Level Risk Factors and Protective Factors for Engaging in IPV

Community factors	High rates of poverty and limited educational and economic opportunities
	High unemployment rates
	High rates of violence and crime
	Neighbors do not know or look out for each other, and residents have low community involvement
	Easy access to drugs and alcohol
	Weak community sanctions against IPV
Societal factors	Traditional gender norms and gender inequality
	Cultural norms that support aggression toward others
	Societal income inequality
	Weak health, educational, economic, and social policies or laws
Protective factors	Strong social support networks and stable, positive relationships with others
	Neighborhood collective efficacy, meaning residents feel connected to each other and are involved in the community
	Coordination of resources and services among community agencies
	Communities with access to safe, stable housing
	Communities with access to medical care and mental health services
	Communities with access to economic and financial help

SOURCES: Modified from Capaldi et al. (2012); CDC (2021).

FACTORS INFLUENCING DISCLOSURE

Barriers to Disclosure

There are several reasons commonly cited by women experiencing IPV to not disclose that they are experiencing IPV to a clinician, including shame and fear of the consequences of reporting, such as retaliation (Heron et al., 2021; Othman et al., 2014). Also, they may not believe a clinician has time or interest in addressing IPV (Narula et al., 2012; Spangaro et al., 2011). People experiencing IPV also cited a lack of awareness of the range of services and supports available to them as a reason they did not disclose (Ravi et al., 2022). Additionally, cultural and religious norms and values can influence a woman's disclosure decision (Hulley et al., 2023).

Parents experiencing IPV may be concerned about the effects of disclosure on their children. Children are present or otherwise members of the household in 59–76 percent of cases of IPV reported to the police (Campbell et al., 2020; Ernst et al., 2006; McDonald et al., 2006). Child maltreatment co-occurs with as many as 30–40 percent of IPV cases (Appel and Holden, 1998; Hamby et al., 2010). Children's experience of witnessing IPV can have long-term adverse effects on their physical and mental health

(Artz et al. 2014; Carpenter and Stacks, 2009; Evans et al., 2008; Felitti, 2009; Kitzmann et al., 2003; Tiyyagura et al., 2018; Vu et al., 2016). While disclosure is a potential way for mothers and their children to separate from these dangerous conditions, the perceived risk of retaliation can be a substantial barrier (Buttell and Ferreira, 2020). Qualitative studies have found that parents experiencing IPV also fear retaliation against their children if they disclose (Cerulli et al., 2014; Meyer, 2010). Another commonly cited concern for parents regarding disclosure of IPV is the possibility that their clinician will file a report of child abuse. This may lead to actions by child protective services, such as removing the child from the home. Most states require clinicians and government employees to report suspected child abuse (Children's Bureau, 2019). Additionally, most states and territories require clinicians to report several types of crime-related injuries, and some states have laws requiring reporting domestic violence in general (Lizdas et al., 2019). Fear of losing custody of their children is a commonly reported barrier for women experiencing IPV who are considering disclosure (DeVoe and Smith, 2003; Heron and Eisma, 2021; Lippy et al., 2019; Varcoe and Irwin, 2004).

Child-related barriers are compounded by additional issues for some populations. Immigration documentation status may also affect the decision to disclose IPV, as some women may not disclose because of a fear of deportation (Kelly, 2009). Women with disabilities are also particularly deterred from disclosure due to biases against them in custody decisions (Ballan et al., 2014; Ortoleva and Lewis, 2012).

While some barriers to IPV disclosure are shared by most women experiencing IPV, some populations face additional challenges that increase their hesitancy to disclose that they are experiencing IPV. A systematic review of 47 articles found that Black women often encounter unique barriers to disclosing IPV that are rooted in harmful racist stereotypes (Hulley et al., 2023; Waller et al., 2022). This reinforces their concern that they will not be believed if they disclose (Hulley et al., 2023; Waller et al., 2022). Other studies have noted that pressure stemming from cultural beliefs about protecting family honor in Latin American and South Asian populations can discourage women in these populations from disclosing IPV (Hulley et al., 2023). In one qualitative study of 83 participants in AI/AN communities, some women who experienced IPV explained that the intergenerational experience of violence can contribute to the normalization of abusive behavior within the family, including intimate partners (Jock et al., 2022). That normalization can make AI/AN people experiencing IPV less likely to disclose because they perceive IPV as normal (Jock et al., 2022). Additionally, some respondents indicated that such intergenerational experiences of violence were related to historical oppression of their communities (Jock et al., 2022).

Stigma and systematic inequities have acted as barriers to disclose for those in the LBTQ population (Calton et al., 2016). Due to existing discrimination toward sexual minorities, there may be reluctance to seek help out of fear of further discrimination. There also may be hesitation to disclose incidents of IPV if the individual has been selective about who they share their sexual orientation with, therefore the fear of being outed may hinder one's likelihood of seeking help (Calton et al., 2016).

CHAPTER SUMMARY

Lifetime IPV prevalence is high for all women in the United States. Frequent inconsistencies in terminology and data collection in IPV epidemiological research limit comparison and applicability of the data. Prevalence rates for women reporting they have experienced IPV are higher among some populations. Understanding the prevalence of IPV, the populations most at risk, factors associated with people engaging in IPV, and barriers to disclosure can enable planning that ensures that the health care needs of women experiencing IPV are addressed, whether during steady state conditions or public health emergencies. The next chapter provides an overview of public health emergencies and discusses their impact on IPV prevalence and access to IPV related health care.

REFERENCES

AbiNader, M. A. 2020. Correlates of intimate partner homicide in the rural United States: Findings from a national sample of rural counties, 2009–2016. *Homicide Studies* 24(4):353-376.

ACOG (American College of Obstetricians and Gynecologists). 2012. ACOG committee opinion no. 518: Intimate partner violence. *Obstet Gynecol* 119(2 Pt 1):412-417.

Adams, E. N., H. M. Clark, M. M. Galano, S. F. Stein, A. Grogan-Kaylor, and S. Graham-Bermann. 2021. Predictors of housing instability in women who have experienced intimate partner violence. *J Interpers Violence* 36(7-8):3459-3481.

Alexander, K. A., T. C. Willie, R. McDonald-Mosley, J. C. Campbell, E. Miller, and M. R. Decker. 2021. Associations between reproductive coercion, partner violence, and mental health symptoms among young black women in Baltimore, Maryland. *J Interpers Violence* 36(17-18):NP9839-NP9863.

Alhusen, J. L., G. Lyons, K. Laughon, and R. B. Hughes. 2023. Intimate partner violence during the perinatal period by disability status: Findings from a united states population-based analysis. *J Adv Nurs* 79(4):1493-1502.

Appel, A. E., and G. W. Holden. 1998. The co-occurrence of spouse and physical child abuse: A review and appraisal. *Journal of Family Psychology* 12(4):578-599.

Artz, S., M. A. Jackson, K. R. Rossiter, A. Nijdam-Jones, I. Géczy, and S. Porteous. 2014. A comprehensive review of the literature on the impact of exposure to intimate partner violence for children and youth. *International Journal of Child, Youth and Family Studies* 5(4):493-587.

Badenes-Ribera, L., A. Bonilla-Campos, D. Frias-Navarro, G. Pons-Salvador, and I. B. H. Monterde. 2016. Intimate partner violence in self-identified lesbians: A systematic review of its prevalence and correlates. *Trauma Violence Abuse* 17(3):284-297.

Bailey, B. A., and R. A. Daugherty. 2007. Intimate partner violence during pregnancy: Incidence and associated health behaviors in a rural population. *Matern Child Health J* 11(5):495-503.

Ballan, M. S., M. B. Freyer, C. N. Marti, J. Perkel, K. A. Webb, and M. Romanelli. 2014. Looking beyond prevalence: A demographic profile of survivors of intimate partner violence with disabilities. *J Interpers Violence* 29(17):3167-3179.

Ballard, J., M. Witham, and M. Mittal. 2019. Chapter 6: Intimate partner violence among immigrants and refugees. In *Immigrant and refugee families*. 2nd Ed ed.

BIA (Bureau of Indian Affairs). 2022. *Tribal leaders directory*. https://www.bia.gov/service/tribal-leaders-directory (accessed 2023).

BIA. n.d. *Missing and murdered indigenous people crisis*. https://www.bia.gov/service/mmu/missing-and-murdered-indigenous-people-crisis (accessed 2023).

Breiding, M. J., and B. S. Armour. 2015. The association between disability and intimate partner violence in the United States. *Ann Epidemiol* 25(6):455-457.

Breiding, M. J., S. G. Smith, K. C. Basile, M. L. Walters, J. Chen, and M. T. Merrick. 2014. Prevalence and characteristics of sexual violence, stalking, and intimate partner violence victimization—National Intimate Partner and Sexual Violence Survey, United States, 2011. *MMWR Surveill Summ* 63(8):1-18.

Breiding, M. J., K. C. Basile, S. G. Smith, M. C. Black, and R. R. Mahendra. 2015. *Intimate partner violence surveillance: Uniform definitions and recommended data elements. Version 2.0*. Edited by Centers for Disease Control and Prevention. Atlanta, GA: National Center for Injury Prevention and Control.

Breiding, M. J., K. C. Basile, J. Klevens, and S. G. Smith. 2017. Economic insecurity and intimate partner and sexual violence victimization. *Am J Prev Med* 53(4):457-464.

Buttell, F., and R. J. Ferreira. 2020. The hidden disaster of COVID-19: Intimate partner violence. *Psychol Trauma* 12(S1):S197-S198.

Calton, J. M., L. B. Cattaneo, and K. T. Gebhard. 2016. Barriers to help seeking for lesbian, gay, bisexual, transgender, and queer survivors of intimate partner violence. *Trauma Violence Abuse* 17(5):585-600.

Campbell, A. M., R. A. Hicks, S. L. Thompson, and S. E. Wiehe. 2020. Characteristics of intimate partner violence incidents and the environments in which they occur: Victim reports to responding law enforcement officers. *Journal of Interpersonal Violence* 35(13-14):2583-2606.

Campbell, J., S. Matoff-Stepp, M. L. Velez, H. H. Cox, and K. Laughon. 2021. Pregnancy-associated deaths from homicide, suicide, and drug overdose: Review of research and the intersection with intimate partner violence. *J Womens Health (Larchmt)* 30(2):236-244.

Campbell, J. C., M. L. Baty, R. M. Ghandour, J. K. Stockman, L. Francisco, and J. Wagman. 2008. The intersection of intimate partner violence against women and HIV/AIDS: A review. *Int J Inj Contr Saf Promot* 15(4):221-231.

Campbell, J. C., D. Webster, J. Koziol-McLain, C. Block, D. Campbell, M. A. Curry, F. Gary, N. Glass, J. McFarlane, C. Sachs, P. Sharps, Y. Ulrich, S. A. Wilt, J. Manganello, X. Xu, J. Schollenberger, V. Frye, and K. Laughon. 2003. Risk factors for femicide in abusive relationships: Results from a multisite case control study. *Am J Public Health* 93(7):1089-1097.

Cao, J., S. G. Silva, M. Quizhpilema Rodriguez, Q. Li, A. M. Stafford, R. C. Cervantes, and R. M. Gonzalez-Guarda. 2023. Acculturation, acculturative stress, adverse childhood experiences, and intimate partner violence among Latinx immigrants in the U.S. *J Interpers Violence* 38(3-4):3711-3736.

Capaldi, D. M., N. B. Knoble, J. W. Shortt, and H. K. Kim. 2012. A systematic review of risk factors for intimate partner violence. *Partner Abuse* 3(2):231-280.

Carpenter, G. L., and A. M. Stacks. 2009. Developmental effects of exposure to intimate partner violence in early childhood: A review of the literature. *Children and Youth Services Review* 31(8):831-839.

CDC (Centers for Disease Control and Prevention). 2021. Risk and protective factors for perpetration. https://www.cdc.gov/violenceprevention/intimatepartnerviolence/riskprotectivefactors.html (accessed August 18, 2023).

Cerulli, C., C. L. Kothari, M. Dichter, S. Marcus, J. Wiley, and K. V. Rhodes. 2014. Victim participation in intimate partner violence prosecution: Implications for safety. *Violence Against Women* 20(5):539-560.

Children's Bureau. 2019. *Mandatory reporters of child abuse and neglect.* https://www.childwelfare.gov/pubPDFs/manda.pdf (accessed 2023).

Cizmeli, C., M. Lobel, K. K. Harland, and A. Saftlas. 2018. Stability and change in types of intimate partner violence across pre-pregnancy, pregnancy, and the postpartum period. *Womens Reprod Health (Phila)* 5(3):153-169.

Corey, J., M. Duggan, and A. Travers. 2023. Risk and protective factors for intimate partner violence against bisexual victims: A systematic scoping review. *Trauma Violence Abuse* 24(4):2130-2142.

D'Angelo, D. V., J. M. Bombard, R. D. Lee, K. Kortsmit, M. Kapaya, and A. Fasula. 2022. Prevalence of experiencing physical, emotional, and sexual violence by a current intimate partner during pregnancy: Population-based estimates from the pregnancy risk assessment monitoring system. *J Fam Violence* 38(1):117-126.

Dardis, C. M., S. E. Ullman, L. M. Rodriguez, E. A. Waterman, E. R. Dworkin, and K. M. Edwards. 2021. Bidirectional associations between alcohol use and intimate partner violence and sexual assault victimization among college women. *Addictive Behaviors* 116:106833.

Decker, M. R., K. T. Grace, C. N. Holliday, K. G. Bevilacqua, A. Kaur, and J. Miller. 2022. Safe and stable housing for intimate partner violence survivors, Maryland, 2019-2020. *Am J Public Health* 112(6):865-870.

DeVoe, E. R., and E. L. Smith. 2003. Don't take my kids: Barriers to service delivery for battered mothers and their young children. *Journal of Emotional Abuse* 3(3-4):277-294.

Devries, K. M., J. C. Child, L. J. Bacchus, J. Mak, G. Falder, K. Graham, C. Watts, and L. Heise. 2014. Intimate partner violence victimization and alcohol consumption in women: A systematic review and meta-analysis. *Addiction* 109(3):379-391.

DuBois, K. O. 2022. Rural isolation, small towns, and the risk of intimate partner violence. *J Interpers Violence* 37(5-6):NP2565-NP2587.

Dunkle, K. L., and M. R. Decker. 2013. Gender-based violence and HIV: Reviewing the evidence for links and causal pathways in the general population and high-risk groups. *Am J Reprod Immunol* 69(Suppl 1):20-26.

Edwards, K. M. 2015. Intimate partner violence and the rural-urban-suburban divide: Myth or reality? A critical review of the literature. *Trauma Violence Abuse* 16(3):359-373.

Edwards, K. M., S. Lim, M. Huff, R. Herrington, L. Leader Charge, and H. Littleton. 2023. Rates and correlates of intimate partner violence among indigenous college students: A multi-campus study. *Journal of Interpersonal Violence* 38(11-12):7852-7866.

El-Bassel, N., L. Gilbert, V. Frye, E. Wu, H. Go, J. Hill, and B. L. Richman. 2004. Physical and sexual intimate partner violence among women in methadone maintenance treatment. *Psychol Addict Behav* Jun;18(2):180-183.

El-Bassel, N., L. Gilbert, E. Wu, H. Go, and J. Hill. 2005. Relationship between drug abuse and intimate partner violence: A longitudinal study among women receiving methadone. *American Journal of Public Health* 95(3):465-470.

Ernst, A. A., S. J. Weiss, and S. Enright-Smith. 2006. Child witnesses and victims in homes with adult intimate partner violence. *Acad Emerg Med* 13(6):696-699.

Evans, S. E., C. Davies, and D. DiLillo. 2008. Exposure to domestic violence: A meta-analysis of child and adolescent outcomes. *Aggression and Violent Behavior* 13(2):131-140.

Fedina, L., Y. Shyrokonis, B. Backes, K. Schultz, L. Ashwell, S. Hafner, and A. Rosay. 2022. Intimate partner violence, economic insecurity, and health outcomes among American Indian and Alaska Native men and women: Findings from a national sample. *Violence Against Women* 29(11):2060-2079. https://doi.org/10.1177/10778012221127725.

Felitti, V. J. 2009. Adverse childhood experiences and adult health. *Acad Pediatr* 9(3):131-132.

Flanagan, J. C., K. C. Gordon, T. M. Moore, and G. L. Stuart. 2015. Women's stress, depression, and relationship adjustment profiles as they relate to intimate partner violence and mental health during pregnancy and postpartum. *Psychol Violence* 5(1):66-73.

Fraga Rizo, C., L. B. Klein, B. Chesworth, R. J. Macy, and R. Dooley. 2022. Intimate partner violence survivors' housing needs and preferences: A brief report. *J Interpers Violence* 37(1-2):958-972.

Gauthier, G. R., S. C. Francisco, B. Khan, and K. Dombrowski. 2021. Social integration and domestic violence support in an indigenous community: Women's recommendations of formal versus informal sources of support. *J Interpers Violence* 36(7-8):3117-3141.

Hagan, J. F., J. S. Shaw, and P. M. Duncan. 2017. *Bright futures: Guidelines for health supervision of infants, children, and adolescents [pocket guide].* 4th ed. American Academy of Pediatrics.

Hahn, C. K., A. K. Gilmore, R. O. Aguayo, and A. A. Rheingold. 2018. Perinatal intimate partner violence. *Obstet Gynecol Clin North Am* 45(3):535-547.

Hahn, J. W., M. C. McCormick, J. G. Silverman, E. B. Robinson, and K. C. Koenen. 2014. Examining the impact of disability status on intimate partner violence victimization in a population sample. *Journal of Interpersonal Violence* 29(17):3063-3085.

Hamby, S., D. Finkelhor, H. Turner, and R. Ormrod. 2010. The overlap of witnessing partner violence with child maltreatment and other victimizations in a nationally representative survey of youth. *Child Abuse Negl* 34(10):734-741.

Harper, S. B. 2022. "I'm just like, you know what, it's now or never": Exploring how women of color experiencing severe abuse and homicide risk journey toward formal help-seeking. *Journal of Interpersonal Violence* 37(15-16):NP13729-NP13765.

Hart, B. J., and A. F. Klein. 2013. *Practical implications of current intimate partner violence research for victim advocates and service providers.* Washington, DC: U.S. Department of Justice Office of Justice Programs.

Heron, R. L., and M. C. Eisma. 2021. Barriers and facilitators of disclosing domestic violence to the healthcare service: A systematic review of qualitative research. *Health Soc Care Community* 29(3):612-630.

Hulley, J., L. Bailey, G. Kirkman, G. R. Gibbs, T. Gomersall, A. Latif, and A. Jones. 2023. Intimate partner violence and barriers to help-seeking among Black, Asian, minority ethnic and immigrant women: A qualitative metasynthesis of global research. *Trauma, Violence, & Abuse* 24(2):1001-1015.

Huyser, K. R., A. J. Y. Horse, A. A. Kuhlemeier, and M. R. Huyser. 2021. COVID-19 pandemic and indigenous representation in public health data. *Am J Public Health* 111(S3):S208-S214.

Jiwatram-Negrón, T., and N. El-Bassel. 2019. Overlapping intimate partner violence and sex trading among high-risk women: Implications for practice. *Women & Health* 59(6):672-686.

Jock, B. W. I., G. Dana-Sacco, J. Arscott, M. E. Bagwell-Gray, E. Loerzel, T. Brockie, G. Packard, V. M. O'Keefe, C. E. McKinley, and J. Campbell. 2022. "We've already endured the trauma, who is going to either end that cycle or continue to feed it?": The influence of family and legal systems on Native American women's intimate partner violence experiences. *Journal of Interpersonal Violence* 37(21-22):NP20602-NP20629.

Keller, P. S., M. El-Sheikh, M. Keiley, and P. J. Liao. 2009. Longitudinal relations between marital aggression and alcohol problems. *Psychol Addict Behav* 23(1):2-13.

Kelly, U. A. 2009. "I'm a mother first": The influence of mothering in the decision-making processes of battered immigrant Latino women. *Research in Nursing & Health* 32(3):286-297.

Kitzmann, K. M., N. K. Gaylord, A. R. Holt, and E. D. Kenny. 2003. Child witnesses to domestic violence: A meta-analytic review. *J Consult Clin Psychol* 71(2):339-352.

Kivisto, A. J., S. Mills, and L. S. Elwood. 2022. Racial disparities in pregnancy-associated intimate partner homicide. *J Interpers Violence* 37(13-14):NP10938-NP10961.

Korngiebel, D. M., M. Taualii, R. Forquera, R. Harris, and D. Buchwald. 2015. Addressing the challenges of research with small populations. *Am J Public Health* 105(9):1744-1747.

Kozhimannil, K. B., V. A. Lewis, J. D. Interrante, P. L. Chastain, and L. Admon. 2023. Screening for and experiences of intimate partner violence in the United States before, during, and after pregnancy, 2016–2019. *Am J Public Health* 113(3):297-305.

Leemis, R. W., N. Friar, S. Khatiwada, M. S. Chen, M.-j. Kresnow, S. G. Smith, S. Caslin, and K. C. Basile. 2022. *The National Intimate Partner and Sexual Violence Survey: 2016/2017 report on intimate partner violence.* https://www.cdc.gov/violenceprevention/pdf/nisvs/nisvsreportonipv_2022.pdf

Li, Y., C. M. Marshall, H. C. Rees, A. Nunez, E. E. Ezeanolue, and J. E. Ehiri. 2014. Intimate partner violence and HIV infection among women: A systematic review and meta-analysis. *J Int AIDS Soc* 17(1):18845.

Lippy, C., S. N. Jumarali, N. A. Nnawulezi, E. P. Williams, and C. Burk. 2019. The impact of mandatory reporting laws on survivors of intimate partner violence: Intersectionality, help-seeking and the need for change. *Journal of Family Violence* 35(3):255-267.

Lipsky, S., R. Caetano, and P. Roy-Byrne. 2009. Racial and ethnic disparities in police-reported intimate partner violence and risk of hospitalization among women. *Women's Health Issues* 19(2):109-118.

Lizdas, K., A. O'Flaherty, N. Durborow, A. Marjavi, and A. Ali. 2019. *Compendium of state and US territory statutes and policies on domestic violence and health care.* Edited by Futures Without Violence. 4th ed. https://ipvhealth.org/wp-content/uploads/2019/09/Compendium-4th-Edition-2019-Final-small-file.pdf.

Maman, S., J. Campbell, M. D. Sweat, and A. C. Gielen. 2000. The intersections of HIV and violence: Directions for future research and interventions. *Soc Sci Med* 50(4):459-478.

Marshall, K. J., D. N. Fowler, M. L. Walters, and A. B. Doreson. 2018. Interventions that address intimate partner violence and HIV among women: A systematic review. *AIDS and Behavior* 22:3244-3263.

McCauley, H. L., R. N. Dick, D. J. Tancredi, S. Goldstein, S. Blackburn, J. G. Silverman, E. Monasterio, L. James, and E. Miller. 2014. Differences by sexual minority status in relationship abuse and sexual and reproductive health among adolescent females. *J Adolesc Health* 55(5):652-658.

McDonald, R., E. N. Jouriles, S. Ramisetty-Mikler, R. Caetano, and C. E. Green. 2006. Estimating the number of American children living in partner-violent families. *J Fam Psychol* 20(1):137-142.

McKinley, C. E., and J. L. Liddell. 2022. "Why I stayed in that relationship": Barriers to indigenous women's ability to leave violent relationships. *Violence Against Women* 28(14):3352-3374.

Meyer, S. 2010. Seeking help to protect the children?: The influence of children on women's decisions to seek help when experiencing intimate partner violence. *Journal of Family Violence* 25(8):713-725.

Miller, E., H. L. McCauley, D. J. Tancredi, M. R. Decker, H. Anderson, and J. G. Silverman. 2014. Recent reproductive coercion and unintended pregnancy among female family planning clients. *Contraception* 89(2):122-128.

Narula, A., G. Agarwal, and L. McCarthy. 2012. Intimate partner violence: Patients' experiences and perceptions in family practice. *Fam Pract* 29(5):593-600.

Noursi, S., J. A. Clayton, J. Campbell, and P. Sharps. 2020. The intersection of maternal morbidity and mortality and intimate partner violence in the United States. *Current Women's Health Reviews* 16(4):298-312.

Ortoleva, S., and H. Lewis. 2012. Forgotten sisters—a report on violence against women with disabilities: An overview of its nature, scope, causes and consequences. *Northeastern University School of Law Research Paper* 104-2012.

Othman, S., C. Goddard, and L. Piterman. 2014. Victims' barriers to discussing domestic violence in clinical consultations: A qualitative enquiry. *J Interpers Violence* 29(8):1497-1513.

Palladino, C. L., V. Singh, J. Campbell, H. Flynn, and K. J. Gold. 2011. Homicide and suicide during the perinatal period: Findings from the national violent death reporting system. *Obstet Gynecol* 118(5):1056-1063.

Pavao, J., J. Alvarez, N. Baumrind, M. Induni, and R. Kimerling. 2007. Intimate partner violence and housing instability. *Am J Prev Med* 32(2):143-146.

Peek-Asa, C., A. Wallis, K. Harland, K. Beyer, P. Dickey, and A. Saftlas. 2011. Rural disparity in domestic violence prevalence and access to resources. *J Womens Health (Larchmt)* 20(11):1743-1749.

Peitzmeier, S. M., M. Malik, S. K. Kattari, E. Marrow, R. Stephenson, M. Agenor, and S. L. Reisner. 2020. Intimate partner violence in transgender populations: Systematic review and meta-analysis of prevalence and correlates. *Am J Public Health* 110(9):e1-e14.

Petrosky, E., L. M. Mercer Kollar, M. C. Kearns, S. G. Smith, C. J. Betz, K. A. Fowler, and D. E. Satter. 2021. Homicides of American Indians/Alaska Natives—national violent death reporting system, United States, 2003-2018. *MMWR Surveill Summ* 70(8):1-19.

Porsch, L. M., M. Xu, C. B. Veldhuis, L. A. Bochicchio, S. S. Zollweg, and T. L. Hughes. 2022. Intimate partner violence among sexual minority women: A scoping review. *Trauma Violence Abuse* 24(5):3014-3036.

Raponi, M. B. G., P. C. Condeles, N. F. Azevedo, and M. T. Ruiz. 2023. Prevalence and risk factors for intimate partner violence and indigenous women: A scoping review. *Int J Nurs Pract* e13159.

Ravi, K. E., S. R. Robinson, and R. V. Schrag. 2022. Facilitators of formal help-seeking for adult survivors of IPV in the United States: A systematic review. *Trauma Violence Abuse* 23(5):1420-1436.

Reckdenwald, A., A. Yohros, and A. Szalewski. 2017. Health care professionals, rurality, and intimate femicide. *Homicide Studies* 22(2):161-187.

Roman-Galven, S., S. Martin-Pelaez, B. M. Fernandez-Felix, J. Zamora, K. S. Khan, and A. Bueno-Cavanillas. 2021. Worldwide prevalence of intimate partner violence in pregnancy. A systematic review and meta-analysis. *Frontiers in Public Health* 9:73859.

Rosay, A. B. 2016. Violence against American Indian and Alaska Native women and men. *NIJ Journal* (277).

Sabina, C., J. L. Schally, and L. Marciniec. 2017. Problematic alcohol and drug use and the risk of partner violence victimization among male and female college students. *Journal of Family Violence* 32(3):305-316.

Salgado, G., and B. Gurm. 2020. *Chapter 21: Relationship violence (IPV) in immigrant and refugee communities, Making sense of a global pandemic: Relationship violence & working together towards a violence free society.* Kwantlen Polytechnic University.

Saltzman, L. E., J. L. Fanslow, P. M. McMahon, and G. A. Shelley. 1999. *Intimate partner violence surveillance: Uniform definitions and recommended data elements. Version 1.0.* Atlanta, GA: Centers for Disease Control and Prevention. National Center for Injury Prevention and Control.

Saltzman, L. E., C. H. Johnson, B. C. Gilbert, and M. M. Goodwin. 2003. Physical abuse around the time of pregnancy: An examination of prevalence and risk factors in 16 states. *Matern Child Health J* 7(1):31-43.

Sareen, J., J. Pagura, and B. Grant. 2009. Is intimate partner violence associated with HIV infection among women in the United States? *General Hospital Psychiatry* 31(3):274-278.

Scheer, J. R., and V. P. Poteat. 2021. Trauma-informed care and health among LGBTQ intimate partner violence survivors. *Journal of Interpersonal Violence* 36(13-14):6670-6692.

Scott, S., D. R. Lavage, G. Acharya, L. Risser, S. G. Bocinski, E. A. Walker, K. A. Randell, M. I. Ragavan, and E. Miller. 2023. Experiences of exploitation and associations with economic abuse in adolescent dating relationships: Findings from a US cross-sectional survey. *Journal of Trauma & Dissociation* 1-17.

Spangaro, J. M., A. B. Zwi, and R. G. Poulos. 2011. "Persist. Persist.": A qualitative study of women's decisions to disclose and their perceptions of the impact of routine screening for intimate partner violence. *Psychology of Violence* 1(2):150.

Stockman, J. K., M. B. Lucea, and J. C. Campbell. 2013. Forced sexual initiation, sexual intimate partner violence and HIV risk in women: A global review of the literature. *AIDS Behav* 17(3):832-847.

Stockman, J. K., H. Hayashi, and J. C. Campbell. 2015. Intimate partner violence and its health impact on disproportionately affected populations, including minorities and impoverished groups. *J Womens Health (Larchmt)* 24(1):62-79.

Stone, R., and E. F. Rothman. 2019. Opioid use and intimate partner violence: A systematic review. *Current Epidemiology Reports* 6(2):215-230.

Taylor, B. G., and E. A. Mumford. 2016. A national descriptive portrait of adolescent relationship abuse: Results from the national survey on teen relationships and intimate violence. *J Interpers Violence* 31(6):963-988.

Temple, J. R., and D. H. Freeman, Jr. 2011. Dating violence and substance use among ethnically diverse adolescents. *J Interpers Violence* 26(4):701-718.

Testa, M., J. A. Livingston, and K. E. Leonard. 2003. Women's substance use and experiences of intimate partner violence: A longitudinal investigation among a community sample. *Addict Behav* 28(9):1649-1664.

Thompson, M. P., and J. B. Kingree. 2006. The roles of victim and perpetrator alcohol use in intimate partner violence outcomes. *Journal of Interpersonal Violence* 21(2):163-177.

Tiyyagura, G., C. Christian, R. Berger, D. Lindberg, and S. I. Ex. 2018. Occult abusive injuries in children brought for care after intimate partner violence: An exploratory study. *Child Abuse Negl* 79:136-143.

Ulibarri, M. D., M. Salazar, J. L. Syvertsen, A. R. Bazzi, M. G. Rangel, H. S. Orozco, and S. A. Strathdee. 2019. Intimate partner violence among female sex workers and their noncommercial male partners in Mexico: A mixed-methods study. *Violence Against Women* 25(5):549-571.

Vagi, K. J., E. O'Malley Olsen, K. C. Basile, and A. M. Vivolo-Kantor. 2015. Teen dating violence (physical and sexual) among US high school students: Findings from the 2013 National Youth Risk Behavior Survey. *JAMA Pediatr* 169(5):474-482.

Varcoe, C., and L. G. Irwin. 2004. "If I killed you, I'd get the kids": Women's survival and protection work with child custody and access in the context of woman abuse. *Qualitative Sociology* 27:77-99.

Vil, N. M. S., M. Sperlich, J. Fitzpatrick, E. Bascug, and J. Elliott. 2022. "I thought it was normal:" perspectives of Black nursing students from high-risk IPV communities on causes and solutions to IPV in the Black community. *Journal of Interpersonal Violence* 37(13-14):NP12260-NP12283.

Vu, N. L., E. N. Jouriles, R. McDonald, and D. Rosenfield. 2016. Children's exposure to intimate partner violence: A meta-analysis of longitudinal associations with child adjustment problems. *Clin Psychol Rev* 46:25-33.

Wahab, S., and L. Olson. 2004. Intimate partner violence and sexual assault in Native American communities. *Trauma Violence Abuse* 5(4):353-366.

Waller, B. Y., J. Harris, and C. R. Quinn. 2022. Caught in the crossroad: An intersectional examination of African American women intimate partner violence survivors' help seeking. *Trauma Violence Abuse* 23(4):1235-1248.

White, H. R., and P. H. Chen. 2002. Problem drinking and intimate partner violence. *J Stud Alcohol* 63(2):205-214.

Willie, T. C., J. K. Stockman, R. Perler, and T. S. Kershaw. 2018. Associations between intimate partner violence, violence-related policies, and HIV diagnosis rate among women in the United States. *Ann Epidemiol* 28(12):881-885.

Yellow Horse, A. J., and K. R. Huyser. 2022. Indigenous data sovereignty and COVID-19 data issues for American Indian and Alaska Native tribes and populations. *J Popul Res (Canberra)* 39(4):527-531.

3

Intimate Partner Violence and Public Health Emergencies

PUBLIC HEALTH EMERGENCIES

The committee defines a *public health emergency* (PHE) for the purposes of this report as a situation with health consequences whose scale, timing, or unpredictability threatens to overwhelm the routine capabilities of the affected geographic area. Examples include infectious disease outbreaks; extreme weather events such as hurricanes, heat waves, or wildfires; earthquakes; and technological disasters such as mass power outages, nuclear incidents, or oil spills.

Terms and Approaches

Five Phases

The five phases or steps of emergency management are prevention, mitigation, preparedness, response, and recovery (DHS, 2015). *Prevention* refers to activities undertaken to avoid these incidents. *Mitigation* involves reducing emergencies' or disasters' impacts and consequences (DHS, 2015). *Preparedness* refers to actions designed to develop resilience and the capability to respond to and recover from the effects of an incident. It involves planning, training, and educational activities (DHS, 2015). Mitigation and preparedness need to occur in advance of an incident. The *response* phase refers to activities undertaken during and immediately after an incident to address its impact directly (DHS, 2015). The *recovery* phase involves restoration efforts during the longer-term aftermath of an event (DHS,

2015). These five phases are used throughout the field of emergency management to guide efforts to address PHEs of all magnitudes.

All-Hazards Approach

An *all-hazards approach*, as defined by the Centers for Medicare & Medicaid (CMS), "is an integrated approach to emergency preparedness planning that focuses on capacities and capabilities that are critical" in order to prepare for, respond to, and recover from the full spectrum of emergencies or disasters, whether human-made or natural (CMS, 2017). The International Federation of the Red Cross and Red Crescent formally defines *disasters* as "serious disruptions to the functioning of a community that exceeds its capacity to cope using its own resources" (IFRC, 2023, para. 1). The shock of a disaster disrupts the health, well-being, and functioning of communities. This includes damage to infrastructure—such as the loss of electrical power or public transportation, supply shortages, and damage to buildings and homes. Notably, the functionality of health care systems may be affected, contributing to a lack of access to health care for the local community (Bayntun, 2012; Bell et al., 2020).

All-hazards planning is based on two core premises:

1. Potential hazards, threats, and vulnerabilities have been assessed in advance and plans are in place to address these; and
2. A uniform approach to response and recovery will be employed regardless of the hazard that occurs.

In other words, an all-hazards approach seeks to be ready for any disaster. The process includes the development of capacities and capabilities essential for effective disaster preparedness for all types of emergencies and disasters (CMS, 2016; FEMA, 2021). However, an all-hazards approach also includes planning specific to the locale of the service provider. It accounts for the different types of hazards that could potentially occur in a given community (FEMA, 2021).

Actors and Roles in Public Health Emergency Response

Initially, all disaster response is local in nature and consists of local emergency services supplemented by state and volunteer entities. All states and territories, as well as some tribal and local governments, have adopted statutes to guide and empower government leaders to respond to PHEs. Provisions relevant to PHEs may be found in statutes developed in preparation for natural disasters, disease outbreaks, civil unrest, and general emergencies. In addition, federal laws provide guidance and authority to federal officials concerning how to support PHE preparedness, response, and recovery.

The response to PHEs may involve different actors and roles depending on the nature of the event and the jurisdiction's organizational structure. In the public sector, federal and state, local, tribal, and territorial (SLTT) governments may be involved. At each of these levels, the response is typically led by the jurisdiction's emergency management official. The emergency manager works under the direction of the chief executive— the president and one or more governors as well as local executives, such as mayors or county executives. In addition, state, territorial, city, and county health officers and agencies as well as officials and agencies responsible for other sectors—such as transportation, housing, agriculture, and others—may also be involved.

At the federal level, key entities involved in PHE response include the cabinet-level departments, especially the Department of Homeland Security (DHS) and the Department of Health and Human Services (HHS), as well as the plethora of sub-entities formed within each department. For example, under DHS, the Federal Emergency Management Agency (FEMA) is responsible for coordinating the response to emergencies and disasters that overwhelm SLTT governments. Under the HHS umbrella, a variety of entities play key roles. The Administration for Strategic Preparedness and Response (ASPR) is responsible for "medical and public health preparedness for, response to, and recovery from disasters and other public health emergencies" (ASPR, n.d.). CMS administers the two largest federal health care programs. The Centers for Disease Control and Prevention (CDC) provides technical and financial support to state and territorial governments for monitoring, controlling, and preventing disease outbreaks and injuries. The Food and Drug Administration (FDA) ensures that drugs, biologics, and medical devices (including some forms of personal protective equipment) are safe and effective. In turn, each of these sub-departmental agencies is populated by additional layers of centers, programs, and offices devoted to particular functions or areas of concern.

In 2008, the World Health Organization recommended that jurisdictions adopt a "whole of society" approach to pandemics (and later, other PHEs), which involves ensuring that partners from across all sectors and functions of society are engaged across all five phases of PHE management (WHO, 2009). This has been echoed through the FEMA publication *A Whole Community Approach to Emergency Management: Principles, Themes, and Pathways for Action* (FEMA, 2011).

U.S. Laws and Regulations Concerning Emergency Response

Several federal laws are principally relevant to PHE response. The Public Health Service Act[1] (PHSA) and its amending legislation[2] authorizes various federal emergency declarations, including PHE declarations, Emergency Use Authorization (EUA) declarations, and Pandemic Readiness and Emergency Preparedness Act[3] (PREP) declarations. The Social Security Act[4] (SSA) includes requirements applicable to Medicare and Medicaid, among other health care regulations. The Robert T. Stafford Disaster Relief and Emergency Assistance Act[5] (Stafford Act) and National Emergencies Act[6] (NEA) authorize emergency and major disaster declarations.

The most relevant federal declarations to ensure access to essential health care services related to IPV during a PHE are made under Section 319 of the PHSA and the various declarations available under the Stafford Act. A Section 319[7] PHE declaration allows HHS and its multiple sub-agencies, including CMS, to suspend or waive specific federal requirements, including requirements rising out of the Health Insurance Portability and Accountability Act (HIPAA) Privacy Rule, various conditions of clinic and clinician participation in Medicare, and various requirements applicable to state Medicaid programs, among other federal regulations.

The president may issue two distinct declarations under the Stafford Act when federal assistance is needed to supplement state, tribal, and local efforts and capabilities: an emergency declaration or a major disaster declaration. Both declarations authorize the distribution of federal relief funds and various forms of direct assistance, but the scope of assistance available under a major disaster declaration is broader than that under an emergency declaration. A state governor or tribal chief executive may only request a disaster declaration and accompanying federal assistance, but the president may issue a declaration unilaterally when an emergency exists for which the primary responsibility rests with the federal government.

---

[1] *Public Health Service Act* 42 USC 247d.

[2] See: *Public Readiness and Emergency Preparedness (PREP) Act of 2005*, Public Law 109-148, 109th Congress (December 30, 2005); *Pandemic All-Hazards Preparedness Act*, Public Law 109-417, 109th Congress (December 19, 2006); *Pandemic and All-Hazards Preparedness Reauthorization Act (PAHPRA)*, Public Law 113-5, 113th Congress (March 13, 2013); *Pandemic and All-Hazards Preparedness and Advancing Innovation Act (PAHPAIA)*, Public Law 116-22, 116th Congress (January 3, 2019), *Public Health Service Act*, Public Law 356, 117th Congress (January 25, 2023).

[3] *Public Readiness and Emergency Preparedness Act of 2005*, Public Law 109-148, 109th Congress (December 30, 2005).

[4] *Social Security Act* 42 USC § 1320b-5.

[5] *Robert T. Stafford Disaster Relief and Emergency Assistance Act*, Public Law 100-707, 100th Congress (May 22, 1974) (November 23, 1988).

[6] *National Emergencies Act*, Public Law 94-412, 94th Congress (September 14, 1976).

[7] *Public Health Service Act* 42 USC 247d § 319.

During declared federal emergencies and disasters, federal authorities collaborate with SLTT authorities to provide emergency and disaster assistance, which may include services and supplies as well as financial assistance. Emergency declarations also act as triggers for provisions under other laws, which allow officials powers that they would not have in steady state conditions. The most well-known of these is found in Section 1135 of the SSA.[8] This authority allows federal officials to temporarily waive or modify requirements under Medicare, Medicaid, and the Children's Health Insurance Program during declared disasters and emergencies. Such *1135 waivers* are designed to ensure the stability and availability of health care services during emergencies.

In March 2020, CMS issued an 1135 waiver modifying the requirements for clinicians under the Emergency Medical Treatment and Active Labor Act[9] (EMTALA) (Brown, 2021). EMTALA ordinarily requires covered medical facilities to screen, stabilize, and appropriately transfer patients presenting to their emergency departments. This mandate, which is a condition for a clinician's participation in Medicare, protects patients regardless of their ability to pay, documentation status, citizenship status, or other circumstances. COVID-19-era 1135 waivers allowed medical facilities to refer patients to alternative locations for screening, including those that were off site. Facilities were also allowed to transfer patients before they were fully stabilized.

During a declared PHE, federal officials may also exercise authorities available under various steady state provisions. For example, the SSA provides the basis for an Emergency Preparedness Rule applicable to health care institutions participating in CMS-funded programs (e.g., Medicare and Medicaid) (CMS, 2016). The PHSA[10] includes communicable disease control powers that are not conditioned on an emergency declaration, such as the power to take measures deemed necessary by the HHS Secretary to prevent or mitigate the spread of communicable disease across international, state, or territorial borders.

CMS Emergency Preparedness Rule

The CMS Emergency Preparedness Requirements for Medicare and Medicaid Participating Providers and Suppliers Final Rule (EP rule) has particular relevance to PHE planning relevant to ensuring access to essential intimate partner violence (IPV) health care services. In 2016, this rule came into effect for all health care institutions participating in CMS-funded

---

[8] *Social Security Act* Section 1135 42 USC § 1320b-5.
[9] *Social Security Act* Section 1867 42 USC § 1395dd.
[10] *Public Health Service Act* 42 USC § 264.

programs (Medicare and Medicaid) (CMS, 2016). The rule mandated the documentation of annual disaster response training; drill exercises; and plans for communicating how to contact local, state, and federal emergency preparedness officials (CMS, 2016). Examples of health care institutions subject to the EP rule and relevant to this report are hospitals, nursing homes, Federally Qualified Health Centers, community mental health centers, psychiatric residential treatment facilities, religious nonmedical health care institutions, and intermediate care facilities for individuals with intellectual disabilities (CMS, 2016).

The EP rule was designed to promote preparedness at the health care organization level, leaving flexibility to the organization in determining the amount and depth of training, drilling, and demonstrating competencies. This flexibility could be used to encourage preparedness activities among facilities with specific IPV care responsibilities.

Effects of Emergency Declarations

A PHE or disaster declaration can rapidly change legal requirements for health care delivery and financing. State emergency and disaster management declarations typically empower a governor to adopt reasonable and necessary measures for protecting life and property and bringing the situation under control. In some states, such as California and Oregon, these powers are far-reaching and may include the entirety of the state's police powers.[11] Disaster declarations open the door for funding and organizational support for the health care entities affected by a disaster, resources without which health care institutions may be unable to mount an effective response (ASPR, 2021a).

At the federal level, the president may issue an NEA[12] declaration, which authorizes federal agencies to waive or suspend requirements and obligations under federal law. These remain in place for 1 year and may be renewed. The HHS Secretary may issue a declaration authorizing FDA to issue EUAs to facilitate the availability and use of medical countermeasures needed during PHEs. Section 564 of the Federal Food, Drug, and Cosmetic Act[13] authorizes the FDA to issue EUAs for medical countermeasures, including personal protective equipment (PPE), diagnostics, therapeutics, and vaccines. EUAs allow the use of a countermeasure before it has met full FDA approval for the specific emergency use in question. Instead, the regulatory procedure for an EUA only requires federal officials to demonstrate that a current emergency justifies its issuance. Additionally, the HHS

---

[11] CAL. GOV. CODE § 8627; OR. REV. STAT. § 401.168(1).
[12] *National Emergencies Act* 50 USC 1601, 1621, 1622.
[13] *Federal Food, Drug, and Cosmetic Act* Section 564 21 USC § 360bbb-3.

Secretary may issue a PREP Act[14] declaration that limits liability for medical countermeasures provided during this time.

Indian Health Service and Tribal Emergency Preparedness

American Indian and Alaska Native (AI/AN) tribes have a unique relationship with the U.S. government. Based on treaties, laws, and court decisions, each of the federally recognized tribal nations maintain a government-to-government relationship with the U.S. federal government. With limited exceptions, state and local governments throughout the United States do not exercise authority over tribal governments (Hershey, 2019). These unique relationships are recognized within the American emergency preparedness and response structure at the federal level through amendments to the Stafford Act.[15] These amendments allow tribal governments to declare emergencies and request presidential disaster declarations independent of the states. Additionally, FEMA policy[16] recognizes the unique relationship between the tribal governments and the federal government and emphasizes specific consultations with tribal nations on issues that impact them (FEMA, 2020).

Given the diversity of AI/AN populations, it is difficult and potentially inappropriate to comprehensively identify the specific emergency preparedness and response challenges they face. Instead, the challenges many AI/AN individuals face are better understood through their general health risks and care limitations. These health factors are compounded due to the often-remote locations of most reservations. The emergency response services available to tribal members are often provided, similar to non-tribal neighbors, through a patchwork of federal (i.e., the Indian Health Service), state, local, and private providers (Genovesi, 2014). These providers, and the communities they serve, face challenges common to rural health care, including insufficient staffing, limited infrastructure, long travel times and distances, and challenging access to certain areas (Genovesi, 2014). In addition, AI/AN communities face the risk of morbidity and mortality and certain disease burdens at rates significantly higher than the national average (Hershey, 2019). This combination of increased risks and service delivery limitations makes the consistent delivery of high-quality care a particularly acute challenge when faced with PHEs.

---

[14] *Department of Defense, Emergency Supplemental Appropriations to Address Hurricanes in the Gulf of Mexico, and Pandemic Influenza Act*, Public Law 109-148 Division C: *Public Readiness and Emergency Preparedness (PREP) Act of 2005* § 2, 109th Congress (December 30, 2005).

[15] See *Sandy Recovery Improvement (SRIA) Act of 2013*, Public Law 113-2, 113th Congress (January 29, 2013).

[16] Federal Emergency Management Agency (FEMA) Policy 101-002-02.

The Indian Health Service (IHS) is an HHS agency that provides health services to AI/AN populations with the goal of "ensur(ing) that comprehensive, culturally appropriate personal and public health services are available and accessible to American Indian and Alaska Native people" (IHS, n.d.). Care in tribal communities is delivered primarily by IHS-supported facilities and, since 1976,[17] in tribal-operated health care entities (referred to as 638 clinics). These facilities provide comprehensive primary care and support services in remote and underserved settings on tribal lands where they are typically the only health care professionals available in the area. In general, IHS clinicians function in a manner similar to health care professionals throughout the United States, building relationships and providing appropriate referrals to patients based on need and services available in the community (IHS, 2017). In a PHE, these entities are the essential health care organizations providing a comprehensive range of health and supportive services, including support and care to individuals experiencing IPV.

Federal Frameworks for Disaster Response

The federal government has established multiple overlapping frameworks and systems for accomplishing defined functions to prepare for and recover from disasters. Under the auspices of the Stafford Act, the PHSA, and other agency authorities, the National Response Framework coordinates federal agency responses to PHEs and other disasters, including providing guidance for organizational structures and preparedness (DHS, 2019a). The National Incident Management System includes and expands beyond federal agencies to support all public and private entities to implement an effective emergency response (FEMA, 2017). The National Response Framework delineates 15 Emergency Support Functions (ESFs), which provide the mechanism for coordination among federal agencies (DHS, 2019a). For example, ESF 8, Public Health and Medical Services, is coordinated by HHS and includes diverse partners such as the federal departments of Energy, Labor, and Defense; the U.S. Postal Service; and the American Red Cross (DHS, 2019a). Many of these agencies have primary or supporting roles in other ESFs. ESF 8 specifically addresses public health and medical services capabilities and is intended to coordinate health and health care in SLTTs and across federal agencies (DHS, 2019a). See Appendix A for additional information about ESFs.

The National Disaster Recovery Framework (NDRF) is a companion to the National Response Framework and provides a roadmap for promoting

---

[17] *Indian Self-determination and Education Assistance Act*, Public Law 93-638, 93rd Congress (January 4, 1975)

successful disaster recovery, particularly from large-scale or catastrophic incidents (DHS, 2016). It provides guidance for coordinating the authorities and missions of federal agencies under the Stafford Act, PHSA, and other applicable statutes. The NDRF may be applied to an incident without a federal emergency or disaster declaration. It provides a flexible structure for disaster recovery managers to work in a unified manner and is intended to foster resilience in U.S. communities (DHS, 2016). Under the NDRF, Recovery Support Functions (RSFs) facilitate local stakeholder participation and promote intergovernmental and public–private partnerships (DHS, 2016). Each RSF is directed by designated federal agencies and supported by public and private entities at national, state, tribal, and local levels. Federal agencies gather pertinent specialists and stakeholders for planning during steady state conditions and then coordinate with the same individuals during post-disaster recovery to execute RSFs (DHS, 2016).

The multiplicity and overlap of these frameworks and functions have resulted in confusion among clinicians and members of the public alike. FEMA sought to reduce confusion when it introduced its Community Lifelines Implementation Toolkit, which enables the "continuous operation of critical government and business functions and are essential to human health and safety or economic security" (FEMA, 2023b). The Lifelines represent "the most fundamental services in the community that, when stabilized, enable all other aspects of society to function" (FEMA, 2023a). All eight lifelines in Figure 3-1 are interdependent and essential to enabling uninterrupted government and business functions essential to human health and safety or economic security (FEMA, 2023b). For example, the Health and Medical Lifeline includes objectives for restoring medical care, public health, patient movement, medical supply chain, and fatality management.

Disaster Response Resources

Much of the human resources operational capacity for larger-scale PHE response is focused at the federal level. Volunteer organizations such as the American Red Cross and faith-based organizations also play an important role. Disaster health responder teams need basic capacities to safely deploy in a PHE: rapid mobility, self-containment, self-sufficiency, and multidisciplinary team composition. These teams are often required to deploy within hours of a disaster or stage in a nearby location when a disaster is expected. These teams are expected to be able to independently set up and staff a field hospital and provide health care within hours of arriving on site. Teams usually arrive with adequate equipment, supplies, food, and water to last at least 72 hours (Weiner and Rosman, 2019). Several federal agencies have structures and plans that can help provide human resources, equipment, and protection for deploying disaster teams.

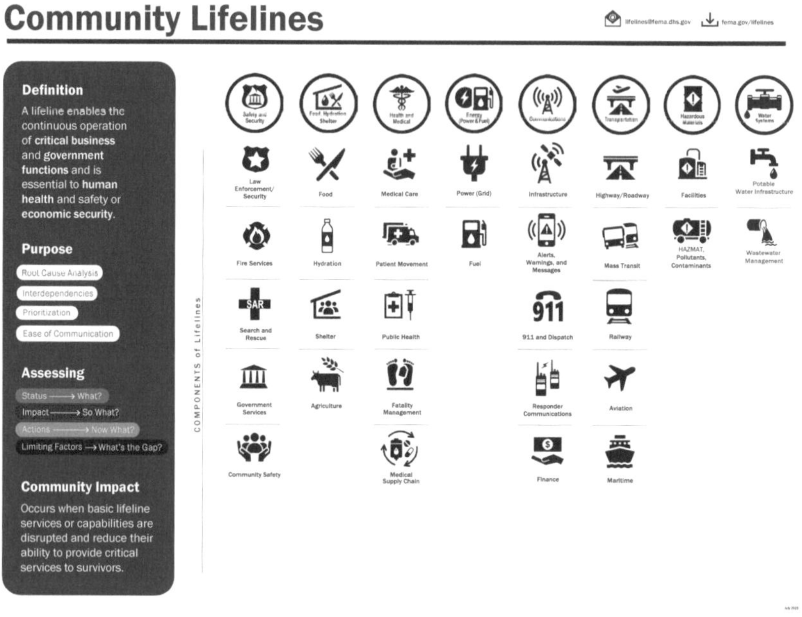

FIGURE 3-1 Federal Emergency Management Agency (FEMA) Community Lifelines. SOURCE: FEMA (2023b).

Additional protections are required for essential health care workers to continue providing care for people experiencing IPV during a PHE. This may include nonpharmaceutical interventions and supplies, such as PPE (gowns, masks, respirators), and pharmaceutical interventions, such as vaccination and pre- and post-exposure prophylaxis. Ensuring the safety of the IPV workforce is essential for maintaining their ability to support those affected by the PHE.

The National Disaster Medical System

The purpose of the National Disaster Medical System (NDMS), overseen by ASPR, is to support SLTTs during PHEs by supplementing existing health and medical systems and response capabilities (ASPR, 2021b). Disaster Medical Assistance Teams (DMATs) are comprised of health care clinicians that provide rapid-response health care when health needs due to disasters or PHEs overwhelm SLTT health resources (ASPR, 2021b). DMAT teams provide patient care in numerous settings and scenarios, including triage and pre-hospital care, general emergency medical care, general medical care, hospital decompression, patient movement and transfer support, and mass prophylaxis and vaccinations (ASPR, 2021b).

Public Health Emergency Response Strike Teams

Public Health Emergency Response Strike Teams are active duty officers with the U.S. Public Health Service (USPHS) who serve as first responders in the event of disasters and PHEs (USPHS, 2022). These teams are designed to deploy rapidly to regional, national, and global emergencies. When not deployed, they support staffing gaps across USPHS-staffed facilities (USPHS, 2022).

Veterans Health Administration

In addition to providing services to veterans during PHEs, the *fourth mission* of the Veterans Health Administration (VHA) includes providing support to nonveteran civilians during times of crisis. Employees of the VHA may be deployed or diverted from their usual roles to provide health care support during federally declared disasters. During disasters, the VHA supports the NDMS (VA, 2021).

Health Care Coalitions

ASPR developed the Hospital Preparedness Program and its associated Health Care Coalitions (HCCs) as part of the response to the September 11, 2001, terror attacks and subsequent anthrax attacks (West Region Health Care Coalition, 2023). The purpose of HCCs is to ensure that local communities can respond to emergencies in an integrated, smooth, and timely manner (ASPR, 2016). Composed of geographically related health care and response organizations, HCCs are generally considered *the* regional organization supporting health care readiness (ASPR, 2016). They are vital for bridging the gap between public health and the health care community (IOM, 2015). The function of this group often depends on the context of the given community. Generally, HCCs are expected to organize stakeholders, medical supplies, real-time communication retrieval, and trained personnel. HCCs are critical for providing logistical guidance during disasters and safeguarding communities from preventable harm (ASPR, 2021b).

A vital role of HCCs is establishing relationships across health care entities on *blue-sky days* to ensure that effective communications are in place before a disaster event. HCCs also serve as a resource to local and regional health care organizations regarding preparedness planning, including coordinating medical response and surge exercises (ASPR, 2016). This unique organizational role could position HCCs as a conduit for ensuring a greater emphasis on IPV care in PHEs, whether through developing and deploying specific protocols or by including IPV scenarios in drills and table-top exercises.

Emergency Management Assistance Compact

The Emergency Management Assistance Compact (EMAC)[18] was cre-ated to better provide support in resource-limited conditions and the com-munities affected by disasters by providing an avenue for assistance between states during disaster declarations. It was signed into law in 1996 under Public Law 104-321. All 50 states and multiple territories have become members via legislation. EMAC's design is intentionally straightforward, allowing responsive action for sharing staff, equipment, and other supplies to support response and recovery in other states. Its governance structure supports building and maintaining relationships across federal and SLTT entities and professional organizations to encourage open communica-tion and sharing of resources. A core strength of EMAC is its ability to move nearly any resource from one state to another (EMAC, 2023).

Building on the successes of EMAC could be an avenue for collabora-tively designing and implementing a system that coordinates access to essen-tial IPV resources through existing protocols and agreements. For example, EMAC supports using and disseminating mission-ready packages, which are "specific response and recovery capabilities that are organized, developed, trained, and exercised prior to an emergency or disaster" (GOHSEP, 2023). Developing a tailored mission-ready package could be of value to IPV care in PHEs.

Public Health Emergencies and Health Disparities

The scientific and lay literature has demonstrated that historically and structurally marginalized populations experience worse outcomes during disasters and PHEs (NASEM, 2019). Specifically, the interaction of weather-and climate-related disasters with the built environment causes damage to critical infrastructure that is essential for the health of communities, such as access to food, water, shelter, health care, transportation, and electrical power (Michaud and Kates, 2017). The current-day consequences associ-ated with structural racism[19] can also influence this interaction. Widening

---

[18] *Emergency Management Assistance Compact*, Public Law 104-321, 104th Congress, (October 19, 1996).

[19] *Structural racism* refers to the ways in which systems such as housing, health care, and education affect and reinforce biases and the discriminatory distribution of resources.

social inequalities, increasing urbanization, and rapid population growth—particularly in coastal areas—further predispose certain groups to disaster-related disparities (Raker et al., 2020).

After a disaster, disruptions in access to health care can be devastating for the 60 percent of American adults living with at least one chronic condition (CDC, 2022). Individuals with chronic health conditions may depend on medical equipment using electrical power, from refrigerators to keep insulin chilled to dialysis to continuous positive airway pressure machines. The careful adherence to the medical treatments needed to keep health conditions under control, such as medication regimens, may be at risk following a PHE. Additionally, mental health practices, substance use disorder treatment practices, health care centers, and dialysis services may experience operational interruptions, and transportation to alternative sources of care may not be possible. Such PHE-related disruptions have been associated with increased hospitalizations among those with chronic and comorbid conditions (Bell et al., 2022). Furthermore, research has described challenges in long-term health care access—specifically the availability of health care professionals—in disaster-affected communities with socioeconomic disparities (Bell et al., 2020).

Older adults are also vulnerable to poor health outcomes during disasters. While age itself does not make an individual at risk, social isolation, frailty, chronic and comorbid diseases (as described above), and cognitive impairment—all issues common to older adults—do. The acute disruption of a disaster can exacerbate these potential vulnerabilities for older adults. Almost 50 percent of deaths attributed to Hurricane Katrina were among adults aged 75 and older (Brunkard et al., 2008). Living through a hurricane has been associated with increased mortality among older adults with dementia, a highly vulnerable group that needs caregiver support for situational awareness during a disaster (Bell et al., 2023).

Racial and ethnic disparities continue to mount after PHEs, despite being documented for decades (Fothergill, 1999). A recent review of multiple studies of heat, extreme cold, hurricanes, flooding, and wildfires finds evidence that minoritized populations, including Black, Hispanic, Native American, Pacific Islander, and Asian communities, are generally at higher risk of climate-related health impacts than are White communities (Berberian et al., 2022). Multiple studies describe racial and ethnic disparities in mental health outcomes after hurricane and flood events, including high rates of depression, anxiety, and post-traumatic stress disorder (Alexander et al., 2017; Ali et al., 2017; Flores, 2020; Ma et al., 2021). While White individuals made up 68 percent of total disaster and extreme weather mortality in a recent study, mortality per 100,000 rates among Black individuals were 1.87 times higher than among White individuals, and for non-Hispanic AI/AN populations mortality per 100,000 was 7.34 times higher (Sharpe and Wolkin,

2022). Extreme heat has also been associated with higher all-cause mortality in the United States, with a greater increase noted among older adults and non-Hispanic Black individuals (Khatana et al., 2022).

Figure 3-2 and Figure 3-3 display Columbia University's Natural Hazards Index (NHI) and CDC's Social Vulnerability Index (SVI), respectively. The NHI shows hazard exposure data at the census tract level for 14 types of natural disasters (NCDP, 2023). The SVI measures the "potential negative effects on communities caused by external stresses on human health" (ATSDR, 2023). Together, these graphics illustrate that the geographic regions that are most socially vulnerable, particularly the Southern and Western United States, are also disproportionately exposed to natural hazards and disasters. In other words, historically and structurally marginalized populations face more harm from natural disasters, but they are also more likely to face them.

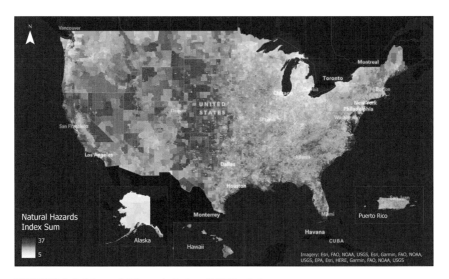

FIGURE 3-2 Natural Hazards Index (NHI) v2.0.
Notes: For detailed documentation including available hazard layers by region, data interpretation and limitations, and views of individual hazard layers, visit the Natural Hazards Index project homepage with live map application at https://bitly. com/hazardsindex. This tool is a hazards map, not a risk map and can be used as a planning tool but does not factor in local mitigation and preparedness efforts or population exposure.
SOURCE: Columbia Climate School National Center for Disaster Preparedness 2023.

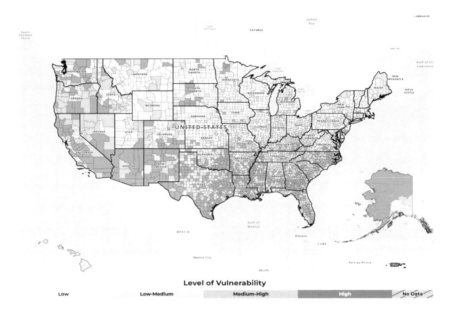

FIGURE 3-3 Social Vulnerability Index (SVI).
SOURCE: ATDSR, 2023.

INTERSECTION OF PUBLIC HEALTH EMERGENCIES AND INTIMATE PARTNER VIOLENCE

Effects of Public Health Emergencies on the Prevalence and Severity of Intimate Partner Violence

PHEs are a time of increased prevalence and severity of IPV. The causes and pathways for these effects overlap and tend to exacerbate inequities. Access to resources and support becomes more challenging for those experiencing IPV. Women experiencing IPV during PHEs can face additional safety risks because of disruptions in the normal function of some government services and lines of communication for measures such as orders of protection. Some mitigation or support efforts focused on the PHE, such as shelter-in-place orders and social distancing, may inadvertently worsen situations for survivors. Those experiencing IPV may be further isolated by abusive partners and structural barriers emerging during the PHE, such as a lack of support services, making it more challenging to connect with care.

Intimate Partner Violence During the COVID-19 Pandemic

The most recent surveillance data and research related to IPV during PHEs comes from the COVID-19 pandemic. The increase in IPV during the COVID-19 pandemic, particularly during the earlier periods of the pandemic, received attention in the media and among the IPV care professionals, advocates, and others who provide care and support for individuals experiencing IPV (Evans et al., 2020; Gupta and Aviva, 2020). Researchers have examined data from IPV hotlines, hospitals and other health care settings, IPV support service providers, and surveys to gain insight into IPV during the COVID-19 pandemic.

In a study by Ragavan and colleagues (2022), victim service advocates shared multiple tactics used to control, frighten, or manipulate IPV survivors. Abusive partners sought to isolate their partners during stay-at-home orders and social distancing that occurred during the COVID-19 pandemic. The inability to seek respite from a violent relationship through work or other activities with friends and family created further stress for survivors of IPV (Ragavan et al., 2022). The advocates explained that blocking or turning off cell phones or internet service was used as a form of coercive control that added to isolation. They also found that partners may withhold health insurance, information about the pandemic, and protective materials including hand sanitizer, as additional ways to create dependence and fear (Ragavan et al., 2022).

Hospital-based studies may not accurately reflect the experiences of those at elevated risk for IPV, as these individuals may not be presenting to hospital settings during infectious disease-related PHEs such as the COVID-19 pandemic. Thus, a systematic review by Beiter and colleagues (2021) found mixed evidence of increases in violent trauma reported by hospitals; two of three studies reported increases in IPV-related trauma as a proportion of all traumas. Gosangi and colleagues (2021) examined health records and clinical and radiological data for patients at a large urban academic medical center in the United States. They found that the number of patients reporting IPV decreased in 2020, but they observed an increased incidence of physical IPV, with a greater number of deep injuries per victim. Some hospital-based studies during the COVID-19 pandemic found reductions in overall emergency room use and IPV-related admissions (Muldoon et al., 2021).

In contrast, a study from a single-site trauma center (using interrupted time-series analysis) found that the IPV incidence nearly doubled compared with before the pandemic (Smith et al., 2022). Smith and colleagues (2022) described a 17 percent increase in IPV-related injury admissions in the weeks following the start of the COVID-19 pandemic shelter-in-place order. Avalos and colleagues (2023) noted a 38 percent increase in the first month of the pandemic in unsafe and unstable living situations among pregnant women.

Holland and colleagues (2021) reported on cross-sectional data from CDC's National Syndromic Surveillance Program that were collected before and during the COVID-19 pandemic. These data, which capture about 70 percent of emergency department encounters in the United States, showed decreases in IPV-related visits to the emergency department during the pandemic (Holland et al., 2021). This underscores the dramatic shifts in care seeking at emergency departments that occurred as a result of the pandemic (Holland et al., 2021). Many studies noted the likelihood of under-reporting and undercounting IPV due to fear of infection and limited hospital and community resources.

A nationally representative online survey in 2020 during the pandemic assessed physical and psychological IPV. An analysis of the results found that people who were infected with COVID-19 or who lost employment were more likely to use and experience IPV (Davis et al., 2021). Similarly, in a cross-sectional online survey in the spring of 2020, 18 percent of respondents reported IPV, with increased odds of experiencing IPV among those with employment or income change due to the pandemic than those without change (Jetelina et al., 2021). Furthermore, IPV worsened in severity among those experiencing physical and sexual IPV (Jetelina et al., 2021).

In an anonymous online survey conducted from May 2020 through July 2020 focusing specifically on lesbian, gay, bisexual, transgender, and queer (LGBTQ+) adults (N=1,090), those who had experienced IPV in their relationship prior to the COVID-19 pandemic (n=98) reported increasing frequency of IPV since the pandemic began (Stults et al., 2022). More than 18 percent of those LGBTQ+ individuals reported an increase of IPV frequency, with 45.9 percent reporting that the instances stayed the same (Stults et al., 2022). A general population online survey of women, transgender, and nonbinary individuals in Michigan in July and August of 2020 found that nearly 10 percent of respondents had reported new or more frequent IPV since the start of the pandemic (Peitzmeier et al., 2022). This study also highlighted key demographic differences for those who identified as sexual/gender minorities, younger, urban or suburban, pregnant, had disabilities, or had less educational attainment, demonstrating that these groups were more likely to report incidents of IPV or exacerbated IPV since the start of the pandemic (Peitzmeier et al., 2022).

According to nationally representative data from the Adolescent Behavior and Experiences Survey (conducted from January to June 2021 among more than 7,000 respondents), 1 in 12 female-identified respondents had experienced non-dating sexual violence, 12.5 percent had experienced sexual dating violence, and 7.7 percent had experienced physical dating violence (Krause et al., 2023).

Intimate Partner Violence During Heat Waves

Extreme heat events can also disrupt routine capabilities. Heat-related health problems can lead to patient volume surges that overwhelm first responders and health care systems (Sanz-Barbero et al., 2018). Patient surges can be compounded by extreme heat or humidity that limits the function of some medical equipment and the first responders themselves. Excessive heat can also exacerbate relationship tensions and contribute to increased aggressive or violent behavior in some people (Sanz-Barbero et al., 2018). Heat waves and prolonged exposure to high temperatures can have serious physiological and psychological repercussions, such as increased irritability, discomfort, and sleep disruption (Vida et al., 2012). When these variables are combined with other stressors, they can exacerbate conflicts and raise the possibility of violence within partnerships.

Extreme heat has been linked to an upsurge in IPV (Henke and Hsu, 2020). Increases in police reports of domestic abuse (including IPV) phone calls and requests for access to shelters have also been documented during episodes of extreme heat (Rotton and Cohn, 2001; Sanz-Barbero et al., 2018). The impact of this violence extends throughout time, with varied lag periods depending on the violence indicators studied. The latency between temperature rising and aggression could be important in establishing strategies to avert catastrophic consequences of IPV (Sanz-Barbero et al., 2018).

Intimate Partner Violence During Hurricanes and Other Storms

A rapid review of 12 studies examining the relationship between IPV and disasters suggests increased severity and frequency of IPV during pandemics and natural disasters (Brabete et al., 2021). Anastario and colleagues (2009) reported increases in the lifetime prevalence of gender-based violence and IPV in the 2 years after Hurricane Katrina, with associated increases in depressive symptoms and suicidal ideation.

Intimate Partner Violence During Technological Disasters

Technological disasters are caused by the breakdown or malfunction of a technological system (Lindsey et al., 2021). They may occur spontaneously due to a natural disaster, mechanical malfunction, human error, or intentional attacks. Technological disasters include blackouts, hazardous waste incidents, oil spills, nuclear or radiological events, and cyberattacks. In addition to the unique logistical pressures presented by technological disasters, evidence shows that they substantially harm survivors' mental health (Longmuir and Agyapong, 2021; Osofsky et al., 2011; Rubin and Rogers, 2019). Women have been shown to be particularly affected by these harms during technological disasters (Rung et al., 2016). Technological disasters also have unique and gendered resilience dynamics (Ferreira et al., 2018; Lightfoot et al., 2020).

There is little evidence on the prevalence of IPV during technological disasters. However, women who experienced exposure to the Deepwater Horizon oil spill were twice as likely to have experienced both emotional and physical IPV (Lauve-Moon and Ferreira, 2017).

Double Survivorship

Women experiencing IPV during PHEs experience *double survivorship*, in the form of enduring IPV (one survivorship experience) within the context of a PHE (another survivorship). Women with current or previous experiences of IPV are often called survivors because they experience psychological and physical trauma and injuries, and they are encouraged to be empowered to recover from their situation (Alexenko et al., n.d.). Given that IPV can result in severe injuries and homicide, the concept of survivor also helps to communicate that individual's ability to outlive that situation. Similarly, individuals experiencing a PHE are also often referred to as survivors because they have been exposed to psychological and physical trauma and injuries related to the event or circumstance of that PHE and have stayed alive (e.g., lived through a disaster, war, or pandemic). Similar terms are used in these different survivorship experiences when referring to necessary resources such as shelter. It is important to consider the context of these resources—for example, whether shelter is needed because of the IPV, PHE, or both—when considering essential services for this population.

Survivors of IPV and PHEs often experience similar sequelae related to their experiences that when combined, are likely to have a cumulative or synergistic effect on their experience of trauma. For example, symptoms of post-traumatic stress disorder (PTSD) are among the most common consequences of IPV and are also common in a PHE such as a natural disaster (Golding et al., 1999; Lai et al., 2017). Research shows that individuals with a history of trauma and PTSD are more likely to have a more severe traumatic stress response in the context of a new stressor and trauma exposure. For example, poly-victimization and exposure to multiple types of child maltreatment have been associated with increased severity of PTSD among pregnant women (Carney et al., 2023). Similarly, female veterans experiencing IPV are likely to have experienced other forms of trauma (e.g., military sexual assault), thus compounding the burden of IPV (Rossi et al., 2020).

Trauma exposure related to PHEs likely exacerbates the risk for IPV. Research conducted in Africa using the Uppsala Conflict Dataset documented that an increase in the frequency and severity of IPV was associated with an increase in the number of battles an individual had experienced (Le and Nguyen, 2022). Similarly, a study of married couples in refugee camps found that IPV exposure among women was associated with increased exposure to war events and the associated psychopathology among their male partners (Goessmann et al., 2019).

Studies of other emergencies have also suggested a link between trauma exposure and IPV risk. One study examining conflict tactics between post-partum women and their partners after Hurricane Katrina found that women who experienced damage to their home or property during the storm were more likely to report experiencing one or more of physical, mental, or sexual violence from their partner (Harville et al., 2011). Similar results were reported after the 2010 earthquake in Haiti. Women who resided in the hardest hit areas of Haiti were more likely to report physical and sexual IPV (Weitzman and Berhman, 2016). Weitzman and Behrman (2016) also found that women who lost a household member, lived in a displacement camp, or whose households were affected by the subsequent Haitian cholera outbreak were more likely to report IPV.

Given the prevalence of IPV and the potential for cumulative trauma during and after a PHE, screening for both IPV and stress responses is needed. However, clinicians should be cautious and use appropriate timing when screening for traumatic and stress responses. For example, receiving a new diagnosis of HIV could constitute another traumatic event for women seeking care for IPV (Williams et al., 2017). On the other hand, some women have reported that comprehensive services during IPV screening and treatment have provided peace of mind and helped them move forward (Gonzalez-Guarda et al., 2021). Similarly, women may have different responses to the cumulative traumas of a PHE and IPV. Therefore, it is crucial to keep the experience of double survivorship in mind when screening for IPV during PHEs. Screening for IPV during PHEs using a trauma-informed approach and being guided by the perspective of the person experiencing IPV facilitates collaborative development of strategies that are feasible, acceptable, and safe (CDC, 2020). Services for women experiencing IPV during PHEs should apply these principles of trauma-informed care and empower those individuals to define their own needs and preferences, set their own goals, and make their own choices about the services they receive, with a focus of promoting physical, psychological, and emotional safety (CDC, 2020). Clinicians may need to seek out opportunities to revisit IPV screening if women report that they are currently unable to discuss their experiences.

Barriers to Accessing Intimate Partner Violence Care During Public Health Emergencies

Barriers to accessing care during PHEs include damage to health care facilities, displacement of survivors and health care staff, dysfunctional health care systems during disasters, and staff burnout. Additionally, as mentioned earlier, regulatory and other measures taken to mitigate the risks associated with PHEs may result in unintended barriers to care. These barriers compound the challenges people experiencing IPV encounter when in need of care during steady state conditions. Officials may institute policies that limit certain health care services during PHEs to reserve limited supplies and staff for the care of individuals with the most severe conditions or injuries. For example, officials and health care system leaders cancelled surgeries and other procedures that were considered elective during the COVID-19 pandemic when hospitals were at risk of being overwhelmed with infected patients (CovidSurg Collaborative, 2020). This limited the health care services that could be provided to people experiencing IPV during those times (see Box 3-1).

In the past, PHEs have been disruptive to substance use treatment programs and hindered access to mental health services. Disruption to substance use treatment can lead to withdrawal symptoms, and potential relapse (Rutkow et al., 2012). Post Hurricane Katrina emergency shelters were reported to be ill equipped to assist those who had been receiving substance use care, leaving those individuals without the necessary proper treatment (Rutkow et al., 2012).

BOX 3-1
Effect of the COVID-19 Pandemic on Health Services Delivery

"The anterior cruciate ligament is a major ligament in the knee that is commonly sprained or torn. Those types of sprains happen in women that have been victims of intimate partner violence. Those types of injuries were felt to be more elective than urgent for care. So while we were able to address most fractures in a fairly expeditious timeframe, other injuries got put on the back burner. Also, non-hospital-based clinics for non-trauma orthopedic surgeons may have been shut down completely depending on the municipality."

—Gregory Della Rocca,
University of Missouri-Columbia
Department of Orthopaedic Surgery

SOURCE: Della Roca, G. 2023. *Orthopaedic surgeons' roles in the identification and management of injuries related to intimate partner violence.* Presented at Sustaining Essential Health Care Services Related to Intimate Partner Violence During Public Health Emergencies Meeting #3B, Washington, D.C.

Shelter-in-place or stay-at-home orders are issued at local, state, tribal, or federal levels because of PHEs such as pandemics, chemical hazards, or winter storms (DHS, 2019b). These orders are put in place to protect people in the affected area from an external hazard. During PHEs involving infectious respiratory diseases, as with COVID 19, officials may also enact physical distancing rules to reduce the spread of illness (NASEM, 2020). While effective at reducing the spread of contagious respiratory viruses, this strategy also creates challenges for IPV shelters (see Box 3-2).

The PHE and the immediate emergency response can create conditions that serve as physical barriers that disrupt the delivery of IPV care services. Disasters ranging from blizzards to wildfires can damage infrastructure critical to delivering care for people experiencing IPV. Road closures due to damage or obstruction from water, snow, or debris can limit or prevent staff and the people needing services from getting to facilities. While hospitals typically have generator support to provide backup power for a limited period in case of power outages, this is often not the case for outpatient facilities, social service facilities, and community-based organizations. Damage to facilities can limit or completely disrupt the provision of services, particularly during the early hours or, in some cases, days of a PHE.

Immigration documentation status can create challenges for accessing IPV-related health care services during a PHE. People who are undocumented are not eligible for government-sponsored insurance programs (e.g., Medicaid or Medicare) and may not meet eligibility requirements for government-supported prevention and support services that are limited to citizens during a PHE (KFF, 2023). For example, during the COVID-19 pandemic, U.S. workers without documentation often worked in essential jobs (construction,

---

BOX 3-2
Effect of Distancing Orders on IPV Shelters

"Sharing a room became a big problem. We had to have only one family per room, which had a very significant impact on our occupancy level."
—Ivon Mesa,
Community Action and Human Services Department,
Miami-Dade County

SOURCE: Mesa, I. 2023. *Miami Dade County Violence Prevention and Intervention Division.* Presented at Sustaining Essential Health Care Services Related to Intimate Partner Violence During Public Health Emergencies Meeting 2, Irvine, CA.

food production, health care) but could not access COVID-19 economic relief (Disney et al., 2022). Additionally, individuals may have been reluctant to access COVID-19 food and housing assistance because they feared doing so would have a negative effect on their applications for residency or citizenship, even if they were eligible for these services (e.g., free testing and vaccinations) (Disney et al., 2022). In much the same way, documentation status can be a real or perceived barrier to accessing care and social services for IPV (Parson et al., 2016; Valdovinos et al., 2021). The disproportionate adverse effects that PHEs have on people without documentation can increase levels of stress and trauma, which may also worsen the severity and frequency of IPV within those populations.

Interventions to address IPV during PHEs may be improved by considering the intersectional ways in which marginalized groups may be at greater risk for experiencing IPV. For example, acculturative stress—the stress associated with adapting to a new culture and context for immigrant groups—is a known contributor to IPV (Cao et al., 2023; Kim, 2019). Family-level stressors, such as disagreements among family members related to cultural practices and an inability to center family needs, appear to be the most influential form of acculturative stress in predicting IPV risk (Cao et al., 2013; Cervantes et al., 2016). In general, interventions that address family stressors and differences in cultural values and perspectives among family members appear promising in improving health outcomes (Leite et al., 2023).

Accessing IPV-related health care services during PHEs requires a workforce to deliver that care. The COVID-19 pandemic placed extreme stress on the U.S. health care workforce, exposing its fragility, a lack of preparedness, and the starkly limited operational capacity for providing basic health care during a national crisis (NASEM, 2020). This increased the likelihood of first responders and other health care professionals exiting the workforce (Hendrickson et al., 2022). This was highlighted in an analysis of data collected from a survey of New York state physicians, nurse practitioners, and physician assistants first in April 2020, then repeated with the same clinicians in February 2021, which found that more than a third of respondents considered leaving their profession at least once monthly (N=978, 35.6%; 95% CI: 31.9–39.4%) (DiMaggio et al., 2023). The insights gleaned during the COVID-19 pandemic and other PHEs create an opportunity to address the ongoing barriers to accessing IPV care during disasters—as well as to address existing underlying challenges exposed by these disasters—to better support those affected by IPV. This includes managing the urgent need to shift from the current reactive approach to disasters to a proactive one. For health care organizations in disaster-affected areas, many of which are under-resourced, addressing mitigation and preparedness while still being in response or recovery mode is an enormous challenge. The 2022

Federal Plan for Equitable Long-Term Recovery and Resilience for Social, Behavioral, and Community Health[20] provides several recommendations that could be beneficial for addressing these challenges.

Support Services

Community-based organizations, neighborhood associations, community outreach workers, and other support service providers are critical for addressing social drivers of health during steady state periods. In the context of PHEs, such community partners, usually trusted community members, can be vital partners (Gilmore et al., 2020). These groups are uniquely positioned to carry out essential functions, including the rapid mobilization of community health champions within harder-to-reach populations, building trust with the emergency response system, communication about available resources and mitigation of risk, data collection for surveillance and tracking, and guiding local response protocols (Gilmore et al., 2020). Although not always specific to IPV, these community partnerships provide vital services that mitigate the risk of poor outcomes for people experiencing IPV. Community-based service providers for IPV can provide critical feedback on developing, funding, implementing, and evaluating services and programs to prevent and respond to IPV during PHEs. Including community voices in preparation for PHEs ensures that the programs are relevant and responsive to community priorities, assets, and challenges. Simultaneously, culturally responsive care and attention to health equity in clinical practices during PHE response can reduce health disparities experienced by populations disproportionately affected by IPV during PHEs.

The increased intensity of IPV during PHEs highlights the need to prioritize support services that ensure the safety of these women (Gosangi et al., 2021). Among people experiencing IPV, access to safer housing (e.g., domestic violence shelters), advocacy services, and counseling have been found to increase a sense of safety (Bennett et al., 2004; Campbell and Glass, 2009; Sullivan, 2012). Economic, housing, and food resources, which aggravate stress in existing abusive relationships, are often disrupted during a PHE (Gilroy et al., 2016; Ricks et al., 2016; Tur-Prats, 2021). Consequently, support services that ensure access to food, water, and shelter can be a primary strategy for preventing the escalation of IPV during a PHE.

In studies conducted among advocacy and service provision organizations during the COVID-19 pandemic, advocates and administrators of victim service and child welfare agencies described using many workarounds and strategies to continue their work (also see Box 3-3) (Garcia et al., 2022;

---

[20] https://health.gov/our-work/national-health-initiatives/equitable-long-term-recovery-and-resilience (accessed August 28, 2023).

BOX 3-3
IPV Service Providers' Adaptations During the COVID-19 Pandemic

"…in 2020 a lot really had changed. In our county, we all had to shelter in place beginning, I think it was March 16th, 2020, when all of our school districts were ordered to go to work remotely from home. We really needed to continue our outreach and prevention work because now students weren't physically at school, so the ability for mandated reporters to identify things sooner, or for students who were more comfortable in person and, maybe, sharing things with school staff, that all had now changed when we all went to distance learning. So some of the trainings that we provided that year—and actually ongoing even into 2021, part of 2022—is these considerations for COVID. They talked about text chat lines that might be more helpful than call-in numbers, because as we know, our students usually tend to be more comfortable doing chat lines."

—Charisma De Los Reyes,
Student Wellness and Student Culture Department,
San Diego County Office of Education

"COVID brought a lot of challenges and concerns that our home visitors expressed about being able to see our clients. A lot of times, what we heard during COVID is that it was really important for the home visitor to have eyes on the family, because that's something they typically could do. So that was a challenge. However, virtual visits were done, phone calls were done, and then they were creative sometimes, too, during COVID. They would just drive to the outside of the house and do a lesson on the lawn or do social distancing where they could visit and provide whatever information that family might need at that time."

—Lisa Martin,
Johns Hopkins University
Center for Indigenous Health

"When the pandemic hit, it opened up opportunities that we have been fighting for for a really long time, like the ability to have phone visits, like the ability to coordinate care virtually, or having shorter visits, having more customized care because of what we could do. All of a sudden, access to care opened up for some of our survivors who had never been able to access care."

—Anita Ravi,
PurpLE Health Foundation

Renov et al., 2022). Advocates needed to adjust their approaches and communication strategies to address and support safety. Virtual service provision was often a key strategy for increasing access to support services (Garcia et al., 2022; Ragavan et al., 2020a,b, 2022; Renov et al., 2022). IPV agencies connected rapidly and informally with other community organizations (e.g., grocery stores, food banks, and aid groups) to help share services and increase awareness of support services. At times, larger (or more well-resourced or experienced) agencies reached out to assist smaller, less connected agencies and to advocate on their behalf for additional resources (Garcia et al., 2022; Renov et al., 2022). Administrators noted a need for flexibility in the administration (and subsequent use) of disaster relief funds to adapt to the changing landscape and better support clients and staff. Additionally, culturally affirming organizations often experienced compounding impacts on their time without receiving equitable compensation (Garcia et al., 2022). Staff and administrators were also personally affected by the pandemic, with disruptions in school, child care, and employment, all contributing to burnout (Garcia et al., 2022; Renov et al., 2022).

EXISTING GUIDANCE FOR INTIMATE PARTNER VIOLENCE HEALTH CARE DURING PUBLIC HEALTH EMERGENCIES

The committee sought to identify existing, widely available guidance or standard protocols for disaster and emergency responders specific to IPV care during PHEs in the United States. In order for a resource to be considered widely available, it had to be public-facing and free to access. These efforts identified federal resources that included general guidance and suggested actions with varying levels of detail but had little success in identifying public-facing standard protocols. Researching federal agency protocols, guidance, and training programs explicitly addressing IPV during PHEs and disasters often required multiple keyword searches of individual documents identified following lengthy searches of numerous sections of various agency websites. In order for guidance to be practical, it should be easily accessed by those who need it, such as busy emergency planners and health care clinic leaders, as well as those working on the front lines during PHE response. Some state emergency operations plans echoed a common theme from various federal guidance items that encouraged emergency responders to have phone numbers for domestic violence hotlines and shelters available.[21] Notably, most guidance referred to domestic violence

---

[21] For example, see the emergency operations plans found on the emergency management department websites for Kentucky (https://kyem.ky.gov/programs/Pages/State-ESP-and-EOP.aspx) and Arizona (https://dema.az.gov/emergency-management/preparedness/planning-branch) (accessed April 2023).

instead of explicitly addressing IPV. In instances when IPV and domestic violence overlap, these resources may offer valuable information and protocols. However, guidance focused on domestic violence often frames IPV in the context of families with children and relationships with both partners residing in the same home. This can lead planners and disaster health responders to overlook the possibility of IPV in families that do not have children, couples that do not live together, or former intimate partners.

The most recent version of FEMA's *Developing and Maintaining Emergency Operations Plans: Comprehensive Preparedness Guide 101* encourages emergency planners to "identify and describe the actions that will be taken to provide alternate shelter accommodations for evacuees from domestic violence shelters" (FEMA, 2021, p. C-17). FEMA's planning guidance for evacuation and shelter-in-place for SLTT partners includes a brief discussion of important considerations for evacuating people who have experienced IPV (DHS, 2019b). The guidance suggests that evacuation site managers post phone numbers for the National Domestic Violence Hotline and for local IPV/domestic violence (DV) shelters in visible places in emergency shelters. It also lists alternative accommodations for residents when an IPV/DV shelter must be evacuated, including other IPV/DV shelters, a safe home of a family member or friend, or time-limited placement in a motel or hotel (DHS, 2019b). The guidance encourages disaster planners to include IPV/DV shelter staff on planning teams. Of note, the guide also highlights the importance of ensuring the confidentiality of records from IPV/DV shelters to protect the safety of residents. However, it does not offer guidance to support shelters in that task (DHS, 2019b).

The *Public Health Emergency Response Guide for State, Local, and Tribal Public Health Directors* from the CDC is designed to provide guidance for the first 24 hours of an emergency (CDC, 2011). CDC's most recent *Public Health Emergency Preparedness and Response Capabilities: National Standards for State, Local, Tribal, and Territorial Public Health*, last updated in 2019, mentions the need to include community-based organizations in planning and the need to prioritize the development of behavioral health services for families (CDC, 2019). However, it does not explicitly address capabilities to support people experiencing IPV (CDC, 2019). Likewise, the most recent version of CDC's *Public Health Workbook to Define, Locate, and Reach Special, Vulnerable, and At-Risk Populations in an Emergency* does not mention people experiencing IPV as an at-risk population (CDC, 2010).

The HHS Administration for Children and Families collaborated with ASPR to create a fact sheet for first responders about supporting pregnant people who have experienced IPV or sexual violence during disasters (HHS, 2017). The document identifies several unique needs for these individuals and provides contact information for national hotlines but has only limited

IPV-specific guidance. The fact sheet suggests that first responders refresh their training in case they need to deliver a baby; encourages them to facilitate private conversations with a nurse or advocate; and suggests that they promote access to continued clinical care, healthy foods and baby items, clean water and formula or breastfeeding supplies, and an emergency birth plan (HHS, 2017).

The *HHS Maternal-Child Health Emergency Planning Toolkit* notes the potential for increased IPV after an emergency. It emphasizes the need to ensure continuity of services and support to keep someone experiencing IPV separate from the person engaging in IPV (ASPR, 2021). The toolkit includes a recommendation that encourages first responders, health care professionals, and social service providers to use a trauma-informed approach for those they encounter who may have experienced "abuse" but does not explicitly refer to IPV (ASPR, 2021).

The National Resource Center on Domestic Violence's online information center, VAWnet, includes a Disaster and Emergency Preparedness and Response collection.[22] The majority of resources and information in the collection are targeted at informing and preparing domestic violence and sexual violence organizations for disasters. The collection includes a downloadable participant guide for a 2014 course for disaster response workers (Sarabandi, 2018). The guide offers information about domestic violence (but does not mention IPV specifically), including the effect of disasters on people experiencing domestic violence, screening scripts, guidance for responding to disclosure, guidance for assessing the level of risk, and critical components and considerations for safety planning. It also includes a section that explains vicarious trauma, compassion fatigue, and burnout. That document was the most comprehensive discussion of domestic violence for first responders that our research identified. Of note, this document was found through a link on VAWnet. This website is familiar to those working in IPV care. However, it is not likely to be familiar to those outside the field, including emergency planners and health care practice administrators. This may be why committee members with disaster response expertise were unfamiliar with this document.

CHAPTER SUMMARY

PHE management and response is governed by an ecosystem of laws and agencies across federal and SLTT jurisdictions. Declared emergencies activate certain powers for officials, allow for modification of specific regulations, and make funding available to support response. Federal

---

[22] https://vawnet.org/sc/disaster-and-emergency-preparedness-and-response (accessed June 30, 2023).

frameworks provide guidance for PHE planning and response and collaboration between federal and SLTT agencies and volunteer organizations active in disasters.

PHEs do not affect all people equally. Populations that experience health inequities are more likely to be disproportionately affected by PHEs. These populations are also more likely to be disproportionately affected by IPV. PHEs worsen the frequency and severity of IPV. Ensuring access to care and support services for IPV becomes even more critical during PHEs.

REFERENCES

Alexander, A. C., J. Ali, M. E. McDevitt-Murphy, D. R. Forde, M. Stockton, M. Read, and K. D. Ward. 2017. Racial differences in posttraumatic stress disorder vulnerability following Hurricane Katrina among a sample of adult cigarette smokers from New Orleans. *J Racial Ethn Health Disparities* 4(1):94-103.

Alexenko, N., J. Satinsky, and M. Simmons. n.d. Victim or survivor: Terminology from investigation through prosecution. https://sakitta.rti.org/toolkit/index.cfm?fuseaction=tool&tool=80 (accessed August 25, 2023).

Ali, J. S., A. S. Farrell, A. C. Alexander, D. R. Forde, M. Stockton, and K. D. Ward. 2017. Race differences in depression vulnerability following Hurricane Katrina. *Psychol Trauma* 9(3):317-324.

Anastario, M., N. Shehab, and L. Lawry. 2009. Increased gender-based violence among women internally displaced in Mississippi 2 years post-Hurricane Katrina. *Disaster Med Public Health Prep* 3(1):18-26.

ASPR (Administration for Strategic Preparedness and Response). n.d. *ASPR program offices.* https://aspr.hhs.gov/AboutASPR/ProgramOffices/Pages/ProgramOffice.aspx (accessed August 17, 2023).

ASPR. 2016. *2017-2022 health care preparedness and response capabilities.* Edited by Office of the Assistant Secretary for Preparedness and Response. Rockville, Maryland: U.S. Department of Health and Human Services.

ASPR. 2021. *HHS maternal-child health emergency planning toolkit, public health emergency.* U.S. Department of Health and Human Services.

ASPR. 2021. *Medical assistance.* https://www.phe.gov/Preparedness/support/medicalassistance/Pages/default.aspx (accessed August 25, 2023).

ATDSR (Agency for Toxic Substances and Disease Registry). 2023. *CDC/ATDSR social vulnerability index.* https://www.atsdr.cdc.gov/placeandhealth/svi/index.html#:~:text=Social%20vulnerability%20refers%20to%20the,human%20suffering%20and%20economic%20loss (accessed August 25, 2023).

Avalos, L. A., G. T. Ray, S. E. Alexeeff, S. R. Adams, M. B. Does, C. Watson, and K. C. Young-Wolff. 2023. Association of the COVID-19 pandemic with unstable and/or unsafe living situations and intimate partner violence among pregnant individuals. *JAMA Netw Open* 6(2):e230172.

Bayntun, C. 2012. A health system approach to all-hazards disaster management: A systematic review. *PLoS Curr* 4:e50081cad55861d.

Beiter, K., E. Hayden, S. Phillippi, E. Conrad, and J. Hunt. 2021. Violent trauma as an indirect impact of the COVID-19 pandemic: A systematic review of hospital reported trauma. *Am J Surg* 222(5):922-932.

Bell, S. A., K. Klasa, T. J. Iwashyna, E. C. Norton, and M. A. Davis. 2020. Long-term healthcare provider availability following large-scale hurricanes: A difference-in-differences study. *PLoS ONE* 15(11):e0242823.

Bell, S. A., J. P. Donnelly, W. Li, and M. A. Davis. 2022. Hospitalizations for chronic conditions following hurricanes among older adults: A self-controlled case series analysis. *J Am Geriatr Soc* 70(6):1695-1703.

Bell, S. A., M. L. Miranda, J. P. W. Bynum, and M. A. Davis. 2023. Mortality after exposure to a hurricane among older adults living with dementia. *JAMA Netw Open* 6(3):e232043.

Bennett, L., S. Riger, P. Schewe, A. Howard, and S. Wasco. 2004. Effectiveness of hotline, advocacy, counseling, and shelter services for victims of domestic violence: A statewide evaluation. *J Interpers Violence* 19(7):815-829.

Berberian, A. G., D. J. X. Gonzalez, and L. J. Cushing. 2022. Racial disparities in climate change-related health effects in the United States. *Curr Environ Health Rep* 9(3):451-464.

Brabete, A. C., L. Wolfson, J. Stinson, N. Poole, S. Allen, and L. Greaves. 2021. Exploring the linkages between substance use, natural disasters, pandemics, and intimate partner violence against women: A rapid review in the context of COVID-19. *Sexes* 2(4):509-522.

Brown, H. L. 2021. Emergency care EMTALA alterations during the COVID-19 pandemic in the United States. *J Emerg Nurs* 47(2):321-325.

Brunkard, J., G. Namulanda, and R. Ratard. 2008. Hurricane Katrina deaths, Louisiana, 2005. *Disaster Med Public Health Prep* 2(4):215-223.

Campbell, J., and N. Glass. 2009. Safety planning, danger, and lethality assessment. In *Intimate partner violence: A health-based perspective*. New York, NY: Oxford University Press. Pp. 319-334.

Cao, J., S. G. Silva, M. Quizhpilema Rodriguez, Q. Li, A. M. Stafford, R. C. Cervantes, and R. M. Gonzalez-Guarda. 2023. Acculturation, acculturative stress, adverse childhood experiences, and intimate partner violence among Latinx immigrants in the US. *J Interpers Violence* 38(3-4):3711-3736.

Carney, J. R., L. E. Miller-Graff, T. R. Napier, and K. H. Howell. 2023. Elucidating the relations between adverse childhood experiences, age of exposure to adversity, and adult posttraumatic stress symptom severity in pregnant women. *Child Abuse Negl* 136:105995.

CDC (Centers for Disease Control and Prevention). 2010. *Public health workbook to define, locate, and reach special, vulnerable, and at-risk populations in an emergency*. Centers for Disease Control and Prevention.

CDC. 2011. *Public health emergency response guide for state, local, and tribal public health directors version 2.0*. U.S. Department of Health and Human Services.

CDC. 2019. *Public health emergency preparedness and response capabilities: National standards for state, local, tribal, and territorial public health*. U.S. Department of Health and Human Services.

CDC. 2020. *Infographic: 6 guiding principles to a trauma-informed approach*. https://www.cdc.gov/orr/infographics/6_principles_trauma_info.htm (accessed August 25, 2023).

CDC. 2022. *About chronic diseases*. https://www.cdc.gov/chronicdisease/about/index.htm (accessed September 6, 2023).

Cervantes, R. C., D. G. Fisher, A. M. Padilla, and L. E. Napper. 2016. The Hispanic stress inventory version 2: Improving the assessment of acculturation stress. *Psychol Assess* 28(5):509-522.

CMS (Centers for Medicare & Medicaid Services). 2016. Emergency preparedness requirements for Medicare and Medicaid participating providers and suppliers. *Federal Register* 81(180):63859-64044.

CMS. 2017. *Frequently asked questions (FAQs): Emergency preparedness regulation*. Centers for Medicare & Medicaid Services.

COVIDSurg Collaborative. 2020. Elective surgery cancellations due to the COVID-19 pandemic: Global predictive modelling to inform surgical recovery plans. *Br J Surg* 107(11):1440-1449.

Davis, M., O. Gilbar, and D. M. Padilla-Medina. 2021. Intimate partner violence victimization and perpetration among U.S. adults during the earliest stage of the COVID-19 pandemic. *Violence Vict* 36(5):583-603.

DHS (Department of Homeland Security). 2015. *National preparedness goal.* 2nd ed. Washington, DC: Federal Emergency Management Agency.

DHS. 2016. *National disaster recovery framework.* 2nd ed. Washington, DC: Federal Emergency Management Agency.

DHS. 2019a. *National response framework.* 4th ed. Washington, DC: Federal Emergency Management Agency.

DHS. 2019b. *Planning considerations: Evacuation and shelter-in-place: Guidance for state, local, tribal, and territorial partners.* Washington, DC: Federal Emergency Management Agency.

DiMaggio, C., E. Susser, S. Frangos, D. Abramson, H. Andrews, C. Hoven, M. Ryan, and G. Li. 2023. The New York state COVID-19 healthcare personnel study: One-year follow-up of physicians, nurse practitioners, and physician assistants, 2020-2021. *Public Health Rep* 138(3):518-525.

Disney, L., J. Koo, S. Carnes, and L. Warner. 2022. Essential but excluded: Using critical race theory to examine COVID-19 economic relief policies for undocumented US workers. *J Hum Rights Soc Work* 7(3):225-235.

EMAC (Emergency Management Assistance Compact). 2023. *What is EMAC?* https://www.emacweb.org/index.php/learn-about-emac/what-is-emac (accessed February 3, 2023).

Evans, M. L., M. Lindauer, and M. E. Farrell. 2020. A pandemic within a pandemic—intimate partner violence during COVID-19. *N Engl J Med* 383(24):2302-2304.

FEMA (Federal Emergency Management Agency). 2011. *A whole community approach to emergency management: Principles, themes, and pathways for action.* Washington, DC: U.S. Department of Homeland Security.

FEMA. 2017. *National incident management system.* https://www.fema.gov/emergency-managers/nims (accessed August 25, 2023).

FEMA. 2020. *FEMA tribal policy (rev. 2).* Washington, DC: U.S. Department of Homeland Security.

FEMA. 2021. *Developing and maintaining emergency operations plans: Comprehensive preparedness guide 101 version 3.0.* Washington, DC: U.S. Department of Homeland Security.

FEMA. 2023a. *Community lifelines fact sheet.* Washington, DC: U.S. Department of Homeland Security.

FEMA. 2023b. *Community lifelines implementation toolkit version 2.1.* Washington, DC: U.S. Department of Homeland Security.

Ferreira, R. J., F. Buttell, and K. Elmhurst. 2018. The deepwater horizon oil spill: Resilience and growth in the aftermath of postdisaster intimate partner violence. *Journal of Family Social Work* 21(1):22-44.

Flores, A. B., T. W. Collins, S. E. Grineski, and J. Chakraborty. 2020. Disparities in health effects and access to health care among Houston area residents after Hurricane Harvey. *Public Health Rep* 135(4):511-523.

Fothergill, A., E. G. Maestas, and J. D. Darlington. 1999. Race, ethnicity and disasters in the United States: A review of the literature. *Disasters* 23(2):156-173.

Garcia, R., C. Henderson, K. Randell, A. Villaveces, A. Katz, F. Abioye, S. DeGue, K. Premo, S. Miller-Wallfish, J. C. Chang, E. Miller, and M. I. Ragavan. 2022. The impact of the COVID-19 pandemic on intimate partner violence advocates and agencies. *J Fam Violence* 37(6):893-906.

Genovesi, A. L., B. Hastings, E. A. Edgerton, and L. M. Olson. 2014. Pediatric emergency care capabilities of Indian health service emergency medical service agencies serving American Indians/Alaska Natives in rural and frontier areas. *Rural Remote Health* 14(2):2688.

Gilmore, B., R. Ndejjo, A. Tchetchia, V. de Claro, E. Mago, A. A. Diallo, C. Lopes, and S. Bhattacharyya. 2020. Community engagement for COVID-19 prevention and control: A rapid evidence synthesis. *BMJ Glob Health* 5(10).

Gilroy, H., J. McFarlane, J. Maddoux, and C. Sullivan. 2016. Homelessness, housing instability, intimate partner violence, mental health, and functioning: A multi-year cohort study of IPV survivors and their children. *Journal of Social Distress and the Homeless* 25(2):86-94.

Goessmann, K., H. Ibrahim, L. B. Saupe, A. A. Ismail, and F. Neuner. 2019. The contribution of mental health and gender attitudes to intimate partner violence in the context of war and displacement: Evidence from a multi-informant couple survey in Iraq. *Soc Sci Med* 237:112457.

GOHSEP (Governor's Office of Homeland Security and Emergency Preparedness). 2023. *IMAC and EMAC.* https://gohsep.la.gov/RESPOND/REQUEST-RESOURCES/IMAC-EMAC#:~:text=Mission%20Ready%20Packages%20(MRPs)%20are,can%20help%20make%20this%20happen (accessed August 25, 2023).

Golding, J. M. 1999. Intimate partner violence as a risk factor for mental disorders: A meta-analysis. *Journal of Family Violence* 14(2):99-132.

Gonzalez-Guarda, R. M., J. Williams, D. Lorenzo, and C. Carrington. 2021. Desired characteristics of HIV testing and counseling among diverse survivors of intimate partner violence receiving social services. *Health Soc Work* 46(2):93-101.

Gosangi, B., H. Park, R. Thomas, R. Gujrathi, C. P. Bay, A. S. Raja, S. E. Seltzer, M. C. Balcom, M. L. McDonald, D. P. Orgill, M. B. Harris, G. W. Boland, K. Rexrode, and B. Khurana. 2021. Exacerbation of physical intimate partner violence during COVID-19 pandemic. *Radiology* 298(1):E38-E45.

Gupta, A., and S. Aviva. 2020. For abused women, a pandemic lockdown holds dangers of its own. *New York Times*, March 24 (updated October 8, 2021). https://www.nytimes.com/2020/03/24/us/coronavirus-lockdown-domestic-violence.html (accessed August 25, 2023).

Harville, E. W., C. A. Taylor, H. Tesfai, X. Xu, and P. Buekens. 2011. Experience of Hurricane Katrina and reported intimate partner violence. *J Interpers Violence* 26(4):833-845.

Hendrickson, R. C., R. A. Slevin, K. D. Hoerster, B. P. Chang, E. Sano, C. A. McCall, G. R. Monty, R. G. Thomas, and M. A. Raskind. 2022. The impact of the COVID-19 pandemic on mental health, occupational functioning, and professional retention among health care workers and first responders. *J Gen Intern Med* 37(2):397-408.

Henke, A., and L.-c. Hsu. 2020. The gender wage gap, weather, and intimate partner violence. *Review of Economics of the Household* 18(2):413-429.

Hershey, T. B. 2019. Collaborating with sovereign tribal nations to legally prepare for public health emergencies. *J Law Med Ethics* 47(2_suppl):55-58.

HHS (U.S Department of Health and Human Services). 2017. First responders: Support for pregnant survivors of abuse or rape during disasters. https://asprtracie.hhs.gov/MasterSearch?qt=support+for+pregnant+survivors+of+abuse (accessed August 25, 2023).

Holland, K. M., C. Jones, A. M. Vivolo-Kantor, N. Idaikkadar, M. Zwald, B. Hoots, E. Yard, A. D'Inverno, E. Swedo, M. S. Chen, E. Petrosky, A. Board, P. Martinez, D. M. Stone, R. Law, M. A. Coletta, J. Adjemian, C. Thomas, R. W. Puddy, G. Peacock, N. F. Dowling, and D. Houry. 2021. Trends in US emergency department visits for mental health, overdose, and violence outcomes before and during the COVID-19 pandemic. *JAMA Psychiatry* 78(4):372-379.

IFRC (International Federation of Red Cross and Red Crescent Societies). 2023. *What is a disaster.* https://www.ifrc.org/our-work/disasters-climate-and-crises/what-disaster#:~:text=Disasters%20are%20serious%20disruptions%20to,and%20\vulnerability%20of%20a%20community (accessed August 27, 2023).

IHS (Indian Health Service). n.d. *Agency overview.* https://www.ihs.gov/aboutihs/overview/ (accessed August 21, 2023).

IHS. 2017. *Indian health manual.* Rockville, Maryland: U.S. Department of Health and Human Services.

IOM (Institute of Medicine). 2015. *Healthy, resilient, and sustainable communities after disasters: Strategies, opportunities, and planning for recovery.* Washington, DC: The National Academies Press.

Jetelina, K. K., G. Knell, and R. J. Molsberry. 2021. Changes in intimate partner violence during the early stages of the COVID-19 pandemic in the USA. *Inj Prev* 27(1):93-97.

KFF. 2023. Health coverage and care of immigrants. https://www.kff.org/racial-equity-and-health-policy/fact-sheet/health-coverage-and-care-of-immigrants/ (accessed September 6, 2023).

Khatana, S. A. M., R. M. Werner, and P. W. Groeneveld. 2022. Association of extreme heat and cardiovascular mortality in the United States: A county-level longitudinal analysis from 2008 to 2017. *Circulation* 146(3):249-261.

Kim, C. 2019. Social isolation, acculturative stress and intimate partner violence (IPV) victimization among Korean immigrant women. *International Journal of Intercultural Relations* 72:87-95.

Krause, K. H., S. DeGue, G. Kilmer, and P. H. Niolon. 2023. Prevalence and correlates of non-dating sexual violence, sexual dating violence, and physical dating violence victimization among US high school students during the COVID-19 pandemic: Adolescent behaviors and experiences survey, United States, 2021. *Journal of Interpersonal Violence* 38(9-10):6961-6984.

Lai, B. S., R. Lewis, M. S. Livings, A. M. La Greca, and A. M. Esnard. 2017. Posttraumatic stress symptom trajectories among children after disaster exposure: A review. *J Trauma Stress* 30(6):571-582.

Lauve-Moon, K., and R. J. Ferreira. 2017. An exploratory investigation: Post-disaster predictors of intimate partner violence. *Clinical Social Work Journal* 45(2):124-135.

Le, K., and M. Nguyen. 2022. War and intimate partner violence in Africa. *SAGE Open* 12(2):21582440221096427.

Leite, R. O., V. Pavia, M. A. Kobayashi, T. Kyoung Lee, G. Prado, S. E. Messiah, and S. M. St. George. 2023. The effects of parent-adolescent acculturation gaps on adolescent life-style behaviors: Moderating role of family communication. *J Lat Psychol* 11(1):21-39.

Lightfoot, E. S., A. E. Lesen, and R. J. Ferreira. 2020. Gender and resilience in gulf coast communities: Risk and protective factors following a technological disaster. *International Journal of Disaster Risk Reduction* 50:101716.

Lindsey, A. B., M. Donovan, S. Smith, H. Radunovich, and M. Gutter. 2021. Impacts of technological disasters. *IFAS Extension.* University of Florida. https://edis.ifas.ufl.edu/publication/FY1230 (accessed August 25, 2023).

Longmuir, C., and V. I. O. Agyapong. 2021. Social and mental health impact of nuclear disaster in survivors: A narrative review. *Behav Sci (Basel)* 11(8):113.

Ma, C., T. E. Smith, and R. R. Iversen. 2021. Mental illness prevalence and disparities among Hurricane Sandy survivors: A 2-year retrospective. *Disaster Med Public Health Prep* 15(5):579-588.

Michaud, J., and J. Kates. 2017. Public health in Puerto Rico after Hurricane Maria. *KFF Issue Briefs*, November 17. https://www.kff.org/mental-health/issue-brief/public-health-in-puerto-rico-after-hurricane-maria/ (accessed August 25, 2023).

Muldoon, K. A., K. M. Denize, R. Talarico, D. B. Fell, A. Sobiesiak, M. Heimerl, and K. Sampsel. 2021. COVID-19 pandemic and violence: Rising risks and decreasing urgent care-seeking for sexual assault and domestic violence survivors. *BMC Med* 19(1):20.

NASEM (National Academies of Sciences, Engineering, and Medicine). 2019. *Building and measuring community resilience: Actions for communities and the Gulf Research Program.* Washington, DC: The National Academies Press.

NASEM. 2020. *Rapid expert consultation on understanding causes of health care worker deaths due to the COVID-19 pandemic (December 10, 2020).* Washington, DC: The National Academies Press.

NCDP (National Center for Disaster Preparedness). 2023. *US Natural Hazards Index v2.0.* https://ncdp.columbia.edu/library/mapsmapping-projects/us-natural-hazards-index/ (accessed August 25, 2023).

Osofsky, H. J., J. D. Osofsky, and T. C. Hansel. 2011. Deepwater horizon oil spill: Mental health effects on residents in heavily affected areas. *Disaster Med Public Health Prep* 5(4):280-286.

Parson, N., R. Escobar, M. Merced, and A. Trautwein. 2016. Health at the intersections of precarious documentation status and gender-based partner violence. *Violence Against Women* 22(1):17-40.

Peitzmeier, S. M., L. Fedina, L. Ashwell, T. I. Herrenkohl, and R. Tolman. 2022. Increases in intimate partner violence during COVID-19: Prevalence and correlates. *J Interpers Violence* 37(21-22):NP20482-NP20512.

Ragavan, M. I., A. J. Culyba, F. L. Muhammad, and E. Miller. 2020a. Supporting adolescents and young adults exposed to or experiencing violence during the COVID-19 pandemic. *J Adolesc Health* 67(1):18-20.

Ragavan, M. I., R. Garcia, R. P. Berger, and E. Miller. 2020b. Supporting intimate partner violence survivors and their children during the COVID-19 pandemic. *Pediatrics* 146(3).

Ragavan, M. I., L. Risser, V. Duplessis, S. DeGue, A. Villaveces, T. P. Hurley, J. Chang, E. Miller, and K. A. Randell. 2022. The impact of the COVID-19 pandemic on the needs and lived experiences of intimate partner violence survivors in the United States: Advocate perspectives. *Violence Against Women* 28(12-13):3114-3134.

Raker, E. J., M. C. Arcaya, S. R. Lowe, M. Zacher, J. Rhodes, and M. C. Waters. 2020. Mitigating health disparities after natural disasters: Lessons from the risk project. *Health Aff (Millwood)* 39(12):2128-2135.

Renov, V., L. Risser, R. Berger, T. Hurley, A. Villaveces, S. DeGue, A. Katz, C. Henderson, K. Premo, J. Talis, J. C. Chang, and M. Ragavan. 2022. The impact of the COVID-19 pandemic on child protective services caseworkers and administrators. *Child Abuse Negl* 130(Pt 1):105431.

Ricks, J. L., S. D. Cochran, O. A. Arah, J. K. Williams, and T. E. Seeman. 2016. Food insecurity and intimate partner violence against women: Results from the California women's health survey. *Public Health Nutr* 19(5):914-923.

Rossi, F. S., M. Shankar, K. Buckholdt, Y. Bailey, S. T. Israni, and K. M. Iverson. 2020. Trying times and trying out solutions: Intimate partner violence screening and support for women veterans during COVID-19. *J Gen Intern Med* 35(9):2728-2731.

Rotton, J., and E. G. Cohn. 2001. Temperature, routine activities, and domestic violence: A reanalysis. *Violence Vict* 16(2):203-215.

Rubin, G. J., and M. B. Rogers. 2019. Behavioural and psychological responses of the public during a major power outage: A literature review. *International Journal of Disaster Risk Reduction* 38:101226.

Rung, A. L., S. Gaston, E. Oral, W. T. Robinson, E. Fontham, D. J. Harrington, E. Trapido, and E. S. Peters. 2016. Depression, mental distress, and domestic conflict among Louisiana women exposed to the Deepwater Horizon oil spill in the watch study. *Environ Health Perspect* 124(9):1429-1435.

Rutkow, L., J. S. Vernick, R. Mojtabai, S. O. Rodman, and C. N. Kaufmann. 2012. Legal challenges for substance abuse treatment during disasters. *Psychiatric Services* 63(1):1-9.

Sanz-Barbero, B., C. Linares, C. Vives-Cases, J. L. Gonzalez, J. J. Lopez-Ossorio, and J. Diaz. 2018. Heat wave and the risk of intimate partner violence. *Sci Total Environ* 644:413-419.

Sarabandi, N. 2018. *Curriculum: Intersection of domestic violence and natural disasters.* https://nnedv.org/resources-library/curriculum-intersection-domestic-violence-natural-disasters/ (accessed February 15, 2023).

Sharpe, J. D., and A. F. Wolkin. 2022. The epidemiology and geographic patterns of natural disaster and extreme weather mortality by race and ethnicity, United States, 1999-2018. *Public Health Rep* 137(6):1118-1125.

Smith, R. N., A. Nyame-Mireku, A. Zeidan, A. Tabaie, C. Meyer, V. Muralidharan, R. Kamaleswaran, K. Williams, A. Grant, J. Nguyen, S. Hurst, D. Hanos, E. Benjamin, R. Sola, Jr., and D. P. Evans. 2022. Intimate partner violence at a level-1 trauma center during the COVID-19 pandemic: An interrupted time series analysis. *Am Surg* 88(7):1551-1553.

Stults, C. B., K. D. Krause, R. J. Martino, M. Griffin, C. E. LoSchiavo, S. G. Lynn, S. A. Brandt, D. Tan, N. Horne, G. Lee, J. Wong, and P. N. Halkitis. 2022. Sociodemographic characteristics, depressive symptoms, and increased frequency of intimate partner violence among LGBTQ people in the United States during the COVID-19 pandemic: A brief report. *Journal of Gay & Lesbian Social Services* 35(2):258-270.

Sullivan, C. M. 2012. Domestic violence shelter services: A review of the empirical evidence. *Domestic Violence Evidence Project.* https://www.dvevidenceproject.org/wp-content/themes/DVEProject/files/research/DVShelterResearchSummary10-2012.pdf.

Tur-Prats, A. 2021. Unemployment and intimate partner violence: A cultural approach. *Journal of Economic Behavior & Organization* 185:27-49.

USPHS (U.S. Public Health Service). 2022. *Public health emergency response strike team.* https://www.usphs.gov/pherst (accessed August 25, 2023).

VA (Veterans Affairs Office of Emergency Management). 2021. *Comprehensive emergency management program.* https://www.va.gov/VHAEMERGENCYMANAGEMENT/CEMP/index.asp (accessed August 25, 2023).

Valdovinos, M. G., S. D. Nightingale, and M. Vasquez Reyes. 2021. Intimate partner violence help-seeking for Latina undocumented immigrant survivors: Feminist intersectional experiences narrated through testimonio. *Affilia* 36(4):533-551.

Vida, S., M. Durocher, T. B. M. J. Ouarda, and P. Gosselin. 2012. Relationship between ambient temperature and humidity and visits to mental health emergency departments in Québec. *Psychiatric Services* 63(11):1150-1153.

Weiner, D. L., and S. L. Rosman. 2019. Just-in-time training for disaster response in the austere environment. *Clinical Pediatric Emergency Medicine* 20(2):95-110.

Weitzman, A., and J. A. Behrman. 2016. Disaster, disruption to family life, and intimate partner violence: The case of the 2010 earthquake in Haiti. *Sociological Science* 3:167-189.

West Region Health Care Coalition. 2023. *History of health care coalitions.* https://www.westregionhcc.com/firm-history (accessed August 25, 2023).

WHO (World Health Organization). 2009. *Whole of society pandemic readiness: WHO guidelines for pandemic preparedness and response in the non-health sector.* Geneva, Switzerland: WHO Press.

Williams, J. R., R. M. Gonzalez-Guarda, and V. Ilias. 2017. Trauma-informed decision-making among providers and victims of intimate partner violence during HIV testing: A qualitative study. *J Assoc Nurses AIDS Care* 28(5):819-831.

4

Health Conditions Related to
Intimate Partner Violence

MOST COMMON HEALTH CONDITIONS RELATED
TO INTIMATE PARTNER VIOLENCE

ACUTE PHYSICAL INJURIES

Intimate partner violence (IPV) is a leading cause of injury among women and is associated with fractures, craniofacial injuries, traumatic brain injuries, and musculoskeletal injuries (Alessandrino et al., 2020; Arosarena et al., 2009; Colantonio and Valera, 2022).

Injuries to the Head, Face, and Neck

Facial fractures and other facial and dental injuries are among the most common forms of IPV-related physical trauma. Wu and colleagues (2010) performed a systematic review and meta-analysis of studies examining injuries in women who disclosed IPV while presenting to an emergency department (ED). Their analysis found that the injuries most frequently associated with IPV were those to the head, neck, and face. These findings have been replicated in several other studies. For example, an analysis of National Electronic Injury Surveillance System–All Injury Program (NEISS–AIP) data from 1.65 million IPV-related ED visits found that the face was the most common fracture site (48 percent of fractures; n=68,973) (Loder and Momper, 2020). Another analysis of patients disclosing IPV who presented to a hospital in Massachusetts found that the most common facial fracture site was the nasal bones, followed by the mandible and orbits, respectively (Gujrathi et al., 2022). Le and colleagues (2001) had similar findings in their review of 236 ED admissions at a Level 1 trauma center in Oregon over 5 years in which IPV was identified (Le et al., 2001). They reported that 81 percent (n=191) of those patients presented with maxillofacial injuries. While the majority of patients (61 percent; n=143) had maxillofacial soft tissue injuries, 30 percent (n=70) had facial fractures, and 40 percent (n=28) of those fractures were nasal fractures (Le et al., 2001).

Traumatic blows to the head and face from IPV also lead to dental injuries (Alessandrino et al., 2020). The most common dental injuries due to experiencing IPV are dental fractures, tooth luxations, and tooth avulsions (Alessandrino et al., 2020). However, there is minimal information available about the prevalence of IPV-related dental injuries in the United States. For example, in an analysis of query results from a large dental data repository containing electronic health records data for over 4 million patients from 11 U.S. dental schools that are part of the Consortium for Oral Health Research and Informatics, researchers did not identify any cases of IPV noted in patient records (Banava et al., 2022). Despite limited data, the prevalence of IPV-related injuries due to trauma to the head, neck, and face suggest that it is reasonable to expect that these individuals also experience dental trauma.

Traumatic Brain Injury

Trauma inflicted to the head, face, and neck can result in traumatic brain injury (TBI). TBI, including concussion, resulting from IPV is gaining attention in the literature. However, prevalence estimates vary. Haag and colleagues (2022) found in their scoping review that reported prevalence rates of TBI due to IPV in the literature ranged from 19 to 75 percent in empirical studies, which highlights that variation. They theorized that variations in estimates may result from the lack of a standardized screening tool for TBI in people who have experienced IPV. Additionally, many studies investigating the connection between TBI and IPV rely on smaller convenience samples (Fedina, 2023).

TBI is usually the result of injury to the brain from a mechanical force that leads to motion of the head and the brain within the skull (Davis, 2000). This motion within the skull occurs more quickly than usual or in an anatomically abnormal direction, leading to injury (Davis, 2000). This force may result from a direct blow to the head or another part of the body (Davis, 2000). TBI-induced alterations in brain function lead to a variety of acute problems and chronic sequelae, including loss of consciousness, behavioral changes, neuropsychiatric disorders, post-traumatic seizures, motor deficits, sensory deficits, cognitive deficits, memory loss, headache, fatigue, insomnia, dizziness, and deficits in attention, concentration, and executive functioning (Blaya et al., 2022; Haag et al., 2022). Given the high prevalence of head, neck, and face injuries from IPV, particularly facial fractures, it is reasonable to expect that the women sustaining those blows may also experience TBI (McCarty et al., 2020; Rajandram et al., 2014). Several studies describe symptoms reported by women experiencing physical IPV consistent with TBI, including recurrent dizziness, headache, memory loss, blackouts, cognitive function difficulty, depression, and sleep disturbances (Haag et al., 2022; Stubbs and Szoeke, 2022). However, a systematic review of 52 studies on the effects of IPV on physical health and health-related behaviors found that certain TBI-linked symptoms, including dizziness, depression, and sleep disturbances, were commonly reported by people experiencing IPV who did not have a history of TBI (Stubbs and Szoeke, 2022). Many of the symptoms related to TBIs are similar to those related to the psychological trauma of experiencing IPV (Mehr et al., 2023). Memory loss secondary to TBI may limit a woman's ability to provide an accurate history of her injuries, which likely contributes to variations in reported prevalence of IPV-related TBI in the literature. TBI is also associated with an increased risk for substance use disorders (McHugo et al., 2017; Mehr et al., 2023). Substance use can also create challenges for obtaining an accurate injury history and mask TBI symptoms, further complicating the diagnosis of TBI (Mehr et al., 2023).

Strangulation

Strangulation is an under-reported source of severe and fatal injury due to IPV (Black, 2011; Patch et al., 2021; Pritchard et al., 2017). The reported prevalence of IPV-related strangulation varies in the research literature. An analysis of data collected from 2006 to 2014 in the Nationwide Emergency Department Sample (NEDS) used diagnosis codes for IPV and non-fatal strangulation to identify prevalence in women over 18 years old who presented to an ED that submitted data to NEDS (Patch et al., 2021). Statistical analysis found that 1.21 percent of visits (602 of 49,675 visits) with an IPV diagnosis code also had a strangulation diagnosis code (Patch et al., 2021). Of note, diagnosis codes for IPV are not consistently used to identify patient visits due to IPV, which may limit the accuracy of epidemiologic estimates based on diagnosis code frequency (Adhia et al., 2023; Schafer et al., 2008). A systematic review of 23 articles investigating the epidemiology of IPV-related nonfatal strangulation in nine different countries using self-reported survey results found that 3.0–9.7 percent of women reported having been strangled by an intimate partner in their lifetime (Sorenson et al., 2014). Researchers have hypothesized that under-reporting and variations in prevalence data are likely due to a lack of clinician awareness of the signs and symptoms of non-fatal strangulation, a lack of visible signs of strangulation (such as contusions) when the woman presents for evaluation by a clinician, fear of retaliation for seeking care for an IPV-related injury, and that the woman may not be aware of the potential negative health consequences of strangulation (Donaldson et al., 2023; Patch et al., 2018, 2021).

Strangulation involves the application of external pressure to the neck that results in occlusion of the airway and blood vessels (Valera et al., 2022). IPV-related non-fatal strangulation results in a variety of adverse outcomes, including carotid artery dissection, carotid artery stenosis, stroke, tracheal perforations, laryngeal cartilage fracture, TBI, hypoxic brain injuries, dysphagia, dysphonia, loss of consciousness, seizures, contusions, cervical musculoskeletal injuries, and post-traumatic stress disorder (PTSD) (Messing et al., 2022; Patch et al., 2018; Sorenson et al., 2014; Tang et al., 2023). IPV-related non-fatal strangulation has been described as the violent physical manifestation of coercive control and is often accompanied by violent threats (Pritchard et al., 2017; Stansfield and Williams, 2021). The most severe outcome of strangulation in IPV is death. A meta-analysis of 17 studies investigated risk factors for intimate partner homicide and found that one of the strongest predictors for intimate partner homicide was previous non-fatal strangulation by an intimate partner (Spencer and Stith, 2020).

Musculoskeletal Injuries

Radiology studies have identified a variety of musculoskeletal injuries frequently associated with IPV. Common IPV-related upper extremity fractures include ulnar shaft and medial hand fractures, which often result from attempts to shield oneself from the physical attack, as well as finger and shoulder fractures (Tang et al., 2023). Loder and Momper's (2020) analysis of NEISS-AIP data found that IPV fractures occurred most frequently in the face, finger, upper trunk, and hand. They also found that 87.5 percent of women who presented to EDs sustained sprains or strains due to IPV (Loder and Momper, 2020). While not as common as head, neck, or upper-extremity fractures; rib, sternal, and clavicle fractures are the most common IPV-related torso fractures. Foot and ankle fractures are the most common in the lower extremities (Loder and Momper, 2020; Tang et al., 2023). The radiology literature also identified IPV-related thoracic injuries that are less common than fractures but that can have more severe consequences, including pneumothorax, hemothorax, and pneumomediastinum (Tang et al., 2023). In addition to fractures, sprains, and strains, other common health sequelae of IPV include arthritis, joint disease, and resulting difficulties with mobility (Black, 2011).

GYNECOLOGIC, REPRODUCTIVE HEALTH, PERINATAL, AND OBSTETRIC CONDITIONS

Gynecologic and Reproductive Health

IPV is associated with several adverse sexual and reproductive health outcomes, including unintended pregnancy, rapid repeat pregnancies, sexually transmitted infections (STIs), and HIV infection (El-Bassel et al., 2022; Ely and Murshid, 2018; Moore et al., 2010). During pregnancy, birth-giving people experiencing IPV have a higher risk of adverse outcomes such as preterm delivery, low birthweight babies, preeclampsia, other obstetric complications, and fetal/neonatal death (Alhusen et al., 2014; Auger et al., 2020; Loeffen et al., 2016).

A systematic review and meta-analysis of 57 studies investigating the signs and symptoms of women experiencing IPV who presented to primary care found that gynecologic infections, STIs, and unwanted pregnancy were the gynecologic and reproductive health conditions most often associated with IPV (Vicard-Olagne et al., 2022). Additional research has found that abnormal vaginal discharge or bleeding, dyspareunia, abnormal cervical screening tests, chronic pelvic pain, STIs, and HIV infections (as well as lower CD4+ counts in those who are HIV+), painful menses, and genital injuries are often associated with IPV (Black, 2011; Dillon et al., 2013; Stubbs and Szoeke, 2022; Vicard-Olagne et al., 2022). Reproductive and sexual health outcomes associated with teen dating violence or IPV among adolescents include unintended pregnancy, STIs, and HIV infection (Decker et al., 2005; Exner-Cortens et al., 2013; Miller et al., 2010b, 2014).

Studies investigating increased abnormal cervical cancer screening tests and increased cervical cancer rates associated with IPV have noted that women experiencing IPV tend to be less likely to undergo cervical cancer screening (Bagwell-Gray and Ramaswamy, 2022). Researchers hypothesize that increased STIs, particularly human papillomavirus, may also be a contributing factor (Stubbs and Szoeke, 2022).

Analysis of data from a survey of 1,262 women seeking care in family planning clinics found that those who had recently experienced IPV were more likely to pursue one or more pregnancy tests and use emergency contraception at least once (Kazmerski et al., 2015). This analysis also found that the combination of experiencing recent IPV and reproductive coercion increased the likelihood of seeking multiple pregnancy tests, using emergency contraception multiple times, and seeking STI testing (Kazmerski et al., 2015). A meta-analysis of 38 studies also found that experiencing IPV was associated with unwanted pregnancy, abortions, and the use of emergency contraception (Vicard-Olagne et al., 2022).

Unintended Pregnancy

An analysis of data collected from 20,252 women who gave birth between 2012 and 2015 and completed the Pregnancy Risk Assessment and Monitoring System (PRAMS) survey within 9 months of giving birth found that those who experienced IPV were almost eight times more likely to experience reproductive coercion than those who did not experience IPV (Samankasikorn et al., 2019). IPV, including reproductive coercion, is associated with unintended pregnancy (Miller et al., 2010a, 2014; Samankasikorn et al., 2019).

Women experiencing IPV are less likely than other women to be in control of their fertility regulation due to manipulation tactics and fear of physical abuse from their partners. A cross-sectional cohort study of women seeking services from an IPV shelter or a district attorney's office in a large U.S. metropolitan area identified several commonly reported barriers to the use of contraception by women reporting experiencing IPV and reproductive coercion (Liu et al., 2016). The most common barriers included partners refusing to use contraception, partners would not allow women to use contraception, fear of discussing contraception, experiencing IPV for discussing using contraception, and experiencing IPV for using contraception (Liu et al., 2016). People engaging in IPV and reproductive coercion also sabotage contraception (Baird et al., 2017). These findings were consistent with barriers identified in a systematic review of 42 studies examining the relationship between IPV and condom and oral contraceptive use (Bergmann and Stockman, 2015).

Unintended pregnancy is significantly associated with adverse maternal and infant outcomes, including maternal depression during pregnancy, postpartum depression, preterm birth, and low birthweight (Nelson et al., 2022). Unintended pregnancy has also been identified as a risk factor for experiencing IPV during pregnancy (D'Angelo et al., 2023; E. J. Smith et al., 2023). Experiencing IPV during pregnancy is associated with several serious adverse maternal and infant health outcomes, as well as intimate partner homicide (D'Angelo et al., 2023; Donovan et al., 2016; Guo et al., 2023). Researchers have found that women who became pregnant as a result of reproductive coercion are more likely to continue to experience abuse throughout their pregnancy and to miscarry or experience a stillbirth (Liu et al., 2016). Roberts and colleagues analyzed data from 956 women who participated in the University of California, San Francisco's Turnaway Study, a prospective study of women seeking abortions at 30 different clinics across the United States from 2008 to 2010 (Roberts et al., 2014). Their analysis found that among women experiencing IPV prior to being pregnant, continuing an unintended pregnancy and giving birth was not associated with a decrease in physical IPV (Roberts et al., 2014). However, among women experiencing IPV prior to being pregnant, terminating an unintended pregnancy was associated with a decrease in physical violence (Roberts et al., 2014).

Sexual Assault

Estimates from the 2016–2017 National Intimate Partner and Sexual Violence Survey (NISVS) data indicated that approximately 19.6 percent of U.S. women had experienced contact sexual violence (in the survey this included rape, sexual coercion, and unwanted sexual contact) by an intimate partner in their lifetime (Leemis et al., 2022). An analysis of the use of ICD-10-CM codes for IPV from 2 years of data from electronic health records from 15 different California hospitals found that 33.3 percent (n=5,773) of visits to the ED and 23.1 percent (n=330) of hospital visits for IPV included the IPV ICD-10-CM code for confirmed sexual abuse (Adhia et al., 2023). An analysis of data from the 2010–2012 NISVS survey found that 26.2 percent of respondents that reported rape-related pregnancy identified a current or former intimate partner as the perpetrator (Basile et al., 2018). Bagwell-Gray and colleagues (2015) noted substantial variation in the reported prevalence of sexual IPV in their systematic review of 43 peer-reviewed articles investigating the prevalence of sexual IPV. They noted that inconsistency in the terminology used in the studies and hesitancy on the part of the person experiencing intimate partner sexual assault due at least in part to the existing intimate relationship may contribute to underestimates of prevalence (Bagwell-Gray et al., 2015). IPV-related sexual assault, including rape, may also be under-reported due to legal and social barriers. Marital rape did not become illegal in all 50 states until the early 1990s, and its definitions continue to vary between states (Wright et al., 2022). Additionally, the false beliefs that sex is a duty within intimate relationships such as marriage or that rape can only be perpetrated by a stranger persist (Wright et al., 2022).

IPV sexual assault, including rape, results in psychological trauma, physical injury, STIs, HIV infection, and unplanned pregnancy (Wright et al., 2022). IPV sexual assault is associated with PTSD, depression symptoms, and suicidality (Wright et al., 2022). It is also associated with adverse gynecological outcomes, such as miscarriage, and STIs and HIV infection (Wright et al., 2022). An analysis of data collected from 741 women by sexual assault nurse examiners in New Hampshire from 1997 to 2007 found that women sexually assaulted by a current or former intimate partner were more likely to experience genital injuries than those assaulted by a stranger (Murphy et al., 2011). Increased frequency, duration, and severity of IPV sexual assault are associated with increased use of legal, medical, and social services (Wright et al., 2022).

HIV Infection

The existence of a relationship between IPV and HIV infection has been well documented in the literature (Campbell et al., 2008; El-Bassel et al., 2022; Gielen et al., 2007; Li et al., 2014; Willie et al., 2018). Women living with HIV are at heightened risk for IPV, and women experiencing IPV are at a greater risk for contracting HIV (Marshall et al., 2018). Women experiencing IPV are less likely to have control over a partner's condom use, a key method for protecting them from HIV infection (Bergmann and Stockman, 2015). State-level IPV prevalence is also positively associated with higher rates of HIV diagnosis among women in the United States (Willie et al., 2018).

An analysis of data from the Medical Monitoring Project survey of adults with HIV in the United States found a lifetime prevalence of IPV of 35.6 percent (n=1,060) and a previous 12-month prevalence of 4.5 percent (n=132) for women with HIV (Lemons-Lyn et al., 2021). This study found statistically significant differences in the lifetime prevalence of IPV in people with HIV by gender/sexuality, with bisexual HIV-positive women more likely to experience IPV than heterosexual women and lesbians (Lemons-Lyn et al., 2021). The analysis also found that treatment for HIV can be affected by experiencing IPV. Those who tested positive for HIV and had experienced IPV in the past 12 months were less likely to be retained in HIV medical care, had lower HIV medication regimen adherence, were less likely to have sustained viral suppression, and were more likely to have missed HIV-related medical appointments in the past year than those who did not experience IPV (Lemons-Lyn et al., 2021).

The most direct mechanism linking IPV to HIV susceptibility is forced sex or sexual IPV (i.e., condomless vaginal or anal sex via physical force, coercion, or threat) with a partner living with HIV (Dunkle and Decker, 2013; Li et al., 2014; Maman et al., 2000; Stockman et al., 2013; Tsuyuki et al., 2019). Researchers have posited that indirect mechanisms occur at the biological (e.g., chronic stress response, chronic inflammation, immune dysfunction), behavioral (e.g., individual and perpetrator sexual- and drug-related risk behaviors), and societal levels (e.g., social norms, gender power imbalances) (Campbell et al., 2008; Dunkle and Decker, 2013; El-Bassel et al., 2022; Maman et al., 2000). The intersection of IPV and HIV particularly affects certain populations, including women engaged in sex work, women who use drugs, transgender women, and adolescent girls and young women (aged 15–24 years) (El-Bassel et al., 2022). IPV often interferes with women's engagement in and adherence to HIV care (Sullivan, 2019). Meta-analysis findings showed IPV to be significantly associated with lower use of antiretroviral therapy (ART), poorer self-reported ART adherence, and worsened viral suppression among women (Hatcher et al., 2015).

Perinatal Health

Experiencing IPV in the perinatal period is associated with an increased risk for numerous adverse maternal, neonatal, and infant health outcomes. Pregnant people who experience IPV are more likely to have high blood pressure, edema, vaginal bleeding in the second or third trimester, severe nausea, vomiting, dehydration, kidney infection or urinary tract infection, premature rupture of membranes, and premature birth. They are less likely to achieve gestational-age-appropriate weight and more likely to give birth to low birthweight babies (Alhusen et al., 2014). A 2020 systematic review of 50 global studies found that IPV during pregnancy was associated with adverse health effects for pregnant and postpartum people, fetuses, and infants (Pastor-Moreno et al., 2020). These health effects include premature rupture of membranes, spontaneous abortion, inadequate weight gain during pregnancy, urinary tract infections, and miscarriage, as well as preterm birth, low birthweight, and neonatal death (Pastor-Moreno et al., 2020). The review also found an association between IPV and health care usage, including late entry into prenatal care, longer postpartum hospitalization, and fewer antenatal visits (Pastor-Moreno et al., 2020). Experiencing IPV is also associated with delayed and inadequate prenatal care, which in turn is associated with preterm delivery and low birthweight infants (Cha and Masho, 2014).

BEHAVIORAL HEALTH CONDITIONS

Mental Health

IPV is associated with adverse mental health outcomes such as anxiety, PTSD, depression, substance misuse, suicidality, and eating disorders (Beydoun et al., 2017; Black, 2011; Dichter et al., 2017; Dokkedahl et al., 2022; Lacey et al., 2015; Termos et al., 2022; White et al., 2023). The relationship between IPV and mental health outcomes is complex and bidirectional (Bacchus et al., 2018; Oram et al., 2022). While exposure to IPV increases the risk of developing mental health problems, mental health problems have also been shown to increase women's vulnerability to experiencing IPV (Bacchus et al., 2018; Oram et al., 2022). A recent systematic review and meta-analysis about mental health outcomes of IPV among women globally found increased odds of adverse mental health outcomes associated with IPV, including depression, PTSD, and suicidality (White et al., 2023). Furthermore, physical violence and sexual violence were associated with an increased likelihood of depression and anxiety, respectively (White et al., 2023). Another systematic review and meta-analysis highlighted the role of psychological IPV, particularly experiences of coercive control, in the development of PTSD among women (Dokkedahl et al., 2022). Of note, researchers have indicated that variations in terminology for psychological IPV and variations in psychologic measurement instruments in many of the research studies limit the ability to make comparisons among the studies and to apply their results broadly (Dokkedahl et al., 2022).

An emerging body of literature explores the mental health impacts of IPV in different groups, such as adolescents, racial and ethnic minorities, and lesbian, bisexual, and transgender people. Mental health consequences for adolescents identified in the literature include depression, suicidality, substance abuse, and disordered eating (Exner-Cortens et al., 2013). A systematic review found that experiencing IPV significantly negatively affects the mental health of Black and Hispanic women (Stockman et al., 2015). A large cross-sectional study examined the relationship between IPV exposure, lethality risk, and mental health outcomes among African American women, African Caribbean women, and Black women of mixed ethnicity in the United States and the U.S. Virgin Islands (Sabri et al., 2013). This study found that while African American and African Caribbean women who experienced severe IPV were more likely to experience substantial adverse mental health outcomes, they were not more likely to use mental health resources (Sabri et al., 2013). The researchers also found that Black women, regardless of ethnicity, with mental health problems tended to underutilize mental health services, which echoes the findings of other studies (Sabri et al., 2013). Several studies have noted that Hispanic women who have experienced IPV tend to exhibit higher rates of mental health problems than non-Hispanic women (Reyes et al., 2023). Several studies of Asian American women have also documented the relationship between IPV experiences and adverse mental health, such as depression, anxiety, and suicidality (Hurwitz et al., 2006; Lee et al., 2007; Maru et al., 2018).

American Indian/Alaska Native (AI/AN) women are disproportionately affected by mental health problems (Brave Heart et al., 2016; Duran et al., 2004). However, research into the effects of experiencing IPV on the mental health of AI/AN women is limited, and many studies rely on small samples. A study that analyzed data collected in the 2010 NISVS survey found that experiencing IPV was related to poor mental health in AI/AN women (Fedina et al., 2022). However, when the additional factors of food insecurity, housing insecurity, and health care access were introduced, the relationship between IPV and poor mental health was no longer statistically significant in this population (Fedina et al., 2022).

Among lesbians and bisexual women, experiencing IPV is associated with multiple adverse mental health outcomes, including depression, anxiety, difficulties with emotional regulation, and internalized homophobia (Porsch et al., 2022). An analysis of 2010 NISVS survey data found that bisexual women who had experienced IPV were significantly more likely to report PTSD symptoms than heterosexual women who had (46.2 vs. 22.1 percent) (Walters et al., 2013). In a systematic review, Peitzmeier and colleagues (2020) found that experiencing IPV was associated with poor mental health among transgender individuals (Peitzmeier et al., 2020). They also found that psychological IPV in the form of leveraging transgender-specific vulnerabilities to gain power and control was associated with excess mental health burden in transgender individuals experiencing IPV (Peitzmeier et al., 2020).

The perinatal period is of particular importance when discussing mental health outcomes related to IPV. Adverse mental health outcomes for people experiencing IPV in the perinatal period include higher rates of PTSD, major depressive disorder, suicide ideation, and problematic substance use (Alhusen et al., 2015; Connelly et al., 2013; Kastello et al., 2015; Martin et al., 2003). IPV in the perinatal period has also been found to be associated with postpartum depression (Garabedian et al., 2011). Prevalence of both postpartum depression and IPV are disproportionately high among AI/AN women (Heck, 2021). However, a scoping review published in 2021 found that many studies do not include postpartum depression when examining the mental health effects of perinatal IPV (Heck, 2021). The authors hypothesized that this may contribute to the inconsistent findings of a relationship between IPV and postpartum depression in the literature (Heck, 2021).

Substance Use

A bidirectional relationship exists between substance use disorder (SUD) and IPV. Women who use drugs may be at greater risk of experiencing IPV because partners may perceive them as vulnerable to victimization and they may not be able to leave violent partners (Burke et al., 2005; Martin et al., 2003; Testa et al., 2003). Some researchers theorize that women with experiences of IPV may engage in drug use as a coping mechanism (Gilbert et al., 2015; P. H. Smith et al., 2012). However, other researchers have found the temporal relationship between SUD and IPV difficult to delineate (Mehr et al., 2023). Partner interference can serve as a barrier for women experiencing IPV to access and remain engaged in SUD treatment programs, increasing the potential for relapse (Ogden et al., 2022). A systematic review that sought to investigate the prevalence of opioid use among people who have experienced IPV noted that a limited number of studies have investigated the prevalence of opioid use among people who had experienced IPV (Stone and Rothman, 2019). The authors noted that opioid use was defined differently in all of the studies and that there was substantial variation in how IPV was reported in all of the studies, which prevented meta-analysis and limited data comparison (Stone and Rothman, 2019). Another systematic review of articles published between 2010 and 2020 also noted that inconsistencies in measurement of both substance use and IPV limited the number of studies that met criteria for inclusion to 10 (Ogden et al., 2022).

Several small studies of women who were in substance abuse treatment programs or reported a history of substance use when they sought care in a hospital or ED have noted high rates of reported prior or current IPV (El-Bassel et al., 2005, 2019). A longitudinal study of 241 women with low incomes receiving care in a Bronx, New York, ED found that women who used heroin were twice as likely to experience IPV and 2.7 times more likely to report IPV-related injury (Gilbert et al., 2012). A study of 81 women admitted to a Level 1 trauma center in rural North Carolina over 6 months found a significant relationship between experiencing IPV during their lifetime and substance use (Hink et al., 2015). Experiencing IPV is also associated with higher alcohol consumption (Mehr et al., 2023; Waller et al., 2012). A study that analyzed survey data from 1,863 women living in a large Midwestern metropolitan area found that a history of experiencing physical IPV was associated with heavy drinking (Ullman and Sigurvinsdottir, 2015).

There are few large population-based studies of prevalence of IPV related to substance use in the United States. The results of one large study that analyzed data from the 2004–2005 wave of the National Epidemiological Study on Alcohol and Related Conditions offered useful insight, despite the age of the data (P. H. Smith et al., 2012). The analysis of data from 25,778 respondents who reported being married, dating, or in a relationship in the past year found that women who had an opioid use disorder were more likely to experience IPV (P. H. Smith et al., 2012). Their analysis also found that marijuana use was associated with experiencing IPV (P. H. Smith et al., 2012). They also found that while cocaine use was not related to experiencing IPV, it was associated with using IPV (P. H. Smith et al., 2012). Another study analyzed data from 4,481 female-identified veterans over the age of 45 who were screened for IPV in Veterans Health Administration clinics in 11 different states between 2014 and 2016 (Makaroun et al., 2020). The analysis found that screening positive for IPV was associated with a subsequent diagnosis of SUD (Makaroun et al., 2020).

Given the limited availability of population-based studies that investigate the prevalence of IPV related to substance abuse and the variations in terminology and measurement related to both in other studies, it is difficult to identify clear evidence of a relationship among IPV, substance use, and different demographics. One population-based study that was identified was an analysis of data collected during the 2001–2002 and 2007–2008 waves of the National Longitudinal Study of Adolescent Health, which investigated the role of race, ethnicity, and temporality in the bidirectional relationship between IPV and substance use among 2,959 White, Black, and Hispanic women in early young adulthood (18–26 years old) and young adulthood (24–32 years old), respectively (Nowotny and Graves, 2013). Their analysis found that experiencing IPV in any form during early young adulthood (18–26 years old) was associated with an increased likelihood of marijuana use during young adulthood (24–32 years old) among Hispanic women (Nowotny and Graves, 2013). They also found that experiencing physical IPV during early young adulthood increased the likelihood of marijuana use in young adulthood among White women. There was no relationship identified between experiencing IPV in early young adulthood and any subsequent substance use among Black women (Nowotny and Graves, 2013). Binge drinking during early young adulthood was associated with an increased likelihood of experiencing an IPV-related injury in young adulthood for Hispanic women, and early young adulthood drug use increased the likelihood of experiencing an IPV-related injury in young adulthood among Black women (Nowotny and Graves, 2013). The limited number of population-based studies investigating the relationship between IPV, substance use, and different demographics highlights the need for additional research in this area to better guide targeted interventions.

The intersection of IPV and substance use or abuse results in adverse health outcomes of varying severity. Substance abuse is associated with adverse health effects including mental health disorders, bacterial infections such as streptococcal and staphylococcal infections, acute and chronic cardiac conditions, stroke, organ damage, seizures, and dental disorders (Fox et al., 2013; Khalsa et al., 2008; Meyer et al., 2011). IPV and substance abuse are associated with a higher likelihood of sexual risk taking behaviors, which in turn is associated with greater risk for STIs and HIV (Meyer et al., 2011).

CHRONIC HEALTH CONDITIONS

Chronic Pain

Chronic pain is one of the most common adverse health effects of IPV (Walker et al., 2022). Among women who have experienced IPV, the most common forms of chronic pain are frequent headaches, migraines, chronic back pain, pelvic and abdominal pain, and fibromyalgia (Poleshuck et al., 2018; Walker et al., 2022). In their systematic review, Stubbs and Szoeke (2022) reported that multiple U.S.-based and international studies found that chronic pain was more common in women who experienced IPV (Stubbs and Szoeke, 2022). The increased prevalence of chronic pain among those experiencing IPV was echoed in another systematic review conducted by Vicard-Olagne and colleagues (2022). While there is a logical relationship between the physical injuries sustained due to IPV and chronic pain, experiencing psychological IPV is also associated with chronic pain (Spencer et al., 2022). Smaller studies have investigated the interaction between experiencing IPV and chronic pain. In a study of 108 women seeking treatment at a Midwestern specialty pain rehabilitation and treatment center, 56 percent (n=60) reported having experienced IPV at some point in their lifetimes, and 28.7 percent (n=31) reported having experienced IPV within the past year (Craner et al., 2020). A recently published Canadian longitudinal study of 309 women who had separated from partners who used IPV found that chronic pain remained at significant levels by the end of the 4-year study (Ford-Gilboe et al., 2023).

Women experiencing chronic pain are less likely to receive appropriate care and more likely to have their reports of pain dismissed or misdiagnosed by health care professionals as being solely of psychological origin (Samulowitz et al., 2018; Walker et al., 2022). Women experiencing chronic pain often do not feel believed or understood, a concern that can be compounded by experiencing IPV. This intersects with other disparities in pain management. For example, patients who are not White are more likely to report discrimination, bias, and unsatisfactory treatment in pain management than White patients (Morales and Yong, 2021; Mossey, 2011, Trost et al., 2019).

A systematic review investigating the relationship between IPV and chronic pain found conflicting findings in the literature about the nature of the role of PTSD and depression in the relationship between experiencing IPV and chronic pain (Walker et al., 2022). However, it did find that the literature was consistent in finding that IPV, chronic pain, and PTSD, depression, and anxiety frequently co-occur (Walker et al., 2022). Of note, IPV-related chronic pain does not necessarily translate into increased use of pain medication, particularly opioids. Wuest and colleagues (2007) found that despite higher levels of chronic pain among those experiencing IPV, those individuals were less likely to take over-the-counter nonsteroidal anti-inflammatory drugs and were no more likely to take opioid pain medications than women in the general Canadian population (Wuest et al., 2007). Dillon and colleagues (2013) and Stubbs and Szoeke (2022) reported similar findings.

Cardiovascular Disease

Some studies have indicated that there may be an association between experiencing IPV and developing cardiovascular disease (Stubbs and Szoeke, 2022; Wright et al., 2019, 2021). In general, the findings in the literature were mixed in regard to identifying a direct relationship between IPV and cardiovascular disease. The committee reviewed studies examining an association between IPV and cardiovascular disease and concluded that there is currently not enough compelling evidence to link the two.

CHAPTER SUMMARY

The most common health conditions related to IPV include acute physical injuries; gynecologic, reproductive, and obstetric conditions; behavioral health conditions; and other chronic conditions. Some health conditions associated with experiencing IPV, such as TBI or the adverse health effects of strangulation, can have serious or fatal outcomes. Unintended pregnancy due to IPV is associated with serious adverse maternal and infant health outcomes. A person experiencing unintended pregnancy is also more likely to experience IPV during that pregnancy, which is also associated with serious adverse maternal and infant health outcomes. The adverse health conditions related to experiencing IPV do not occur in isolation. Treating these conditions is key to treating IPV in steady state conditions and in PHEs. The next chapter will discuss the essential health care services related to IPV.

REFERENCES

Adhia, A., R. Rebbe, A. Lane Eastman, R. Foust, and E. Putnam-Hornstein. 2023. Intimate partner violence-related emergency department and hospital visits in California following the ICD-10-CM transition, 2016–2018. *Journal of Interpersonal Violence* 38(7-8):6230-6241.

Alessandrino, F., A. Keraliya, J. Lebovic, G. S. M. Dyer, M. B. Harris, P. Tornetta, G. W. L. Boland, S. E. Seltzer, and B. Khurana. 2020. Intimate partner violence: A primer for radiologists to make the "invisible" visible. *Radiographics* 40(7):2080-2097.

Alhusen, J. L., L. Bullock, P. Sharps, D. Schminkey, E. Comstock, and J. Campbell. 2014. Intimate partner violence during pregnancy and adverse neonatal outcomes in low-income women. *J Womens Health (Larchmont)* 23(11):920-926.

Alhusen, J. L., N. Frohman, and G. Purcell. 2015. Intimate partner violence and suicidal ideation in pregnant women. *Archive Womens Ment Health* 18(4):573-578.

Arosarena, O. A., T. A. Fritsch, Y. Hsueh, B. Aynehci, and R. Haug. 2009. Maxillofacial injuries and violence against women. *Archive Facial Plast Surg* 11(1):48-52.

Auger, N., B. J. Potter, S. He, J. Healy-Profitós, M. E. Schnitzer, and G. Paradis. 2020. Maternal cardiovascular disease 3 decades after preterm birth: Longitudinal cohort study of pregnancy vascular disorders. *Hypertension* 75(3):788-795.

Bacchus, L. J., M. Ranganathan, C. Watts, and K. Devries. 2018. Recent intimate partner violence against women and health: A systematic review and meta-analysis of cohort studies. *BMJ Open* 8(7):e019995.

Bagwell-Gray, M. E., J. T. Messing, and A. Baldwin-White. 2015. Intimate partner sexual violence: A review of terms, definitions, and prevalence. *Trauma Violence Abuse* 16(3):316-335.

Bagwell-Gray, M. E., and M. Ramaswamy. 2022. Cervical cancer screening and prevention among survivors of intimate partner violence. *Health Soc Work* 47(2):102-112.

Baird, K., D. Creedy, and T. Mitchell. 2017. Intimate partner violence and pregnancy intentions: A qualitative study. *J Clin Nurs* 26(15-16):2399-2408.

Banava, S., S. A. Lippman, G. Schenk, and S. A. Gansky. 2022. Intimate partner violence and orofacial injuries in a multi-school dental data repository. *J Dent Educ* 87(Suppl 3):1827–1831. https://doi.org/10.1002/jdd.13016.

Basile, K. C., S. G. Smith, Y. Liu, M. J. Kresnow, A. M. Fasula, L. Gilbert, and J. Chen. 2018. Rape-related pregnancy and association with reproductive coercion in the US. *American Journal of Preventive Medicine* 55(6):770-776.

Bergmann, J. N., and J. K. Stockman. 2015. How does intimate partner violence affect condom and oral contraceptive use in the United States?: A systematic review of the literature. *Contraception* 91(6):438-455.

Beydoun, H. A., M. Williams, M. A. Beydoun, S. M. Eid, and A. B. Zonderman. 2017. Relationship of physical intimate partner violence with mental health diagnoses in the nationwide emergency department sample. *J Womens Health (Larchmont)* 26(2):141-151.

Black, M. C. 2011. Intimate partner violence and adverse health consequences: Implications for clinicians. *American Journal of Lifestyle Medicine* 5(5):428-439.

Blaya, M. O., A. P. Raval, and H. M. Bramlett. 2022. Traumatic brain injury in women across lifespan. *Neurobiology of Disease* 164:105613.

Brave Heart, M. Y., R. Lewis-Fernandez, J. Beals, D. S. Hasin, L. Sugaya, S. Wang, B. F. Grant, and C. Blanco. 2016. Psychiatric disorders and mental health treatment in American Indians and Alaska Natives: Results of the National Epidemiologic Survey on Alcohol and Related Conditions. *Soc Psychiatry Psychiatr Epidemiol* 51(7):1033-1046.

Burke, J. G., L. K. Thieman, A. C. Gielen, P. O'Campo, and K. A. McDonnell. 2005. Intimate partner violence, substance use, and HIV among low-income women: Taking a closer look. *Violence Against Women* 11(9):1140-1161.

Campbell, J. C., M. L. Baty, R. M. Ghandour, J. K. Stockman, L. Francisco, and J. Wagman. 2008. The intersection of intimate partner violence against women and HIV/AIDS: A review. *Int J Inj Contr Saf Promot* 15(4):221-231.

Cha, S., and S. W. Masho. 2014. Intimate partner violence and utilization of prenatal care in the United States. *J Interpers Violence* 29(5):911-927.

Colantonio, A., and E. M. Valera. 2022. Preface to brain injury and intimate partner violence. *J Head Trauma Rehabil* 37(1):2-4.

Connelly, C. D., A. L. Hazen, M. J. Baker-Ericzén, J. Landsverk, and S. M. Horwitz. 2013. Is screening for depression in the perinatal period enough? The co-occurrence of depression, substance abuse, and intimate partner violence in culturally diverse pregnant women. *J Womens Health (Larchmont)* 22(10):844-852.

Craner, J. R., E. S. Lake, K. E. Bancroft, and K. M. Hanson. 2020. Partner abuse among treatment-seeking individuals with chronic pain: Prevalence, characteristics, and association with pain-related outcomes. *Pain Medicine* 21(11):2789-2798.

D'Angelo, D. V., J. M. Bombard, R. D. Lee, K. Kortsmit, M. Kapaya, and A. Fasula. 2023. Prevalence of experiencing physical, emotional, and sexual violence by a current intimate partner during pregnancy: Population-based estimates from the pregnancy risk assessment monitoring system. *Journal of Family Violence* 38(1):117-126.

Davis, A. E. 2000. Mechanisms of traumatic brain injury: Biomechanical, structural and cellular considerations. *Crit Care Nurs Q* 23(3):1-13.

Decker, M. R., J. G. Silverman, and A. Raj. 2005. Dating violence and sexually transmitted disease/HIV testing and diagnosis among adolescent females. *Pediatrics* 116(2):e272-e276.

Dichter, M. E., A. Sorrentino, S. Bellamy, E. Medvedeva, C. B. Roberts, and K. M. Iverson. 2017. Disproportionate mental health burden associated with past-year intimate partner violence among women receiving care in the Veterans Health Administration. *Journal of Traumatic Stress* 30(6):555-563.

Dillon, G., R. Hussain, D. Loxton, and S. Rahman. 2013. Mental and physical health and intimate partner violence against women: A review of the literature. *Int J Family Med* 2013:313909.

Dokkedahl, S. B., R. Kirubakaran, D. Bech-Hansen, T. R. Kristensen, and A. Elklit. 2022. The psychological subtype of intimate partner violence and its effect on mental health: A systematic review with meta-analyses. *Syst Rev* 11(1):163.

Donaldson, A. E., E. Hurren, C. Harvey, A. Baldwin, and B. Solomon. 2023. Front-line health professionals' recognition and responses to nonfatal strangulation events: An integrative review. *J Adv Nurs* 79(4):1290-1302.

Donovan, B. M., C. N. Spracklen, M. L. Schweizer, K. K. Ryckman, and A. F. Saftlas. 2016. Intimate partner violence during pregnancy and the risk for adverse infant outcomes: A systematic review and meta-analysis. *Bjog* 123(8):1289-1299.

Dunkle, K. L., and M. R. Decker. 2013. Gender-based violence and HIV: Reviewing the evidence for links and causal pathways in the general population and high-risk groups. *Am J Reprod Immunol* 69 Suppl 1:20-26.

Duran, B., M. Sanders, B. Skipper, H. Waitzkin, L. H. Malcoe, S. Paine, and J. Yager. 2004. Prevalence and correlates of mental disorders among Native American women in primary care. *American Journal of Public Health* 94(1):71-77.

El-Bassel, N., L. Gilbert, E. Wu, H. Go, and J. Hill. 2005. Relationship between drug abuse and intimate partner violence: A longitudinal study among women receiving methadone. *Am J Public Health* 95(3):465-470.

El-Bassel, N., P. L. Marotta, D. Goddard-Eckrich, M. Chang, T. Hunt, E. Wu, and L. Gilbert. 2019. Drug overdose among women in intimate relationships: The role of partner violence, adversity and relationship dependencies. *PLoS ONE* 14(12):e0225854.

El-Bassel, N., T. I. Mukherjee, C. Stoicescu, L. E. Starbird, J. K. Stockman, V. Frye, and L. Gilbert. 2022. Intertwined epidemics: Progress, gaps, and opportunities to address intimate partner violence and HIV among key populations of women. *Lancet HIV* 9(3):E202-E213.

Ely, G. E., and N. S. Murshid. 2018. The relationship between partner violence and number of abortions in a national sample of abortion patients. *Violence Vict* 33(4):585-603.

Exner-Cortens, D., J. Eckenrode, and E. Rothman. 2013. Longitudinal associations between teen dating violence victimization and adverse health outcomes. *Pediatrics* 131(1):71-78.

Fedina, L. 2023. *Health effects of IPV on individuals experiencing IPV across the lifespan.* Paper commissioned by the Committee on Sustaining Essential Health Care Services Related to Intimate Partner Violence During Public Health Emergencies (see Appendix B).

Fedina, L., Y. Shyrokonis, B. Backes, K. Schultz, L. Ashwell, S. Hafner, and A. Rosay. 2022. Intimate partner violence, economic insecurity, and health outcomes among American Indian and Alaska Native men and women: Findings from a national sample. *Violence Against Women* 29(11):2060-2079. https://doi.org/10.1177/10778012221127725.

Ford-Gilboe, M., C. Varcoe, J. Wuest, J. Campbell, M. Pajot, L. Heslop, and N. Perrin. 2023. Trajectories of depression, post-traumatic stress, and chronic pain among women who have separated from an abusive partner: A longitudinal analysis. *Journal of Interpersonal Violence* 38(1-2):1540-1568.

Fox, T. P., G. Oliver, and S. M. Ellis. 2013. The destructive capacity of drug abuse: An overview exploring the harmful potential of drug abuse both to the individual and to society. *International Scholarly Research Notices* 2013.

Garabedian, M. J., K. Y. Lain, W. F. Hansen, L. S. Garcia, C. M. Williams, and L. J. Crofford. 2011. Violence against women and postpartum depression. *J Womens Health (Larchmont)* 20(3):447-453.

Gielen, A. C., R. M. Ghandour, J. G. Burke, P. Mahoney, K. A. McDonnell, and P. O'Campo. 2007. HIV/AIDS and intimate partner violence: Intersecting women's health issues in the United States. *Trauma Violence Abuse* 8(2):178-198.

Gilbert, L., N. El-Bassel, M. Chang, E. Wu, and L. Roy. 2012. Substance use and partner violence among urban women seeking emergency care. *Psychol Addict Behav* 26(2):226-235.

Gilbert, L., A. Raj, D. Hien, J. Stockman, A. Terlikbayeva, and G. Wyatt. 2015. Targeting the SAVA (substance abuse, violence, and AIDS) syndemic among women and girls: A global review of epidemiology and integrated interventions. *J Acquir Immune Defic Syndr* 69(0 2):S118-S127.

Gujrathi, R., A. Tang, R. Thomas, H. Park, B. Gosangi, H. M. Stoklosa, A. Lewis-O'Connor, S. E. Seltzer, G. W. Boland, K. M. Rexrode, D. P. Orgill, and B. Khurana. 2022. Facial injury patterns in victims of intimate partner violence. *Emerg Radiol* 29(4):697-707.

Guo, C. C., M. T. Wan, Y. Wang, P. J. Wang, M. Tousey-Pfarrer, H. Y. Liu, L. M. Yu, L. Q. Jian, M. T. Zhang, Z. Q. Yang, F. F. Ge, and J. Zhang. 2023. Associations between intimate partner violence and adverse birth outcomes during pregnancy: A systematic review and meta-analysis. *Frontiers in Medicine* 10:1140787.

Haag, H., D. Jones, T. Joseph, and A. Colantonio. 2022. Battered and brain injured: Traumatic brain injury among women survivors of intimate partner violence—a scoping review. *Trauma, Violence, & Abuse* 23(4):1270-1287.

Hatcher, A. M., E. M. Smout, J. M. Turan, N. Christofides, and H. Stöckl. 2015. Intimate partner violence and engagement in HIV care and treatment among women: A systematic review and meta-analysis. *AIDS* 29(16):2183-2194.

Heck, J. L. 2021. Postpartum depression in American Indian/Alaska Native women: A scoping review. *MCN Am J Matern Child Nurs* 46(1):6-13.

Hink, A. B., E. Toschlog, B. Waibel, and M. Bard. 2015. Risks go beyond the violence: Association between intimate partner violence, mental illness, and substance abuse among females admitted to a rural level I trauma center. *Journal of Trauma and Acute Care Surgery* 79(5):709-714.

Hurwitz, E. J. H., J. Gupta, R. Liu, J. G. Silverman, and A. Raj. 2006. Intimate partner violence associated with poor health outcomes in US south Asian women. *Journal of Immigrant and Minority Health* 8:251-261.

Kastello, J. C., K. H. Jacobsen, K. F. Gaffney, M. P. Kodadek, L. C. Bullock, and P. W. Sharps. 2015. Self-rated mental health: Screening for depression and posttraumatic stress disorder among women exposed to perinatal intimate partner violence. *J Psychosoc Nurs Ment Health Serv* 53(11):32-38.

Kazmerski, T., H. L. McCauley, K. Jones, S. Borrero, J. G. Silverman, M. R. Decker, D. Tancredi, and E. Miller. 2015. Use of reproductive and sexual health services among female family planning clinic clients exposed to partner violence and reproductive coercion. *Maternal and Child Health Journal* 19:1490-1496.

Khalsa, J. H., G. Treisman, E. McCance-Katz, and E. Tedaldi. 2008. Medical consequences of drug abuse and co-occurring infections: Research at the National Institute on Drug Abuse. *Substance Abuse* 29(3):5-16.

Lacey, K. K., R. Parnell, D. M. Mouzon, N. Matusko, D. Head, J. M. Abelson, and J. S. Jackson. 2015. The mental health of US Black women: The roles of social context and severe intimate partner violence. *BMJ Open* 5(10):e008415.

Le, B. T., E. J. Dierks, B. A. Ueeck, L. D. Homer, and B. E. Potter. 2001. Maxillofacial injuries associated with domestic violence. *J Oral Maxillofac Surg* 59(11):1277-1283; discussion 1283-1274.

Lee, J., E. C. Pomeroy, and T. M. Bohman. 2007. Intimate partner violence and psychological health in a sample of Asian and Caucasian women: The roles of social support and coping. *Journal of Family Violence* 22:709-720.

Leemis, R. W., N. Friar, S. Khatiwada, M. S. Chen, M.-j. Kresnow, S. G. Smith, S. Caslin, and K. C. Basile. 2022. *The National Intimate Partner and Sexual Violence Survey: 2016/2017 report on intimate partner violence*. Atlanta, GA: Centers for Disease Control and Prevention.

Lemons-Lyn, A. B., A. R. Baugher, S. Dasgupta, J. L. Fagan, S. G. Smith, and R. L. Shouse. 2021. Intimate partner violence experienced by adults with diagnosed HIV in the US. *American Journal of Preventive Medicine* 60(6):747-756.

Li, Y., C. M. Marshall, H. C. Rees, A. Nunez, E. E. Ezeanolue, and J. E. Ehiri. 2014. Intimate partner violence and HIV infection among women: A systematic review and meta-analysis. *Journal of the International AIDS Society* 17(1):18845.

Liu, F., J. McFarlane, J. A. Maddoux, S. Cesario, H. Gilroy, and A. Nava. 2016. Perceived fertility control and pregnancy outcomes among abused women. *Jognn-Journal of Obstetric Gynecologic and Neonatal Nursing* 45(4):592-600.

Loder, R. T., and L. Momper. 2020. Demographics and fracture patterns of patients presenting to US emergency departments for intimate partner violence. *J Am Academy Orthopaedic Surg Global Research Reviews* 4(2).

Loeffen, M. J., S. H. Lo Fo Wong, F. P. Wester, M. G. Laurant, and A. L. Lagro-Janssen. 2016. Are gynaecological and pregnancy-associated conditions in family practice indicators of intimate partner violence? *Fam Pract* 33(4):354-359.

Makaroun, L. K., E. Brignone, A. M. Rosland, and M. E. Dichter. 2020. Association of health conditions and health service utilization with intimate partner violence identified via routine screening among middle-aged and older women. *JAMA Network Open* 3(4):e203138-e203138.

Maman, S., J. Campbell, M. D. Sweat, and A. C. Gielen. 2000. The intersections of HIV and violence: Directions for future research and interventions. *Soc Sci Med* 50(4):459-478.

Marshall, K. J., D. N. Fowler, M. L. Walters, and A. B. Doreson. 2018. Interventions that address intimate partner violence and HIV among women: A systematic review. *AIDS Behav* 22(10):3244-3263.

Martin, S. L., J. L. Beaumont, and L. L. Kupper. 2003. Substance use before and during pregnancy: Links to intimate partner violence. *The American Journal of Drug and Alcohol Abuse* 29(3):599-617.

Maru, M., T. Saraiya, C. S. Lee, O. Meghani, D. Hien, and H. C. Hahm. 2018. The relationship between intimate partner violence and suicidal ideation among young Chinese, Korean, and Vietnamese American women. *Women & Therapy* 41(3-4):339-355.

McCarty, J. C., E. Kiwanuka, S. Gadkaree, J. M. Siu, and E. J. Caterson. 2020. Traumatic brain injury in trauma patients with isolated facial fractures. *J Craniofacial Surg* 31(5):1182-1185.

McHugo, G. J., S. Krassenbaum, S. Donley, J. D. Corrigan, J. Bogner, and R. E. Drake. 2017. The prevalence of traumatic brain injury among people with co-occurring mental health and substance use disorders. *J Head Trauma Rehabil* 32(3):E65-E74.

Mehr, J. B., E. R. Bennett, J. L. Price, N. L. de Souza, J. F. Buckman, E. A. Wilde, D. F. Tate, A. D. Marshall, K. Dams-O'Connor, and C. Esopenko. 2023. Intimate partner violence, substance use, and health comorbidities among women: A narrative review. *Frontiers in Psychology* 13:1028375.

Messing, J. T., J. Campbell, M. A. AbiNader, and R. Bolyard. 2022. Accounting for multiple nonfatal strangulation in intimate partner violence risk assessment. *J Interpers Violence* 37(11-12):NP8430-NP8453.

Meyer, J. P., S. A. Springer, and F. L. Altice. 2011. Substance abuse, violence, and HIV in women: A literature review of the syndemic. *J Womens Health (Larchmont)* 20(7):991-1006.

Miller, E., M. R. Decker, H. L. McCauley, D. J. Tancredi, R. R. Levenson, J. Waldman, P. Schoenwald, and J. G. Silverman. 2010a. Pregnancy coercion, intimate partner violence and unintended pregnancy. *Contraception* 81(4):316-322.

Miller, E., B. Jordan, R. Levenson, and J. G. Silverman. 2010b. Reproductive coercion: Connecting the dots between partner violence and unintended pregnancy. *Contraception* 81(6):457-459.

Miller, E., H. L. McCauley, D. J. Tancredi, M. R. Decker, H. Anderson, and J. G. Silverman. 2014. Recent reproductive coercion and unintended pregnancy among female family planning clients. *Contraception* 89(2):122-128.

Moore, A. M., L. Frohwirth, and E. Miller. 2010. Male reproductive control of women who have experienced intimate partner violence in the United States. *Social Science & Medicine* 70(11):1737-1744.

Morales, M. E., and R. J. Yong. 2021. Racial and ethnic disparities in the treatment of chronic pain. *Pain Med* 22(1):75-90.

Mossey, J. M. 2011. Defining racial and ethnic disparities in pain management. *Clin Orthopaedics and Related Research* 469(7):1859-1870.

Murphy, S. B., S. J. Potter, J. Pierce-Weeks, J. G. Stapleton, and D. Wiesen-Martin. 2011. An examination of sane data: Clinical considerations based on victim-assailant relationship. *J Forensic Nurs* 7(3):137-144.

Nelson, H. D., B. G. Darney, K. Ahrens, A. Burgess, R. M. Jungbauer, A. Cantor, C. Atchison, K. B. Eden, R. Goueth, and R. Fu. 2022. Associations of unintended pregnancy with maternal and infant health outcomes: A systematic review and meta-analysis. *JAMA* 328(17):1714-1729.

Nowotny, K. M., and J. L. Graves. 2013. Substance use and intimate partner violence victimization among White, African American, and Latina women. *Journal of Interpersonal Violence* 28(17):3301-3318.

Ogden, S. N., M. E. Dichter, and A. R. Bazzi. 2022. Intimate partner violence as a predictor of substance use outcomes among women: A systematic review. *Addictive Behaviors* 127:107214.

Oram, S., H. L. Fisher, H. Minnis, S. Seedat, S. Walby, K. Hegarty, K. Rouf, C. Angenieux, F. Callard, P. S. Chandra, S. Fazel, C. Garcia-Moreno, M. Henderson, E. Howarth, H. L. MacMillan, L. K. Murray, S. Othman, D. Robotham, M. B. Rondon, A. Sweeney, D. Taggart, and L. M. Howard. 2022. The Lancet Psychiatry Commission on Intimate Partner Violence and Mental Health: Advancing mental health services, research, and policy. *Lancet Psychiatry* 9(6):487-524.

Pastor-Moreno, G., I. Ruiz-Perez, J. Henares-Montiel, V. Escriba-Aguir, C. Higueras-Callejon, and I. Ricci-Cabello. 2020. Intimate partner violence and perinatal health: A systematic review. *Bjog* 127(5):537-547.

Patch, M., J. C. Anderson, and J. C. Campbell. 2018. Injuries of women surviving intimate partner strangulation and subsequent emergency health care seeking: An integrative evidence review. *J Emerg Nurs* 44(4):384-393.

Patch, M., Y. M. K. Farag, J. C. Anderson, N. Perrin, G. Kelen, and J. C. Campbell. 2021. United States emergency department visits by adult women for nonfatal intimate partner strangulation, 2006 to 2014: Prevalence and associated characteristics. *J Emerg Nurs* 47(3):437-448.

Peitzmeier, S. M., M. Malik, S. K. Kattari, E. Marrow, R. Stephenson, M. Agenor, and S. L. Reisner. 2020. Intimate partner violence in transgender populations: Systematic review and meta-analysis of prevalence and correlates. *Am J Public Health* 110(9):e1-e14.

Poleshuck, E., C. Mazzotta, K. Resch, A. Rogachefsky, K. Bellenger, C. Raimondi, J. Thompson Stone, and C. Cerulli. 2018. Development of an innovative treatment paradigm for intimate partner violence victims with depression and pain using community-based participatory research. *J Interpers Violence* 33(17):2704-2724.

Porsch, L. M., M. Xu, C. B. Veldhuis, L. A. Bochicchio, S. S. Zollweg, and T. L. Hughes. 2022. Intimate partner violence among sexual minority women: A scoping review. *Trauma, Violence, & Abuse* 24(5):3014-3036. https://doi.org/10.1177/15248380221122815.

Pritchard, A. J., A. Reckdenwald, and C. Nordham. 2017. Nonfatal strangulation as part of domestic violence: A review of research. *Trauma, Violence, & Abuse* 18(4):407-424.

Rajandram, R. K., S. N. Syed Omar, M. F. Rashdi, and M. N. Abdul Jabar. 2014. Maxillofacial injuries and traumatic brain injury—a pilot study. *Dental Traumatology* 30(2):128-132.

Reyes, M. E., L. Simpson, T. P. Sullivan, A. A. Contractor, and N. H. Weiss. 2023. Intimate partner violence and mental health outcomes among Hispanic women in the United States: A scoping review. *Trauma, Violence, & Abuse* 24(2):809-827.

Roberts, S., M. A. Biggs, K. S. Chibber, H. Gould, C. H. Rocca, and D. G. Foster. 2014. Risk of violence from the man involved in the pregnancy after receiving or being denied an abortion. *BMC Medicine* 12(1):1-7.

Sabri, B., R. Bolyard, A. L. McFadgion, J. K. Stockman, M. B. Lucea, G. B. Callwood, C. R. Coverston, and J. C. Campbell. 2013. Intimate partner violence, depression, PTSD, and use of mental health resources among ethnically diverse Black women. *Social Work in Health Care* 52(4):351-369.

Samankasikorn, W., J. Alhusen, G. Yan, D. L. Schminkey, and L. Bullock. 2019. Relationships of reproductive coercion and intimate partner violence to unintended pregnancy. *J Obstet Gynecol Neonatal Nurs* 48(1):50-58.

Samulowitz, A., I. Gremyr, E. Eriksson, and G. Hensing. 2018. "Brave men" and "emotional women": A theory-guided literature review on gender bias in health care and gendered norms towards patients with chronic pain. *Pain Research & Management* 2018.

Schafer, S. D., L. L. Drach, K. Hedberg, and M. A. Kohn. 2008. Using diagnostic codes to screen for intimate partner violence in Oregon emergency departments and hospitals. *Public Health Rep* 123(5):628-635.

Smith, P. H., G. G. Homish, K. E. Leonard, and J. R. Cornelius. 2012. Intimate partner violence and specific substance use disorders: Findings from the National Epidemiologic Survey on Alcohol and Related Conditions. *Psychol Addict Behav* 26(2):236-245.

Smith, E. J., B. A. Bailey, and A. Cascio. 2023. Sexual coercion, intimate partner violence, and homicide: A scoping literature review. *Trauma Violence Abuse* 25(1):341-353. https://doi.org/10.1177/15248380221150474.

Sorenson, S. B., M. Joshi, and E. Sivitz. 2014. A systematic review of the epidemiology of nonfatal strangulation, a human rights and health concern. *Am J Public Health* 104(11):e54-e61.

Spencer, C. M., and S. M. Stith. 2020. Risk factors for male perpetration and female victimization of intimate partner homicide: A meta-analysis. *Trauma Violence Abuse* 21(3):527-540.

Spencer, C. M., B. M. Keilholtz, M. Palmer, and S. L. Vail. 2022. Mental and physical health correlates for emotional intimate partner violence perpetration and victimization: A meta-analysis. *Trauma Violence Abuse* 25(1):41-53. https://doi.org/10.1177/15248380221137686.

Stansfield, R., and K. R. Williams. 2021. Coercive control between intimate partners: An application to nonfatal strangulation. *Journal of Interpersonal Violence* 36(9-10):NP5105-NP5124.

Stockman, J. K., H. Hayashi, and J. C. Campbell. 2015. Intimate partner violence and its health impact on disproportionately affected populations, including minorities and impoverished groups. *J Womens Health (Larchmont)* 24(1):62-79.

Stockman, J. K., M. B. Lucea, and J. C. Campbell. 2013. Forced sexual initiation, sexual intimate partner violence and HIV risk in women: A global review of the literature. *AIDS Behav* 17(3):832-847.

Stone, R., and E. F. Rothman. 2019. Opioid use and intimate partner violence: A systematic review. *Current Epidemiology Reports* 6(2):215-230.

Stubbs, A., and C. Szoeke. 2022. The effect of intimate partner violence on the physical health and health-related behaviors of women: A systematic review of the literature. *Trauma Violence Abuse* 23(4):1157-1172.

Sullivan, T. P. 2019. The intersection of intimate partner violence and HIV: Detection, disclosure, discussion, and implications for treatment adherence. *Topics Antiviral Med* 27(2):84-87.

Sutton, A., H. Beech, B. Ozturk, and D. Nelson-Gardell. 2020. Preparing mental health professionals to work with survivors of intimate partner violence: A comprehensive systematic review of the literature. *Affilia* 36(3):426-440.

Tang, A., A. Wong, and B. Khurana. 2023. Imaging of intimate partner violence, from the AJR special series on emergency radiology. *AJR Am J Roentgenology* 220(4):476-485.

Termos, M., V. Murugan, and J. J. Helton. 2022. IPV and health consequences among CPS-involved caregivers: A fixed effects analysis stratified by race and ethnicity. *Violence Against Women* 28(6-7):1610-1630.

Testa, M., J. A. Livingston, and K. E. Leonard. 2003. Women's substance use and experiences of intimate partner violence: A longitudinal investigation among a community sample. *Addictive Behaviors* 28(9):1649-1664.

Trost, Z., J. Sturgeon, A. Guck, M. Ziadni, L. Nowlin, B. Goodin, and W. Scott. 2019. Examining injustice appraisals in a racially diverse sample of individuals with chronic low back pain. *J Pain* 20(1):83-96.

Tsuyuki, K., A. N. Cimino, C. N. Holliday, J. C. Campbell, N. A. Al-Alusi, and J. K. Stockman. 2019. Physiological changes from violence-induced stress and trauma enhance HIV susceptibility among women. *Curr HIV/AIDS Rep* 16(1):57-65.

Ullman, S. E., and R. Sigurvinsdottir. 2015. Intimate partner violence and drinking among victims of adult sexual assault. *Journal of Aggression, Maltreatment & Trauma* 24(2):117-130.

Valera, E. M., J. C. Daugherty, O. C. Scott, and H. Berenbaum. 2022. Strangulation as an acquired brain injury in intimate-partner violence and its relationship to cognitive and psychological functioning: A preliminary study. *Journal of Head Trauma Rehabilitation* 37(1):15-23.

Vicard-Olagne, M., B. Pereira, L. Rouge, A. Cabaillot, P. Vorilhon, G. Lazimi, and C. Laporte. 2022. Signs and symptoms of intimate partner violence in women attending primary care in Europe, North America and Australia: A systematic review and meta-analysis. *Fam Pract* 39(1):190-199.

Walker, N., K. Beek, H. Chen, J. Shang, S. Stevenson, K. Williams, H. Herzog, J. Ahmed, and P. Cullen. 2022. The experiences of persistent pain among women with a history of intimate partner violence: A systematic review. *Trauma, Violence, & Abuse* 23(2):490-505.

Waller, M. W., B. J. Iritani, S. L. Christ, H. K. Clark, K. E. Moracco, C. T. Halpern, and R. L. Flewelling. 2012. Relationships among alcohol outlet density, alcohol use, and intimate partner violence victimization among young women in the United States. *J Interpers Violence* 27(10):2062-2086.

Walters, M. L., M. J. Breiding, and J. Chen. 2013. *The National Intimate Partner and Sexual Violence Survey: 2010 findings on victimization by sexual orientation.* National Center for Injury Prevention and Control of the Centers for Disease Control and Prevention. Atlanta, GA: National Center for Injury Prevention and Control, Centers for Disease Control and Prevention.

White, S. J., J. Sin, A. Sweeney, T. Salisbury, C. Wahlich, C. M. Montesinos Guevara, S. Gillard, E. Brett, L. Allwright, and N. Iqbal. 2023. Global prevalence and mental health outcomes of intimate partner violence among women: A systematic review and meta-analysis. *Trauma, Violence, & Abuse* 25(1):494-511. https://doi.org/10.1177/15248380231155529.

Willie, T. C., J. K. Stockman, R. Perler, and T. S. Kershaw. 2018. Associations between intimate partner violence, violence-related policies, and HIV diagnosis rate among women in the United States. *Annals of Epidemiology* 28(12):881-885.

Wright, E. N., A. Hanlon, A. Lozano, and A. M. Teitelman. 2019. The impact of intimate partner violence, depressive symptoms, alcohol dependence, and perceived stress on 30-year cardiovascular disease risk among young adult women: A multiple mediation analysis. *Preventive Medicine* 121:47-54.

Wright, E. N., A. Hanlon, A. Lozano, and A. M. Teitelman. 2021. The association between intimate partner violence and 30-year cardiovascular disease risk among young adult women. *Journal of Interpersonal Violence* 36(11-12):NP6643-NP6660.

Wright, E. N., J. Anderson, K. Phillips, and S. Miyamoto. 2022. Help-seeking and barriers to care in intimate partner sexual violence: A systematic review. *Trauma Violence Abuse* 23(5):1510-1528.

Wu, V., H. Huff, and M. Bhandari. 2010. Pattern of physical injury associated with intimate partner violence in women presenting to the emergency department: A systematic review and meta-analysis. *Trauma Violence Abuse* 11(2):71-82.

Wuest, J., M. Merritt-Gray, B. Lent, C. Varcoe, A. J. Connors, and M. Ford-Gilboe. 2007. Patterns of medication use among women survivors of intimate partner violence. *Canadian Journal of Public Health* 98:460-464.

5

Essential Health Care Services
for Intimate Partner Violence

ESSENTIAL HEALTH CARE SERVICES RELATED
TO INTIMATE PARTNER VIOLENCE

The committee defines *health care services* as care delivered in or referrable from a health care setting. Therefore, essential health care services related to intimate partner violence (IPV) refer to essential care delivered in or referrable from a health care setting. This reflects the committee's understanding that the health consequences of IPV may require care that extends beyond the traditional health care system. Essential health care services related to IPV include those that address the most prevalent and serious physical and behavioral health conditions related to IPV, which are discussed in Chapter 4. Essential health care services related to IPV also facilitate identification of IPV, protect the safety of the person experiencing IPV (and their children if needed), and meet their basic needs for food and shelter.

Essential Explained

The committee's process for identifying essential health care services related to IPV in steady state conditions was informed by an extensive review of high-quality evidence from several literature searches; recommendations from the U.S. Preventive Services Task Force (USPSTF), the Women's Preventive Services Initiative (WPSI), and the World Health Organization (WHO); and insight gleaned from a commissioned paper and presentations to the committee by experts in IPV-related care.

The committee identified the following criteria for identifying essential health care services related to IPV:

- Evidence-based health care services that address the most common and most serious health outcomes related to experiencing IPV;
- Preventive services recommended by USPSTF and WPSI; and
- Specific support services required to meet the basic safety and housing needs of people experiencing IPV.

Essential Intimate Partner Violence–Related Health Care Services

The many adverse health effects related to experiencing IPV do not occur in isolation. Women experiencing IPV need care for multiple physical and psychological conditions concurrently. The list of essential health care services in the recommendation below should not be considered exhaustive. Each woman's experience of IPV is different, as are her needs for health care services related to IPV.

Recommendation 1: The committee recommends that the Health Resources and Services Administration and all U.S. health care systems classify the following as essential health care services related to intimate partner violence (IPV):

- **Universal IPV screening and inquiry**
- **Universal IPV education**
- **Safety planning**
- **Forensic medical examinations**
- **Emergency medical care**
- **Treatment of physical injuries**
- **Gynecologic and reproductive health care, including all forms of Food and Drug Administration-approved contraception and pregnancy termination**
- **Screening and treatment of sexually transmitted infections and HIV**
- **Treatment for substance use disorders and addiction care**
- **Pharmacy and medication management**
- **Obstetric care, including perinatal home visits**
- **Primary and specialty care**
- **Mental health care**
- **Support services, including shelter, nutritional assistance, and child care**
- **Dental care**

Universal Screening and Education

Screening in health care generally refers to delivering preventive health services that identify a condition or risk for a condition to patients without signs or symptoms of the condition being screened, as opposed to *diagnosing* patients with indications of the condition. Universal screening for IPV includes all patients, regardless of the presence of signs, symptoms, or health conditions related to IPV, to identify those with subclinical experiences of previous or ongoing IPV and those at risk for future IPV. The goal of IPV screening in health care settings is to provide support and patient specific interventions, including referrals, that reduce exposure to IPV and improve health outcomes. Screening for IPV is included for coverage under preventive service mandates of the Patient Protection and Affordable Care Act (ACA).[1]

Periodic universal screening for IPV is an established standard of routine preventive health care for women aged 13 years and older in the United States. The USPSTF recommends screening all women of reproductive age for IPV and providing ongoing support services to women who have a positive screening outcome or referring them to those services (USPSTF et al., 2018). The WPSI recommends screening adolescents and adults with biological or other identification as a woman at least annually and providing women with—or referring them to—intervention and support services if needed (WPSI, 2022). The WPSI recommendation notes that intervention services "include, but are not limited to, counseling, education, harm reduction strategies, and referral to appropriate supportive services" (WPSI, 2022, p. 52). The second part of both the USPSTF and WPSI screening recommendations highlight that providing or referring women to support services is a critical component of screening for IPV.

Routine screening is usually implemented during primary care and maternity care visits, although it also occurs in other settings. Screening in health care settings is generally acceptable to women when done privately and safely, and some prefer self-administered methods, including computerized screening (Ahmad et al., 2009; Kapur and Windish, 2011; MacMillan et al., 2006). A coding guide developed by the WPSI assists clinical practices with coding and billing for IPV screening services. The coding guide includes ICD-10 codes, coding scenarios, and Medicare and Medicaid resources (WPSI, 2022).[2]

Screening generally involves the administration of a validated screening instrument composed of a brief set of questions that may include questions about physical, sexual, and psychological abuse (see Table 5-1).

---

[1] *Patient Protection and Affordable Care Act*, Public Law 118-148, 111th Congress (March 23, 2010).

[2] ICD-10 refers to *International Classification of Diseases*, 10th edition.

TABLE 5-1 Validated Tools for Screening for IPV

Measure	Components	Sensitivity; specificity
Hurt/Insult/Threaten/ Scream tool (HITS)	Four items (hurt, insult, threaten, scream), 5-point Likert scale, self-report or clinician administered survey; score ranges from 4 to 20 points, ≥10 indicates abuse.	86%; 99%
Ongoing Violence Assessment Tool (OVAT)	Four items (threaten, beaten, would like to kill you, no respect), dichotomous scale; score ranges from 0 to 4.	86%; 83%
Partner Violence Screen (PVS)	Three items (past physical violence, perceived personal safety), dichotomous scale, clinician administered; score ranges from 0 to 3, ≥1 indicates IPV.	49–71%; 80–94%
Woman Abuse Screening Tool (WAST)	Eight items (physical, sexual, emotional abuse), 3-point response scale (0 = never, 1 = sometimes, 2 = often); scores range from 0 to 16, and ≥4 indicates exposure to IPV. Short form includes two questions about tension in the relationship and how arguments are resolved.	47–88%; 89–96%
Slapped, Threatened, and Throw (STaT) Measure	Three items (pushed or slapped; threatened with violence; partner has thrown, broken, or punched things), dichotomous, self-report scale; score ranges from 0 to 3.	96%; 75%
Abuse Assessment Screen (AAS)	Five items (sexual coercion, lifetime abuse, current abuse, abuse during pregnancy), dichotomous scale, clinician administered survey; scores range from 0 to 5, with any positive response considered a positive screen.	92%; 55%
Humiliation, Afraid, Rape, Kick (HARK) Tool	Four items (humiliation, afraid, rape, kick), dichotomous scale, self-report survey, adapted from AAS; scoring ranges from 0 to 4.	81%; 95%
Ongoing Abuse Screen (OAS)	Five items (threaten, beaten, would like to kill you, no respect), dichotomous scale; scores range from 0 to 5.	60%; 90%

SOURCE: Feltner et al., 2018.

Some instruments, such as the Ongoing Violence Assessment Tool, focus on physical violence and personal safety (Feltner et al., 2018). In contrast, others, such as the Women Abuse Screening Tool, include additional types of abuse (Feltner et al., 2018). Most instruments identify current IPV or IPV occurring within the previous 12 months, while some collect information about past IPV, such as the Abuse Assessment Screen (AAS) (Feltner et al.,

2018). Validated instruments may not apply to all patient populations, such as non-English speakers, and other screening approaches may be necessary.

Screening tools have also been developed to specifically assess IPV lethality or the risk of intimate partner homicide (Campbell, 1986; Campbell et al., 2009; Echeburúa et al., 2009; López-Ossorio et al., 2019; Messing et al., 2013, 2017, 2020). Sensitivity, specificity, and reliability for these metrics are mixed (Garcia-Vergara et al., 2022; Messing et al., 2017). They are not evaluated or included in the USPSTF or WPSI screening recommendations.

IPV screening may be appropriate for patients and settings outside those specified in routine screening recommendations. These include screening in emergency departments, orthopedic clinics, and other health care settings where IPV-related conditions commonly present but may go unrecognized. In these cases, the use of IPV screening instruments may extend beyond universal screening to detect IPV in the context of coexisting health conditions associated with IPV.

Some researchers and practitioners have raised concerns that screening for IPV may cause harm to women (Chisholm et al., 2017; McLennan and MacMillan, 2016). Potential harms discussed in the literature include opportunity costs regarding other health services, child protection investigation, false positives, increased abuse, retaliation, labeling, and stigma (Feltner et al., 2018; McLennan and MacMillan, 2016). However, a USPSTF evidence review did not find evidence that IPV screening presents a statistically significant risk of harm (Feltner et al., 2018). A separate Cochrane review also found no evidence that screening for IPV poses a significant risk of harm (O'Doherty et al., 2015). However, both reviews indicated that there were few robust studies examining the harms of screening and noted methodological heterogeneity across the literature (Feltner et al., 2018; O'Doherty et al., 2015).

The perinatal period is a critical time to offer screening and health care for IPV. Women access health care more frequently during this period and are more likely to implement suggested health behaviors than in other situations. Therefore, screening during regular perinatal care is important, and attention to the health effects and care needs related to IPV in this population is necessary. Despite the recommendation from the USPSTF calling for universal screening for those of reproductive age, screening practices remain inconsistent throughout perinatal care. Analysis of data from the 2016–2019 Pregnancy Risk Assessment Monitoring System found that of the respondents who reported experiencing physical IPV during pregnancy and received prenatal care, 25.5 percent (n = 1,326, N = 6,124) were not screened for IPV at any prenatal care visits (Kozhimannil et al., 2023).[3]

---

[3]Additional context has been added to the sentence to ensure an accurate representation of the data presented, after initial release of the report.

Within the group of people receiving prenatal care, those who lived in rural districts and those who were covered through private insurance were less likely to be screened for IPV than those in urban areas and those covered through Medicaid (Kozhimannil et al., 2023). Universal screening for IPV in the health care setting not only aids in identifying those who are at risk of or experiencing IPV but can lead to interventions to improve maternal and fetal outcomes. There is a particularly large window of opportunity for screening during perinatal care, as pregnant and postpartum people typically have more regular office visits with their clinicians and have the chance to build trusting relationships with their clinicians during this time (Alhusen et al., 2015). Not all IPV screening assessments screen for physical, psychological, and sexual violence (Chisholm et al., 2017). The American College of Obstetricians and Gynecologists provides guidance for IPV screening in the perinatal period (ACOG, 2012).

Universal education involves offering information about healthy relationships, the intersections of IPV and health, and relevant supports and services during all clinical encounters (McKay, 2021). This approach addresses a limitation of screening often noted by advocates—that a woman experiencing IPV must be ready to disclose in order to receive information about IPV and relevant resources (McKay, 2021). Research directed at identifying barriers to IPV disclosure has highlighted the role of knowledge about IPV and available supports in disclosure and help seeking. A systematic review of 29 studies investigating barriers to disclosing IPV found that two of the most commonly reported reasons women reported for not disclosing IPV during screening were a lack of knowledge about IPV and a lack of awareness of available services to support them (Robinson et al., 2021). This was echoed by Ravi and colleagues in their systematic review of 24 studies investigating facilitators of formal help seeking among people experiencing IPV (Ravi et al., 2022). By highlighting that this information may be relevant to themselves or someone they know, clinicians and front line responders can reduce feelings of shame and isolation that some women experience. A core component of essential health care services is ensuring that information about IPV (including how a public health emergency [PHE] may escalate abusive behaviors in a relationship) is readily available in all settings where individuals seek help.

Safety Planning

Safety planning is the process of collaborating with the woman experiencing IPV to empower her to develop strategies that increase safety by increasing her situational awareness of IPV-related risks (Sabri et al., 2021). The process is centered on the woman experiencing IPV and informed by her identified concerns and priorities. Once those are identified, planning includes identifying and connecting the woman to resources consistent with her needs (Sabri et al., 2021). In some situations, the person experiencing IPV may not want to or may not feel that they can leave an abusive relationship. Research has found that in situations where the person engaging in IPV is highly dangerous, the act of leaving the relationship may increase the woman's level of danger (Campbell et al., 2003, 2009). In that situation, safety planning focuses on strategies to enhance her safety and reduce risk while remaining in the relationship (Sabri et al., 2021). The literature has identified elements of safety plans that are most effective, including:

- Assessing individual needs and circumstances;
- Providing education about the different forms of IPV;
- Helping women identify their safety risks;
- Developing concrete safety plans;
- Directly connecting women to resources and support services;
- Establishing long-term support, including continued safety check-ins during follow-up IPV care and services;
- Focusing on empowerment to enhance women's safety strategies and strengthening support networks to help manage safety threats; and
- Including interventions to address co-occurring conditions, including mental health issues, substance use, and sexual risk behaviors that may put them at risk for sexually transmitted infections (STIs), including HIV (Sabri et al., 2021).

TREATMENT OF CONDITIONS RELATED TO ACUTE INTIMATE PARTNER VIOLENCE

Injuries to the Head, Neck, and Face

Treatment for injuries to the head, neck, and face require different essential health care services depending on the severity of the injury. Fractures to the head, neck, and face can be life-threatening and require emergency medical care to stabilize the fracture and address any associated airway obstruction, spinal cord injury, brain injury, or secondary trauma that can affect vision, hearing, speaking, or jaw function (Chouinard et al., 2016; Jose et al., 2016). These fractures may require surgical intervention, and all fractures will require post-reduction follow-up in the form of specialty medical care. Soft tissue injuries to the head, neck, and face will require treatment for acute trauma and may require surgical intervention and follow-up specialty medical care.

Women with a traumatic brain injury (TBI) related to IPV require multiple health care services and may seek care in a variety of settings. Many of the acute injuries associated with TBI, such as skull fracture, cervical fracture, and intracranial hemorrhage, require emergency medical care and may require surgical intervention (Galgano et al., 2017; Taylor et al., 2017). Women who have sustained an IPV-related TBI may also require hospitalization, depending on the severity of the TBI and associated injuries (Taylor et al., 2017). Women who have sustained an IPV-related TBI may initially seek care for another concomitant physical injury, such as an extremity fracture or dental injury (Ellis et al., 2019; Turkstra et al., 2023). Women who have experienced an IPV-related TBI will require multiple essential health care services, including primary and specialty medical care, mental health care, and pharmacy/medication management to support recovery and long-term management of chronic TBI sequelae. The cognitive sequelae of TBI, such as impaired judgement and executive function deficits, can make it difficult for women with IPV-related TBI to complete both simple everyday tasks and more complex tasks, such as those that may be necessary to access health care or support services, or to separate from a person using IPV (Haag et al., 2022).

Women who sustain a TBI or hypoxic brain injuries due to IPV-related strangulation can reasonably be expected to experience acute and chronic adverse physical, psychological, and cognitive effects that are similar to those associated with sustaining a TBI not due to strangulation (Anderson and Archiniegas, 2010; Valera et al., 2022). As a result, the same categories of IPV-related essential health care services are required for women that have survived IPV-related strangulation.

Musculoskeletal Injuries

Women experiencing IPV-related musculoskeletal injuries will have differing essential health care service needs depending on the severity of their injuries. Severe acute injuries such as dislocations and some fractures are associated with an elevated risk for dangerous complications, such as damage to adjacent vasculature, and require emergency medical care. Those injuries as well as other musculoskeletal injuries require specialty medical care. A growing body of research suggests that a large number of women experiencing IPV-related musculoskeletal injuries seek care in outpatient orthopedic clinics and fracture clinics, highlighting the importance of this setting to essential IPV health care services (Logue et al., 2021; Sprague et al., 2013a,b; Velonis et al., 2019).

Gynecologic and Reproductive Health Issues

Women experiencing IPV have complex gynecologic and reproductive health problems that require multiple essential health care services related to IPV. Emergency medical care is required for severe gynecologic injuries and infections. Gynecologic and reproductive health services, screening and treatment for STIs and HIV, and primary and specialty medical care are needed to address IPV-related injuries, infections, and other disorders. Those services may be delivered in a variety of settings, including primary care clinics, obstetric and gynecology clinics, and other medical specialty clinics such as oncology, family planning, and reproductive health clinics.

Women experiencing reproductive coercion or an unplanned pregnancy related to IPV have unique needs for essential health care services related to IPV. They need gynecologic and reproductive health care services, which include all forms of FDA-approved contraception. Access will reduce the likelihood of unintended pregnancy, particularly in light of the well-documented barriers to accessing some forms of contraception, such as emergency contraception, for those experiencing IPV (Bergmann and Stockman, 2015; Gee et al., 2009; Miller et al., 2014; Smith et al., 2022). In light of the substantial risks to maternal and infant health as well as increased risk to women's safety associated with an IPV-related unintended pregnancy, the essential gynecologic and reproductive health care services related to IPV include pregnancy termination when the woman and her health care professional determine that is appropriate (Auger et al., 2022; Mogos et al., 2016; Nelson et al., 2022; Smith et al., 2023). Some adverse health effects related to unintended pregnancy and IPV are serious and can be life threatening, requiring emergency medical care. Additionally, individuals who experience IPV-related unplanned pregnancies also need access to obstetric care for both standard pregnancy care and to address the adverse health effects associated with IPV and unplanned pregnancy.

Additionally, women experiencing IPV-related sexual assault require several essential health care services related to IPV. They should have access to treatment for physical injuries sustained during the assault and, depending on the severity of their injuries, may need emergency medical care. Their care needs will vary, from needing primary care to needing specialty clinical care, depending on the nature of the injuries or disorders. The needs of women experiencing IPV-related sexual assault include access to gynecologic and reproductive health care services to address both acute and chronic gynecologic injuries and disorders. They also need access to STI and HIV screening and treatment. Mental health care is also important for addressing the psychological trauma associated with experiencing violent acts, such as rape. This array of services should also be available for women who have been raped by an intimate partner. They have time-sensitive needs for essential health care services. Emergency contraception should be available to reduce the risk of unintended pregnancy within 5 days of the rape (Basile et al., 2018; Smith et al., 2023). Additionally, it is possible that a woman who has experienced IPV rape will not know the HIV and STI status of her partner, which makes access to STI and HIV screening and treatment, including post-exposure prophylaxis, an urgent need (Gilmore et al., 2022).

The forensic medical examination, also referred to as a sexual assault medical forensic examination, is an essential health care service related to IPV that facilitates access to time-sensitive care needs related to IPV sexual assault and rape (Gilmore et al., 2021). Individuals who undergo a sexual assault forensic medical examination at a facility with a sexual assault nurse examiner (SANE) also receive crucial medical care, including STI and HIV testing and prophylaxis, as well as emergency contraception (Gilmore et al., 2021). SANEs have specialized training in evaluating and caring for a person who has experienced sexual assault using a trauma-informed approach (Thiede and Miyamoto, 2021). SANE-led care is associated with a high quality of care as well as with more thorough examinations, high-quality evidence collection, and more positive prosecutorial outcomes (Thiede and Miyamoto, 2021). In addition to sexual assault, forensic medical examinations for people who have experienced IPV can be used to document injuries from physical IPV, including strangulation (Pritchard et al., 2017).

In May 2023, the U.S. Department of Justice's Office on Violence Against Women released a National Protocol for Intimate Partner Violence Medical Forensic Examinations (DOJ, 2023). The protocol emphasizes the importance of a warm handoff of the person experiencing IPV to service providers and community-based organizations, in which the clinician connects the individual to the appropriate resource instead of simply providing a telephone number or website address (DOJ, 2023). The protocol also stresses that IPV care providers need to engage in a trauma-informed approach when caring for people experiencing IPV. According to the protocol, a medical forensic examination for people experiencing IPV includes:

- Medical forensic history gathering,
- Comprehensive physical assessment,
- Treatment of injuries,
- Provision of care for other health concerns identified during the examination,
- Sample and evidence collection,
- Photographic documentation of findings,
- Written documentation of the patient encounter, and
- Safety and discharge planning, including targeted referrals based on the patient's specific needs. (DOJ, 2023)

Chronic Pain

Chronic pain is a complex condition that is further confounded in the setting of experiencing IPV. Its complex nature requires individualized and multimodal treatment. These include, but are not limited to, treatment of traumatic physical injuries, gynecologic and reproductive health care, mental health care, pharmacy/medication management, and primary care and specialty medical care.

Mental and Behavioral Health

Given the substantial adverse effects that experiencing IPV has on mental and behavioral health, mental health care is an essential health care service related to IPV. Women experiencing IPV and substance use disorder have broad needs for essential health care services related to IPV, including access to substance use treatment and addiction care, pharmacy/medication management, mental health care, STI and HIV testing and treatment, primary and specialty medical care, and emergency medical care. The syndemic of IPV, substance abuse, and HIV among women in the United States is well documented in the literature (González-Guarda et al., 2011; Meyer et al., 2011; Vavala et al., 2022). Therefore, the essential health care services related to IPV for substance use and HIV are likely to be needed concurrently.

INTIMATE PARTNER VIOLENCE HEALTH CARE ACCESS AND DELIVERY

Essential health care services for IPV are delivered in multiple settings across health care systems, including primary care, practices related to women's health (e.g., Planned Parenthood), perinatal-specific care settings, and settings supported by federal funding. Community-based care settings also serve to provide many of these essential services. One analysis of survey data from 3,333 women in Washington state and Idaho found that women experiencing IPV reported at least 20 percent more health care utilization than those that had not reported experiencing IPV, even after their experiences of IPV have ended (Rivara et al., 2007). Given the higher frequency of health care use among women experiencing IPV, primary care and other specialty care professionals can play an important role in interrupting IPV and promoting women's health and well-being.

A systematic review of IPV interventions in primary care found that most of the reviewed studies (10 of 17) recruited women from reproductive health care settings in obstetrics–gynecology and family planning (Bair-Merritt et al., 2014). Most of the interventions were conducted entirely in the primary care office setting. Most interventions included outside office contact, including case management, phone calls, and home visits. The interventions ranged in length from 10 minutes to 16 hours (eight 2-hour weekly sessions). Nonphysicians delivered the majority of the care, which focused on empowerment, empathetic listening, discussion of the cycle of

violence and safety, and referral to community-based resources. It is important to note that none of the interventions were conducted in a pediatric
setting. Since more than one in six youth in the United States report being
exposed to IPV as children, much still needs to be learned about youth
interventions (Hamby et al., 2011).

As noted earlier, because essential health care services for IPV encompass a wide range of health care settings, specialties, resources, and personnel, services interface not only with the patient and health system but also
with the community and society. Patients access health care services for
IPV through multiple pathways (see Figure 5-1). Most health care services
are accessed through the health care system itself, including health care
provided by first responders, community health workers, and telemedicine
programs, in addition to clinics and hospitals.

Health Care System Settings

IPV is associated with increased health care utilization (Rivara et al.,
2007). Care for patients experiencing IPV involves clinicians and staff
across various settings in health care systems, including outpatient primary
care clinics, specialty clinics, emergency and urgent care settings, and
inpatient facilities.

Emergency department (ED) staff and clinicians routinely serve women
who have experienced IPV. A review of nationwide insurance claims data
found that women with a documented history of experiencing IPV had
4.5 times more ED visits than those without a documented history of
IPV (Kishton et al., 2022). Several studies have noted high reported rates
of IPV, including reproductive coercion, among women seeking care in
family planning and women's health clinics (Miller et al., 2014; Rickert et
al., 2002). In these settings, women with IPV are more likely to seek emergency contraception, treatment for STIs, and pregnancy tests (Kazmerski
et al., 2015; Miller et al., 2010). In an analysis of survey data collected
in eight Canadian and U.S. orthopedic fracture clinics, the prevalence of
IPV within the past year was 18 percent and the lifetime prevalence was
40 percent (Sprague et al., 2013a). Clinicians serving those with chronic
health conditions may see patients whose conditions are directly related
to IPV or exacerbated by new episodes of IPV. In contrast, chronic conditions associated with IPV are common. However, they may go undetected
or under-treated in the health care system (Wilson et al., 2007).

Clinicians in diverse settings, especially those in which confidentiality is ensured are likely to encounter adolescents who have experienced
IPV (Miller et al., 2010). However, adolescents are unlikely to mention
relationship or sexual abuse as the reason for their visit. Instead, they may
present with trauma symptoms, injuries, or mental health problems. They

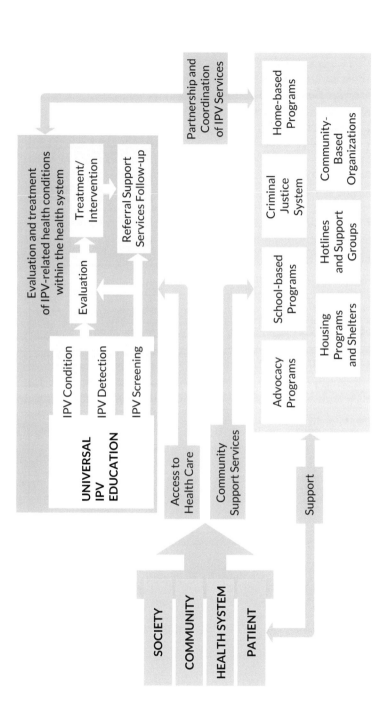

FIGURE 5-1 Access to essential health care services for those experiencing IPV.

NOTES: Patients access health care services through multiple pathways, including treatment of recognized IPV-related health conditions (e.g., acute trauma from IPV assault). IPV is typically detected during the course of health care (e.g., injury identified during a maternity care visit) or through inquiry (e.g., routine IPV screening without current signs or symptoms).

may also present with nonspecific complaints, such as recurrent headaches, poor sleep, abdominal pain, or fatigue (Miller et al., 2010). Requests for pregnancy or STI testing and emergency contraception may suggest that relationship abuse or sexual violence has occurred.

Clinical settings that provide pediatric care are confidential and safe spaces that can support parents and caregivers experiencing IPV who may be more likely to seek care for their children than for themselves (Ragavan and Miller, 2022). Studies in pediatric care settings during the COVID-19 pandemic found that parents reported partners engaging in IPV employed coercive control tactics including social isolation, manipulating child custody, taking stimulus money, and a myriad of other tactics (Kourti et al., 2023; Ragavan et al., 2022). The American Academy of Pediatrics has encouraged pediatric clinicians to engage in training and education about IPV and to consider incorporating universal IPV education into their practices (Thackeray et al., 2023).

Positive and Negative Experiences in Health Care Settings

In its recently released 2023–2025 Strategy to Address Intimate Partner Violence, HRSA notes that an equitable, community-driven approach necessitates seeking input from communities and individuals being served (HRSA, 2023a). People who have experienced IPV can provide critical feedback on developing, funding, implementing, and evaluating services and programs to prevent and respond to IPV. Centering community voices in preparation for public health emergencies ensures that programs are relevant and responsive to community priorities, assets, and challenges. Simultaneously, culturally responsive care and attention to health equity in clinical practices can reduce health disparities experienced by populations disproportionately affected by IPV.

Experiences of Patients

A systematic review of studies of health care for IPV in emergency departments identified several factors contributing to positive and negative experiences with clinicians (Duchesne et al., 2022). Patients reported positive experiences with clinicians who were nonjudgmental and compassionate, validated their experience, and focused on the whole person and not just specific injuries. In addition, the health care system provided access to effective resources and referrals and delivered timely and private care (Duchesne et al., 2022). Patients also identified factors contributing to a negative experience, such as clinicians who minimized patients' concerns; seemed unconcerned, judgmental, or blaming; were uncomfortable with IPV; and lacked knowledge or experience with IPV. Ways in which health care systems have failed to adequately support patients included lacking adequate referrals or services, making the patient feel hopeless, and allowing the partner engaging in IPV to stay in the exam room (Duchesne et al., 2022). In negative encounters, patients experienced long wait times and felt belittled or stereotyped. Negative experiences related to system- and clinician-level factors can lead to avoidance and distrust of the health care system, as illustrated in Figure 5-2. These effects can drive patients experiencing IPV away from the health care settings that could help them. Alternatively, factors related to positive experiences can improve engagement with the health care system.

Experiences of Clinicians

Health care professionals in emergency departments have identified positive and negative factors associated with providing high-quality care for people experiencing IPV. Positive factors include being knowledgeable and well-equipped to care for patients experiencing IPV, having supportive policies and protocols, providing adequate time and private clinical space, and collaborating with a trained interdisciplinary team (Duchesne et al., 2022). Negative factors reported by clinicians included reluctance to address the

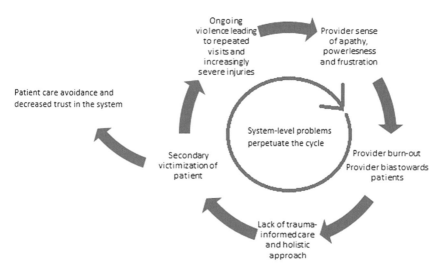

FIGURE 5-2 Health care cycle leading to avoidance and distrust by patients seeking care for intimate partner violence.
NOTE: Patients seeking care for IPV may encounter negative experiences in the health care system related to multiple system-level and health care provider–level factors.
SOURCE: Duchesne et al. (2022).

complexity of IPV in the context of acute care; beliefs that IPV was a social not medical issue and outside their scope; frustration and powerlessness when patients returned to violent environments; lack of training, infrastructure, and support services; working in under-resourced environments; and personal stereotypes and biases about IPV. Many of these issues were also described in studies of barriers to effective IPV interventions in other settings (Rivas et al., 2019).

Patient Preferences in Intimate Partner Violence Care

Studies with women who have experienced IPV indicate that most want clinicians to talk to them about IPV in a safe and private setting, to discuss the possibility of IPV exposure without pushing for disclosure, and to offer tangible medical and social resources for support (Chang et al., 2005; Feder et al., 2006). Patients may not connect the symptoms they are experiencing, such as recurrent headaches, pain, heart palpitations, and insomnia, to stressors associated with IPV. Printed information about linkages between challenging relationships and personal health and information about available supports can be helpful for patients and can help build trust with the practitioner and practice (Miller et al., 2017).

A meta-synthesis of qualitative data focused on women's experiences and expectations of disclosing IPV experiences to a clinician highlighted the importance of delivering woman-centered care (Tarzia et al., 2020). The authors reviewed 31 manuscripts and identified four critical areas related to women's expectations of health care professionals after disclosing IPV. These included emotional connection through kindness and care, recognition and understanding of women's experiences, action and advocacy (doing more than listening), and giving women choice and control in making their own decisions. Similarly, a study of people who have experienced IPV asked what they wanted from professionals in a helping role. Study participants identified three key characteristics: preserving respect for autonomy, offering support and information about existing resources (regardless of disclosure), and not pushing for disclosure (Chang et al., 2005).

Community-Based Care Settings

Community-based services play an important role in addressing IPV. Many IPV-related health care services are provided outside health care systems (e.g., hospitals, clinics, and primary care). In some cases, people experiencing IPV may be referred to community-based care from the health care system. In other cases, these community-based settings may be the first site of care. Additionally, community-based services can provide the primary response to IPV for individuals who do not access health care or do not disclose their experiences to clinicians. Examples of such community-based services include:

- Advocacy programs, which help people experiencing IPV navigate the legal system or access supports such as housing, education, counseling, financial planning, and job placement (Shorey et al., 2014). Advocacy programs may be community-based organizations or may be housed in domestic violence shelters or law schools.
- Criminal justice system, including police and legal offices, enables people experiencing IPV to obtain civil protection orders (Shorey et al., 2014). Some police departments have programs in which individuals with expertise in domestic violence accompany officers on calls of reported IPV to provide crisis intervention and referrals to support services (Shorey et al., 2014).
- Housing programs, which can include crisis violence shelters (also referred to as safe houses), transitional supportive housing, and permanent housing. Shelters, in addition to providing food and a place to live, may also offer counseling, advocacy services, and supports for children of people experiencing IPV, including transportation to and from school and tutoring (Shorey et al., 2014).
- Assistance hotlines, such as the National Domestic Violence Hotline, national and local sexual assault or rape crisis hotlines, the StrongHearts Native Helpline, National Dating Abuse Helpline, and others (NCADV, n.d.).
- Home-based care programs, which are typically associated with home visitation programs for maternal and infant care (Sharps et al., 2016).
- Peer-led support groups (Shorey et al., 2014).

Researchers have examined the effectiveness of community-based approaches for IPV. However, these studies have limitations that make comparison of the effectiveness of different interventions difficult. Individual studies vary in the types of outcomes that are measured, making accurate comparison difficult. Analysis of these studies through the lens of the many challenges associated with conducting IPV intervention research is critical. While inconsistencies in study design make it difficult to determine whether one intervention is more effective than another, it is apparent that community-based interventions play a key role in providing care for women experiencing IPV.

Domestic Violence Advocacy Programs

Many community-based domestic violence advocacy programs serve individuals and families experiencing IPV. These programs often use an empowerment model with a gendered approach by contextualizing IPV within gender oppression (Kasturirangan, 2008). They partner with clients to identify goals, assess risk and engage in safety planning, and connect clients to needed community resources. The resources often include opportunities for individuals experiencing IPV to connect with one another through support groups and other strategies for promoting social support (Kasturirangan, 2008). Offering individuals affected by IPV social support has been found to contribute to improvements in mental health (Ogbe et al., 2020).

Shelters and Housing Programs

Shelters and other housing programs are important for people experiencing IPV. Women who have experienced IPV are at greater risk of experiencing homelessness and housing insecurity than women who have not (Adams et al., 2021; Gilroy et al., 2016; Pavao et al., 2007). Housing insecurity has been linked to worse outcomes with regard to physical safety and mental health (Gilroy ct al., 2016; Rollins et al., 2012). Shelters also allow people experiencing IPV to separate from the person perpetrating the violence.

Critical IPV services are also provided in shelters and other housing programs, spanning emergency, transitional, and permanent housing. Advocacy services are often delivered through IPV shelters and housing programs (Shorey et al., 2014). Although leaders in the field have defined these services as critical in the response to IPV, more studies are needed to evaluate the impact of housing interventions on outcomes for people experiencing IPV (Klein et al., 2021).

Nurse-Family Partnership Home Visit Programs

Nurse–Family Partnership programs are home visitation programs in which nurses provide health promotion interventions for new mothers. This model has positively affected infants and mothers, including showing promise for reducing IPV (Olds and Yost, 2020). Various adaptations of nurse-led interventions delivered at home for mothers, including the Domestic Violence Enhanced Home Visitation Program, have demonstrated promise for improving identification and intervention for mothers experiencing IPV and reducing IPV over time (Burnett et al., 2021; Sharps et al., 2016).

School- and College-Based Health Centers

An estimated 6.3 million students have received services from a school-based health center (SBHC), most of which are located in underserved, low-resource neighborhoods (Love et al., 2019). Features of these centers include access to services for students without health insurance, confidential psychosocial assessments occur routinely, and students can connect with other students through peer-to-peer outreach (Britto et al., 2001; Clayton et al., 2010; Gibson et al., 2013; Juszczak et al., 2003). Adolescent relationship abuse is prevalent among youth seeking care in SBHCs (Miller et al., 2015). IPV is not uncommon among women attending college (Coker et al., 2016; Sutherland et al., 2021). Many of these women seek care at college health and counseling centers (Grace et al., 2023). College health and counseling centers are also helpful as a confidential setting for offering preventive services and connecting survivors to supports and safety.

Federally Supported Care Settings

Several federal programs have been established to meet the needs of under-resourced communities. These include Federally Qualified Health Centers and centers for family planning and reproductive health supported by Title X provisions.

Federally Qualified Health Centers

Federally Qualified Health Centers (FQHCs) are critical sites in the health care safety net. Typically, FQHCs serve medically underserved areas or populations and offer services on a sliding scale to individuals who have low incomes or are uninsured (HRSA, 2023b). In 2022, 66 percent of patients seen at HRSA health centers had incomes at or below the federal poverty level, and 18 percent were uninsured (HRSA, 2023b). FQHCs offer a range of primary health care services to adults and children, referrals to specialty care, and support services such as health education, translation, and transportation that address the social determinants of health. Many FQHCs provide dental care, mental health services, and substance use services. Services may be provided for free or on a sliding scale basis. HRSA requires that FQHCs be governed by a board of directors that includes community members. HRSA's strategy for addressing IPV identifies four priorities for staff and its network of clinics:

- Train the health care and public health workforce to address IPV at community and health-system levels;

- Develop partnerships to raise awareness about IPV within HRSA and the U.S. Department of Health and Human Services (HHS);
- Increase access to high-quality IPV-informed health care services across all populations; and
- Address gaps in knowledge about IPV risks, impacts, and interventions (HRSA, 2023a).

Additionally, one of HRSA's National Training and Technical Assistance Partners, Health Partners on IPV and Exploitation, offers training to health centers about addressing IPV.[4] The training addresses providing trauma-informed services, developing partnerships, policy development, IPV prevention and identification, and referral to support services. Training is also available about IPV among specific populations, including adolescents, pregnant people, victims of human trafficking, and unhoused individuals.

Title X Network of Clinicians

Title X[5] is the federal program administered by the Office of Population Affairs (OPA) that supports the delivery of family planning and related health services to individuals with low incomes. The program is implemented through grants awarded to various organizations, including health departments, family planning clinics, community health centers, and nonprofit agencies, which award subgrants to family planning clinics and other entities that offer family planning services for free or on a sliding scale. In 2021, Title X funds supported more than 3,000 service sites across the United States (Fowler et al., 2022).

Title X–funded clinics serve a diverse population and include many historically underserved communities. Nationally in 2021, 85 percent (1,419,731) of the program's family planning clients were female, 65 percent (1,080,935) had incomes below the poverty level, over one-third (36 percent; 594,416) were uninsured, and 15 percent (255,554) were under 20 years of age. In 2021, more than half (58 percent; 958,762) of clients were White, 25 percent (418,397) were Black, 2 percent (30,637) were Asian, 1 percent (19,349) were American Indian/Alaska Native, and 1 percent (13,195) were Native Hawaiian or Pacific Islander. In addition, 38 percent (626,784) were Hispanic or Latino (OASH, 2022).

The tenets of the Title X program include maintaining confidentiality, advancing equity, and delivering client-centered and trauma-informed care (HHS, 2021). These tenets are consistent with key characteristics of quality IPV-related care. In addition to funding the delivery of family planning

---

[4] https://healthpartnersipve.org/ (accessed August 28, 2023).
[5] *Title X* of the *Public Health Service Act* 42 USC § 300 to 300a-6.

services, the OPA and the Centers for Disease Control and Prevention (CDC) developed the Quality Family Planning Services Recommendations, which provide clinical recommendations for family planning and related services (Gavin et al., 2017). The guidelines specifically recommend that clinicians consider the impact of IPV on contraceptive use, access, and needs (Gavin et al., 2017). Oral contraceptives are the most commonly used reversible contraceptive among women in the United States, and extended supply has been associated with higher continuation rates and lower rates of unintended pregnancy (Judge-Golden et al., 2019; White and Westhoff, 2011).

Staff at family planning clinics often have extensive experience caring for people who have experienced IPV, particularly sexual violence and reproductive coercion. Title X family planning clinics provide a range of essential health care services related to IPV, including FDA-approved contraceptive methods and contraceptive counseling; cervical cancer screening; testing, referrals, and prevention education for STIs and HIV; and diagnosis, counseling, and referrals for pregnancy (Fowler et al., 2022). Smith and colleagues conducted a scoping review and analysis of data from the Colorado Family Planning Initiative (CFPI) and the Colorado National Violent Deaths Reporting System from 2009–2015 (Smith et al., 2023). This analysis demonstrated promising findings for a family planning centered approach to reducing the rates of intimate partner homicide related to unplanned pregnancy (Smith et al., 2023). From 2009 to 2015, the CFPI provided 36,762 long-acting reversible contraceptives (LARCs) to women. LARCs are discrete, tamper resistant, and usable without coordination from other partners. Smith and colleagues (2023) found that, over the same time period, intimate partner homicide in Colorado had a net decline as compared with the 5 years prior to LARC distribution (Smith et al., 2023).

EXISTING AND PROMISING MODELS FOR INTIMATE PARTNER VIOLENCE CARE

Telehealth and Digital Interventions

Telehealth describes health care services delivered using communication technology to supplement or replace in-person visits. These technologies most often include telephone, e-mail, or video, which can be synchronous (i.e., occur at the same time for all participants) or asynchronous (i.e., occur at different times). While telehealth has been well integrated into various health care practices, its use expanded greatly during the COVID-19 pandemic (Acharya et al., 2023; McBain et al., 2023; Uscher-Pines et al., 2023). This increase in telehealth use was also demonstrated for IPV services (Krishnamurti et al., 2021).

Telehealth can have a role in providing IPV care when privacy and safety are assured. A recent systematic review of trials comparing interventions for IPV services using telehealth versus usual care showed similar outcomes for each group. The systematic review included 2,663 women in six randomized controlled trials (RCTs) and one nonrandomized trial investigating telehealth strategies for delivery of women's health and IPV care in the United States (Cantor et al., 2023). The trials enrolled women with positive responses to IPV screening questions or recent IPV experiences (Ford-Gilboe et al., 2020; Gilbert et al., 2015; Glass et al., 2017; Hegarty et al., 2019; Koziol-McLain et al., 2018; McFarlane et al., 2004; Saftlas et al., 2014). Telehealth interventions varied across trials and included personalized online tools, interactive websites, or telephone-based support to supplement or replace in-person care for IPV (Ford-Gilboe et al., 2020; Gilbert et al., 2015; Glass et al., 2017; Hegarty et al., 2019; Koziol-McLain et al., 2018; McFarlane et al., 2004; Saftlas et al., 2014). The outcomes also varied across trials. Compared with usual care, telehealth interventions for IPV services resulted in similar rates of repeat IPV, symptoms of depression, fear of partner, coercive control, self-efficacy, post-traumatic stress disorder, and safety behaviors in studies assessing these outcomes (Cantor et al., 2023). The studies did not adequately evaluate potential harms, but they did note barriers to telehealth including limited internet access, digital literacy, technical challenges, and confidentiality concerns (Cantor et al., 2023). Given the small body of studies in this area, more research is needed to understand access barriers and safety concerns among women experiencing IPV when accessing telehealth medical services.

Futures Without Violence offers a guide for community health centers and advocacy programs about how to best prepare for a telehealth visit while keeping the continuity of care for people who have or are experiencing IPV.[6] The guidance highlights preparing a script to integrate information about IPV throughout the call, prioritizing confidentiality, offering universal education, and offering encouragement as key factors to incorporate during a visit (Futures Without Violence, n.d.). Telehealth visits may not always be a safe place to discuss IPV as others may be in the same room or able to hear the conversation. Futures Without Violence offers some suggested language to help navigate conversations and ensure safety for the patient (Futures Without Violence, n.d.).

---

[6] https://healthpartnersipve.org/telehealth-covid-19-intimate-partner-violence-and-human-trafficking/ (accessed August 25, 2023).

App-Based Interventions for Identifying Risk and Connecting to Resources

App-based interventions are emerging as an important strategy for addressing IPV. A longitudinal study of an app-based screening and safety planning program, MyPlan, found it to be effective for improving safety behaviors and reducing IPV among young adults over time (Glass et al., 2022). During the COVID-19 pandemic, when individuals needed to shelter in place, an app-based intervention that screened for IPV and provided support services appeared to show promise (Krishnamurti et al., 2021).

Programs in Primary Care Settings

Health Care Can Change From Within is a systems-change intervention aimed at improving the identification of women experiencing IPV and caring for their health and well-being (Hamberger et al., 2014). Results of an 18-month longitudinal study of the intervention among women patients seeking care in four different Midwestern primary care clinics showed that the intervention increased IPV inquiry, discussion, and disclosure compared with usual care. Women in intervention clinics made fewer doctor visits and received more prescriptions over time. Notably, researchers did not observe between group differences in levels of physical abuse, psychological abuse, use of safety behaviors, connection to the community, patient-reported satisfaction, or quality of health. However, over the course of the study, both the intervention and usual care groups showed a significant increase in safety behaviors and were less likely to experience severe physical or minor violence, suggesting that participating in the research may have affected both groups (Hamberger et al., 2014).

Multisector Partnerships and Coordinated Community Responses

Multisector partnerships are vital for addressing major public health problems and are relevant for addressing IPV. Multisector partnerships with a clear purpose and structures that support coordination, information sharing, and evaluation have been found to be central to effective public health efforts (Wiggins et al., 2021).

Several multisector models that address IPV appear promising. There are indications that this approach fosters survivorship and growth among people experiencing IPV (Gwinn et al., 2007; Hellman et al., 2021). These vary from local to statewide efforts and are intended to improve the coordination of needed services for individuals and families affected by IPV. Often referred to as Coordinated Community Responses (CCRs), these include the critical role of advocates who ensure that clients have access to a wide range of services, such as advocacy, shelter, and legal protection (Shorey et al., 2014). Although there is no standard protocol for CCRs, they typically involve a coordinating council with representatives from across sectors and services that form relationships among one another and can identify and fill in service gaps (Shorey et al., 2014). Similarly, statewide initiatives, such as Project Catalyst, have engaged leaders from primary care, public health, and domestic violence coalitions and have demonstrated improved collaboration between health centers and domestic violence agencies (Brown et al., 2023).[7]

Domestic Violence and Health Care Partnership

The Domestic Violence and Health Care Partnership initiative, sponsored by Blue Shield of CA Foundation and Futures Without Violence, offers a model for collaboration between community health care centers (including FQHCs) and victim service agencies.[8] The demonstration project focused on strategies for improving the health care delivery system's capacity to collaborate with victim service agencies to address IPV. This included formal referral processes for patients identified in health care settings to rapidly connect with advocacy services and for survivors seeking care in advocacy agencies to receive health care expeditiously (Miller-Walfish et al., 2021).

Integrating Intimate Partner Violence Care into HIV Clinics

Integrating IPV screening, care, and delivery services into HIV clinics can facilitate reductions in repeat or co-occurring victimization (Marshall et al., 2018). Recognizing the critical need for integrated IPV–HIV services, in 2012 the White House established an Interagency Federal Working Group to address issues involving the intersection of IPV and HIV prevention and care (White House, 2013). One of the working group's tasks was to coordinate government agency efforts to integrate sexual and reproductive health services with gender-based violence services and HIV/AIDS services (White House, 2013).

Currently, few states have guidelines for integrating IPV screening into HIV prevention and care. Published guidelines set forth by the New York State Department of Health indicate that domestic violence risk assessment is a standard of care. This guidance notes that "domestic violence as a standard of care" means that discussing domestic violence is encouraged

---

[7] https://www.futureswithoutviolence.org/health-2/project-catalyst/ (accessed August 28, 2023).

[8] https://blueshieldcafoundation.org/grants/legacy-projects/domestic-violence-health-care-partnerships-0 (accessed August 28, 2023).

during pretest counseling for HIV and domestic violence risk assessment is required during post-test counseling of HIV-infected individuals (NYSDOH, 2013). However, the extent to which these guidelines have been implemented or evaluated is unknown.

The Women's HIV Program at the University of California, San Francisco is one of the few HIV clinics that provide integrated IPV–HIV care guided by trauma-informed care principles identified by the Center for Health Care Strategies (Center for Health Care Strategies, 2018; Dawson-Rose et al., 2019). The delivery of trauma-informed care includes the below core components:

- A foundation based in trauma-informed principles and a team approach,
- An empowering environment that supports a sense of calm and safety,
- Education about the health effects of current and past trauma, and
- Inquiry about and response to recent and prior trauma that integrates on-site or community-based resources and care (Machtinger et al., 2019).

Patients in the Women's HIV Program receive universal education about healthy and unhealthy relationships, how IPV affects health, and resources such as a safety card created by Futures Without Violence. Patients who disclose being in an abusive relationship are immediately seen by a clinic social worker who can create a safety plan and connect them with IPV resources as needed. Researchers are still collecting and analyzing data to determine the outcomes of this unique care model.

Some of the limited intervention efforts that have taken place to date have provided domestic violence advocates with HIV prevention knowledge to facilitate prevention and care for women with experiences of IPV. An example of one such effort was a small pilot study of a group-based two-session HIV prevention education intervention for domestic violence advocates conducted in Mississippi (Willie et al., 2022). Key components of the intervention included education on the IPV–HIV relationship, HIV prevention for IPV survivors (e.g., pre-exposure prophylaxis [PrEP]), the barriers that women with experiences of IPV face, and the benefits of PrEP for women with experiences of IPV (Willie et al., 2022). Compared with pre-intervention, investigators found improvements both immediately and at 3 months post-intervention in advocates' knowledge about PrEP and reported self-efficacy for several HIV prevention and information-sharing behaviors all increased (Willie et al., 2022). However, due to high staff turnover, while the pilot began with 25 participants, only 9 were retained by the 3-month post-intervention point.

Veterans Administration Intimate Partner Violence Program

The Veterans Health Administration (VHA) began formally encouraging IPV screening in Veterans Affairs (VA) medical centers in 2014 and issued a national directive calling for routine IPV screening and provision of interventions throughout VHA facilities in 2019 (Miller et al., 2022; Rossi et al., 2020). The VA's Intimate Partner Violence Assistance Program (IPVAP), which began in 2014, provides comprehensive, trauma-informed, recovery-oriented services to veterans, their intimate partners, and VA staff experiencing IPV (Iverson et al., 2022; Rossi et al., 2020). Connecting all individuals who screen positive for IPV in VHA facilities with interventions and supports is a key component of IPVAP (Iverson et al., 2022; Rossi et al., 2020).

All women veterans seeking health services in a VA center are asked about IPV using the five item Extended-Hurt/Insult/Threaten/Scream (E-HITS) screener along with a sexual violence screening question (Miller et al., 2022). A 2022 study analyzing VHA administrative data from 2014 to 2020 investigated the reach of the program and the prevalence of positive screens among women ages 18–44 (Miller et al., 2022). The analysis found that the deployment of IPVAP was associated with a steady increase in the number of women screened for IPV in VHA primary care settings (Miller et al., 2022). The analysis also found that the average percentage of women aged 18–44 who screened positive was 8.1 percent (Miller et al., 2022).

Each VA facility and most units within large VA facilities have an IPV Assistance Program Coordinator (referred to as an IPV Champion)—a staff member assigned to make sure staff are trained in the use of the protocol, help clinicians with particularly challenging cases, and compile reports of screening (Adjognon et al., 2021; Iverson et al., 2019, 2022). At early adoption sites, these IPV Champions were integral in implementing the IPVAP, particularly the screening component (Adjognon et al., 2021; Iverson et al., 2019). In addition to training and supporting staff, IPV Champions develop relationships with community-based organizations, which develops the resources available for veterans experiencing IPV (Adjognon et al., 2021). They also collaborate with their counterparts across the VA to develop clinical guidelines and adapt risk assessment and management processes for diverse populations, including groups minoritized by race, ethnicity, lesbian, gay, bisexual, transgender, or queer status, and immigration status (Adjognon et al., 2021). Studies investigating implementation of IPVAP across VA facilities have highlighted the IPV Champion as a key factor in its success (Adjognon et al., 2021; Rossi et al., 2020).

Recovering from IPV through Strengths and Empowerment (RISE) is an evidence-based, trauma-informed, person-centered, brief psychosocial counseling intervention for people experiencing IPV that has been piloted at several VHA facilities (Iverson et al., 2022). RISE focuses on understanding individuals' values and supporting them in improving their general self-efficacy and personal empowerment. It is designed to maximize flexibility, choice, and autonomy to better meet both patient and clinician needs (Iverson et al., 2022). Modules in the intervention include safety planning, education about the warning signs of IPV and its adverse health effects, coping and self-care skills, building social support, improving decision-making skills, and connecting to resources (Iverson et al., 2022). Evaluations of the pilot program in the literature have had promising findings. A 2022 analysis of data from a cohort of 45 patients who participated in the pilot program found a statistically significant decrease in depressive symptoms and high participant satisfaction scores (Iverson et al., 2022). A randomized clinical trial investigated outcomes of RISE versus "enhanced care as usual" among 59 women recruited from an urban VHA hospital (Iverson et al., 2021). Women who participated in RISE had greater increases in empowerment and self-efficacy than those who received enhanced care as usual (Iverson et al., 2021).

Care Models for Intimate Partner Violence in the Perinatal Period

Women experiencing IPV in the perinatal period require many of the essential health care services related to IPV. Women experiencing perinatal IPV need additional obstetric care and specialty medical care to address the multiple adverse health effects of experiencing IPV in the perinatal period. Some adverse health effects associated with perinatal IPV are life threatening, such as preeclampsia, and require emergency medical services. These women also need treatment for traumatic physical injuries due to IPV. Women experiencing IPV in the perinatal period also require mental health care to address the psychological effects of perinatal IPV. Referrals to treatments, interventions, and additional resources are imperative during the perinatal period, as people are most likely to adopt interventions when receiving perinatal care as compared with other care contexts (Hahn et al., 2018).

Perinatal home visit programs using interventions focused on Dutton's empowerment model have shown promising results in decreasing the incidence of IPV. One example is the Domestic Violence Enhanced Home Visitation Program (DOVE) (Sharps et al., 2016). The DOVE program is a brochure-based intervention developed to be integrated and implemented within existing home visit programs. Nurses or community health workers are trained to use the DOVE brochure to share information and resources about IPV during their home visits and can modify this intervention to meet the individual woman's needs. The DOVE brochure includes educational information about the cycle of violence; the Danger Assessment, which assesses the woman's risk for intimate partner homicide; options available to the woman; safety planning information that is consistent with the context and level of danger; community-specific IPV resources; and national hotline information (Sharps et al., 2016). A pragmatic trial of the DOVE intervention found that participants in the group that received the DOVE intervention experienced a greater decrease in IPV than those that did not receive the DOVE intervention (Sharps et al., 2016). The greater reduction in IPV was sustained at 2 years postpartum, despite the intervention ending 3 months postpartum (Sharps et al., 2016). Prior research on home visit programs found that the nurses and community health workers felt underprepared to assist a woman if she disclosed that she was experiencing IPV (Dyer and Abildsco, 2019). Programs such as DOVE offer needed guidance for those conducting home visits, providing them with resources for supporting the pregnant or postpartum person experiencing IPV.

Existing Intimate Partner Violence Prevention Guidance and Strategies

CDC developed evidence-based prevention strategies with the greatest potential to prevent IPV for communities and states (Table 5-2) (Niolon et al., 2017). These include strategies for teaching safe and healthy relationship skills and engaging influential adults and peers in IPV education and prevention programs. Strategies for disrupting the developmental pathway toward IPV include early childhood programs, parenting programs, and

TABLE 5-2 CDC IPV Prevention Strategies

Risk or Protective Factors*	Strategy	Approach
• Cultural norms that support aggression toward others • Anger, hostility, and other antisocial behavior • Lack of nonviolent social problem-solving skills • Traditional gender norms and gender inequality	Teach safe and healthy relationship skills	• Social–emotional learning programs for youth • Healthy relationship programs for couples
	Engage influential adults and peers	• Men and boys as allies in prevention • Bystander empowerment and education • Family-based programs

TABLE 5-2 Continued

Risk or Protective Factors*	Strategy	Approach
• Low self-esteem • Depression and suicide attempts • Aggressive or delinquent behavior as a youth • Heavy alcohol and drug use • History of physical and emotional abuse in childhood	Disrupt the developmental pathway toward partner violence	• Early childhood home visitation • Preschool enrichment with family engagement • Parenting skills and family relationship programs • Treatment for at-risk children, youth, and families
• Strong social support networks and stable, positive relationships with others • Neighborhood collective efficacy • Coordination of resources and services among community agencies • High rates of violence and crime • Easy access to drugs and alcohol • Weak community sanctions against IPV • Weak health, educational, economic, and social policies or laws	Create protective environments	• Improve school climate and safety • Improve organizational policies and workplace climate • Modify the physical and social environments of neighborhoods
• Low education or income • Societal income inequality	Strengthen economic supports for families	• Strengthen household financial security • Strengthen work–family supports
• Communities with access to medical care and mental health services • Communities with access to economic and financial help • Communities with access to safe, stable housing	Support survivors to increase safety and lessen harms	• Victim-centered services • Housing programs • First responder and civil legal protections • Patient-centered approaches • Treatment and support for survivors of IPV

*Risk and protective factors may apply to multiple strategies.
SOURCE: Niolon et al. (2017).

treatment for at-risk children, youth, and families. Strategies for creating protective environments, including schools, work, and neighborhoods, could reduce IPV risk related to established risk factors. Services for supporting survivors that increase safety and reduce harm provide an additional secondary prevention strategy. Together, these strategies provide a comprehensive plan for IPV prevention that particularly targets prevention at the community level.

Promoting Healthy Families and Communities

Primary prevention of IPV is crucial for preventing IPV and its consequences across the lifespan and for promoting healthy families and communities. One of the key ways to accomplish this is by promoting healthy, respectful, and nonviolent relationships. Initiatives in this area include social–emotional learning programs for youth and programs that focus on forming healthy couple relationships before violence occurs. Safe Dates is a school-based program designed to promote healthy relationships that in a randomized controlled trial (RCT) was found to reduce the likelihood of engaging in teen dating violence among participants without a history of engaging in abuse and prevent teen relationship violence (Foshee et al., 2004). Expect Respect Support Groups is another evidence-based intervention designed for teens who are at high risk for teen relationship violence and have a history of exposure to violence (Reidy et al., 2017). A study of the program in 36 Texas high schools found that among boys, participation in the program was associated with a decrease in psychological and sexual teen dating violence (Reidy et al., 2017). Healthy relationship programs for couples, such as the Prevention and Relationship Enhancement Program, can be helpful for addressing factors such as relationship satisfaction and anger management among adult couples and have shown evidence of preventing later-life IPV (Anderson et al., 2013; Braithwaite and Fincham, 2014; Markman et al., 1993).

There are several promising programs targeted at bystander education. One example is Coaching Boys Into Men, a program that trained high school coaches to educate their male athletes in grades 9–12 in healthy relationship skills (Miller et al., 2013). A cluster-randomized controlled trial of 2,006 student athletes at 16 California schools found that athletes who received the coach-led education reported they were less likely to laugh at or go along with peers' abusive behaviors. However, the study did not find a difference between the intervention and control group for intention to intervene in observed IPV, recognition of abusive behaviors, or gender-equitable attitudes (Miller et al., 2013). Bystander programs among college students, such as Bring in the Bystander and the Green Dot program, aim to educate and empower college students to engage in reactive and proactive responses to IPV and to reduce the likelihood of assault (Coker et al.,

2015; Moynihan et al., 2015). Analyses of the outcomes of these programs have found mixed results, particularly in long-term follow ups. However, lessons learned through studies of these programs represent an opportunity for future intervention development.

Results from research conducted outside the United States have had promising findings regarding the effect of interventions at the community level that focus on addressing the effect of gender inequities on IPV prevalence. For example, the SASA! Study, an RCT conducted in Uganda that investigated a multilevel community intervention designed to prevent violence against women and reduce HIV risk, found that after 3 years of intervention programming, women in participating communities were less likely to report experiencing physical IPV in the past year (Abramsky et al., 2016).

Healing-Centered Engagement

Healing-centered engagement (HCE) is a holistic approach that emphasizes the importance of culture to well-being and integrates empowering the individual that has experienced trauma to understand their strengths and take an active role in their healing with an understanding of healing as a collective experience (Gupta, 2021). HCE approaches have shown promise in studies of application of the intervention with youth and adults from minoritized populations (Condon et al., 2022; Maleku, et al., 2022; Pearce et al., 2019). Clinicians and other frontline health workers could benefit from learning about a community's history, its collective trauma experiences, and how to use strengths-based approaches to encourage patients and clients to problem solve together. A healing-centered approach that focuses on universal education shifts away from an overemphasis on disclosure to building a trusting relationship with the patient that is compassionate, relational, and centers the autonomy and strengths of patients.

Universal Prevention and Harm Reduction Education

Universal prevention and harm reduction education related to IPV during clinical encounters shifts the emphasis away from eliciting a disclosure and mitigates against the assumption that a "no" response to a screening question about abuse means the patient has not experienced or is not currently experiencing violent or controlling behaviors. This approach has been evaluated in reproductive, college, and adolescent health settings and has been shown to increase patients' knowledge of resources and strategies for harm reduction and to reduce reproductive coercion and abuse victimization among adolescent and young adult women (Miller et al., 2011, 2015, 2016, 2020).

Firearm Violence Prevention

Women are more likely to be shot and killed by a male intimate partner than they are to be killed by a stranger (Sorenson, 2017; Sorenson and Schut, 2018). A 2020 meta-analysis of results from 17 studies investigating risk factors for intimate partner homicide found that the greatest risk factor for women to experience intimate partner homicide was the person engaging in IPV having direct access to a firearm (Spencer and Stith, 2020). Extreme-risk protection orders, also known as *red flag laws*, may provide an avenue for health professionals to intervene in situations where they determine that an individual poses a significant risk of IPV-related gun violence. In Maryland,[9] Colorado,[10] Hawaii,[11] Michigan,[12] and New York,[13] as well as the District of Columbia,[14] a medical, mental health, or other health professional may initiate a court petition that could ultimately authorize law enforcement officials to temporarily remove firearms from a person who poses a significant danger of firearm violence to themselves or others.[15] Requirements governing who is qualified to file a petition vary by state. For example, to initiate a petition in Maryland, the clinician must have examined the individual who poses a threat.[16] To initiate a petition in Colorado, the clinician must have examined either the individual who poses a threat or that individual's child within 6 months. In the District of Columbia, any mental health professional who is in a position to state facts in support of the risk assessment may initiate a petition.[17] In several other states, health professionals are ineligible to file a petition but may advise patients of their right to do so.

Preventing Intimate Partner Violence Among Adolescents

Efficacious, easily implementable, and scalable interventions for preventing adolescent relationship abuse are essential for promoting adolescent health and wellness (Piolanti and Foran, 2022). Core components of evidence-based and research-informed IPV prevention programs for adolescents include gender equity transformative programming, adult social supports and mentoring, parent–adolescent communication, promoting social norms to protect against violence, bystander interventions, and creating

---

[9] Maryland Code Ann. Pub. Safety § 5-601(e).
[10] Colorado Revised Statutes, title 13, article 14.5.
[11] Hawaii Revised Statutes §134-67.
[12] Michigan Public Act 38 of 2023.
[13] New York Civil Practice Law and Rules article 63-a § 6340-6348.
[14] District of Columbia Code § 7-2510.
[15] List of states and laws current as of August 2023.
[16] Maryland Code Ann. Pub. Safety § 5-601(e).
[17] District of Columbia Code § 7-2510.

protective environments (Finnie et al., 2022; Niolon et al., 2019). Several interventions and strategies have demonstrated positive effects, including family-, community-, and school-based prevention programs (Basile et al., 2016; Niolon et al., 2019). Open parent–adolescent communication is associated with less exposure to and use of adolescent relationship abuse (Kast et al., 2016; Ombayo et al., 2019). School- and clinic-based education and assessment programs can increase youth recognition of abusive behaviors (Finnie et al., 2022; Foshee et al., 2004). The School Health Center Healthy Adolescent Relationships Program (SHARP) is a provider-delivered, brief universal education and counseling intervention created to be used with all students seeking care in school-based health centers (Miller et al., 2015). The intervention was designed to be inclusive of all gender and sexual identities and clinic visit types, and it addresses a range of adolescent relationship abuse, including cyber dating abuse and reproductive coercion (Miller et al., 2015). A study of 939 students aged 14–19 found that those who received the SHARP intervention and filled out surveys 3 months after a clinic visit demonstrated greater recognition of sexual coercion and reduced victimization (Miller et al., 2015).

ADDRESSING HEALTH DISPARITIES AND BARRIERS SPECIFIC TO PEOPLE EXPERIENCING INTIMATE PARTNER VIOLENCE

Individual-Level Barriers

Individual-level barriers—sociodemographic characteristics that intersect culture and behavior—affect the delivery of essential services for IPV. Women in some communities are often pressured to maintain the privacy of IPV experiences to avoid community shame and adhere to traditional gender norms. This barrier is compounded by insufficient accessibility of IPV resources within those communities (Schmidt et al., 2023). Nuanced cultural differences within racial and ethnic groups (e.g., African American and Caribbean Black women) can hinder access to IPV services. Women who are immigrants or refugees often express confidentiality concerns related to inadequate access to linguistically appropriate services (Guruge and Humphreys, 2009). Women who are immigrants also experience confusion over their legal rights, social isolation, and disparities in economic and social resources (between a woman and her partner), further impeding IPV service use (Stockman et al., 2015). Intersecting racial, ethnic, and gender stereotypes (e.g., the strong Black woman) contribute to decreased use of formal essential services (Bent-Goodley, 2007; Monterrosa, 2021). Cultural stigmas or ideologies that delegitimize experiences of IPV and that promote acceptance of violence as a norm combined with various stereotypes collectively reduce the uptake of services (Overstreet and Quinn, 2013; Stockman et al., 2014).

General feelings of social disconnectedness and hopelessness can also serve as barriers for Black women with IPV experiences who also have had a history of involvement with the legal system (Gutowski et al., 2023). The interaction of behavioral health problems (e.g., substance use) with IPV may create additional barriers to engagement with needed services (Ponce et al., 2014).

Some women experiencing IPV distrust service organizations, the health care system, and the legal system, among other essential services. This is often rooted in intergenerational trauma related to historical events involving abuse and atrocities against certain populations (e.g., forced sterilization among American Indian/Alaska Native women) and discriminatory practices embedded in services and service delivery (Robinson et al., 2021; Stockman et al., 2015). In general, a less representative physician workforce can reduce patient trust in the medical system and in their personal physician. This, in turn, may lead to worse health outcomes (Mcintosh-Clarke et al., 2019; Schoenthaler et al, 2014; Snyder et al., 2023). IPV services that are culturally specific or culturally tailored are not broadly available (Guruge and Humphreys, 2009; Kulkarni, 2018). Moreover, access to specialized IPV services is lacking for marginalized women, including those with disabilities (e.g., the deaf community) and women who identify as LBTQ+ (Calton et al., 2016; Mastrocinque et al., 2017). Client/patient–provider communication can also be less than optimal for women, which can create barriers to both disclosure and connection to the essential health care services that match their needs (Stockman et al., 2015).

LBTQ+ women face unique barriers while seeking essential services for IPV. Stigma can present a barrier to disclosure (Ard and Makadon, 2011; Calton et al., 2016; Scheer et al., 2020). In particular, the fear of being outed, or having their identity revealed to others such as family, friends, coworkers, or medical professionals, may pose a strong barrier to disclosure (Ollen et al., 2017; Porsch et al., 2022; Scheer et al., 2023). This stigma is sometimes reinforced via bias from physicians and other resources, which reduces both disclosure and the effectiveness of services (Calton et al., 2016; Guadalupe-Diaz and Jasinski, 2017).

Transgender women also report stigma and discrimination as barriers to disclosing IPV (Gray et al., 2023; Kurdyla et al., 2021). In particular, transgender women have reported experiencing discrimination when seeking access to gendered shelters (Ezie, 2023; James et al., 2016). They are far less likely to report or seek help from help-giving resources, including police officers, hotlines, shelters, or legal support when compared to cisgendered individuals. When reporting or seeking help after an IPV experience, transgender women are far more likely to report to friends, family, or a mental health professional (Kurdyla et al., 2021).

Other individual-level factors may influence access to IPV care. For example, given that animal maltreatment is a strategy that partners engaging in IPV use to control and intimidate their partners, concern for the safety of pets can be a barrier to disclosure and care seeking. Access to shelters that allow women experiencing IPV to bring their pets can reduce this barrier (Campbell and Glass, 2009; Collins et al., 2018). Concern surrounding animal abuse can delay women from entering a shelter. A study conducted in Utah found that 22.8 percent (N=101, n=23) of women who had entered a shelter delayed going due to concern for their pets (Ascione et al., 2007). Some studies have noted that women have left shelters to check on pets or returned to abusive relationships because their pet was still with the partner who engaged in IPV (Barrett et al., 2020). An analysis of data from a Canadian survey of 128 human services professionals and 43 veterinarians and other animal welfare professionals noted that respondents emphasized the need for pet-friendly IPV shelters and long-term housing options (Giesbrecht, 2022). Having a safety plan and alternative resources for housing a pet is an important barrier to be addressed when women are seeking shelter services (Hageman et al., 2018).

Additionally, there is a general lack of availability and accessibility of essential IPV services for women who are homeless or marginally housed, reside in rural geographic or low-income areas, or reside in tribal communities or reservations (Edwards, 2015; Jock et al., 2022; Ponce et al., 2014; Rodriguez et al., 2009). Lack of resources, including transportation and child care, can pose additional challenges to accessing essential IPV services, further contributing to preexisting disparities (Robinson et al., 2021; Wadsworth et al., 2018). IPV care approaches that prioritize women's sense of agency, culture, and mutual respect while acknowledging experiences of cumulative trauma can help reduce their barriers to accessing IPV-related care.

Health Care Deserts

Health care provider maldistribution, in which the distribution of clinicians does not match the health care needs of a geographic area, has led to health care deserts across the United States. These health care deserts have created additional barriers for people experiencing IPV to access needed care.

Primary Care Clinicians

A large body of literature reports that the nation faces a worsening shortage in the availability of primary care clinicians, including physicians and nurses, who are major providers of preventive services, including screening and education for IPV. The challenges and burnout presented by the COVID-19 pandemic have hastened and exacerbated workforce shortages, which have been building for several years.

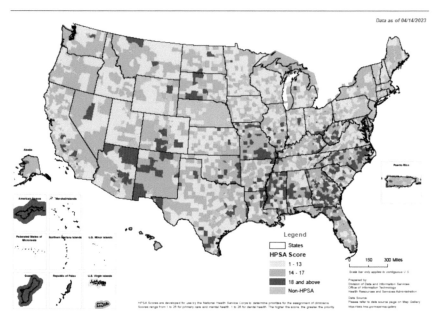

FIGURE 5-3 Health Resources and Services Administration (HRSA) Primary Care Health Professional Shortage Area Map.
SOURCE: HRSA (2023e).

HRSA (2023a) estimates that 100 million people live in a federally designated Health Professional Shortage Area for primary care services, and these gaps are expected to grow (see Figure 5-3). HRSA (2023d) projects that between 2020 and 2035, the supply of primary care physicians will grow by 12 percent, but demand will grow by 16 percent.[18] HRSA projects a 13 percent increase in supply for general internal physicians, short of the expected 24 percent increase in demand[19] between 2020 and 2035 (HRSA, 2023d). The Bureau of Labor Statistics projects approximately 193,100 job openings for registered nurses annually between 2022 and 2032 (BLS, 2023). Clinician shortages are spread unevenly and are particularly pronounced in rural areas, which have had longstanding challenges with provider recruitment and retention as well as with hospital closures.

---

[18] Projection data as of September 13, 2023.
[19] Projection data as of September 13, 2023.

Maternity Care Professionals

The March of Dimes categorizes maternity care deserts as counties that have no hospitals or birth centers offering obstetric care and no obstetricians/gynecologists (OB-GYNs) or certified nurse midwives providing deliveries (Brigance et al., 2022). Their analysis used data from HRSA, the CDC National Center for Health Statistics, and the U.S. Census Bureau (see Figure 5-4). In 2022 approximately one-third (35.6 percent) of counties in the United States were classified as maternity care deserts, and another 11.9 percent were considered to have low access to maternity care (Brigance et al., 2022). As with primary care, shortages in the perinatal workforce are particularly stark in rural communities, especially the most remote areas. More than half of rural counties do not have obstetric services, and more than half of women who live in rural communities must travel at least 30 minutes to reach a hospital that offers obstetric care services (Brigance et al., 2022; Hung et al., 2017). Gaps in maternity care have been associated with increases in emergency department births and preterm births (Kozhimannil et al., 2020; Wallace et al., 2021).

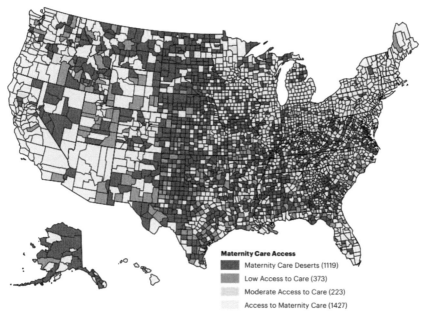

FIGURE 5-4 March of Dimes Maternity Care Deserts by county in the United States. SOURCE: Brigance, C., R. Lucas, E. Jones, A. Davis, M. Oinuma, K. Mishkin, and Z. Henderson. 2022. *Nowhere to Go: Maternity Care Deserts Across the U.S.* (Report No. 3). March of Dimes. https://www. marchofdimes.org/research/maternity-care-deserts-report.aspx (accessed August 25, 2023).

Sexual and Reproductive Health Care Professionals

In some regions there are major shortages and gaps in the availability and distribution of clinicians providing the full range of sexual and reproductive health care. Contraception is a fundamental element of women's health care, and federal law[20] requires full coverage of contraceptives for those with private insurance or Medicaid. Additionally, the federal Title X program, administered by the Office of Population Affairs, provides free and low-cost contraceptives at approximately 3,000 sites across the United States (Fowler et al., 2022). Despite these protections, not all individuals have ready access to the full range of contraceptive options. A study analyzing data from 2019 found that many counties and states in the United States lack a clinic that provides comprehensive contraception services under Title X (Smith et al., 2022). This translates to millions without access to this care (Smith et al., 2022). The rapidly changing regulatory environment in the wake of the Supreme Court ruling in *Dobbs v. Jackson Women's Health Organization*[21] makes it challenging to estimate how many people lack access to comprehensive contraception services under Title X at the time of this report. For women who are uninsured, most of whom are low-income, out-of-pocket costs may make contraception unaffordable. Given that according to an analysis of data from the 2022 KFF Women's Health Survey, 90 percent of female respondents reported using contraception at some point and 76 percent of respondents reported using more than one method over the course of their lifespan, access to the full range of methods is an important aspect of women's control over their family planning and reproductive health (Frederiksen et al., 2022).

In addition to the shortages and uneven distribution of clinicians, there are gaps in the availability of some services. In 2020, a nationally representative survey of OB-GYNs found that just over a quarter (28 percent) work at practices that provide gender-affirming care, including hormone therapy or surgery (Weigel et al., 2021). While the vast majority of OB-GYNs reported that they felt somewhat or very prepared to meet the sexual reproductive health care needs of patients who are lesbian, gay, bisexual, and queer, only about half (56 percent) felt the same about providing care to transgender patients (Weigel et al., 2021). Shortages are particularly stark for abortion services. Abortion care is delivered primarily in outpatient clinics, but there are vast differences in clinic availability across the country. As noted earlier in this report, pregnancy coercion and interference with contraception are associated with unintended pregnancies among women

---

[20] *Patient Protection and Affordable Care Act*, Public Law 118-148, 111th Congress (March 23, 2010).
[21] *Dobbs, State Health Officer of the Mississippi Department of Health et al. v. Jackson Women's Health Organization et al.* 597 US_ (2022).

experiencing IPV. Pregnancy testing and abortion services are essential for those who experience sexual IPV and reproductive coercion (Grace and Anderson, 2018). The June 2022 Supreme Court ruling in *Dobbs v. Jackson Women's Health Organization*[22] overturned the precedents in *Roe v. Wade*[23] and *Planned Parenthood v. Casey.*[24] It eliminated the longstanding federal standards regarding abortion access. As of August 2023, abortion is banned in 15 states (KFF, 2023a). No clinicians offer abortion in these states except for under a minimal set of circumstances (KFF, 2023a). An additional 10 states have gestational limits ranging from 6 to 22 weeks as of August 2023 (KFF, 2023a). Several other states have a variety of regulations such as mandatory waiting periods, restrictions on the use of telehealth, and restrictions on the type of provider that can prescribe the medications used in medication abortion (KFF, 2023b). The lack of abortion availability is widest in the South and Plains states, where many states have banned or imposed gestational limits on abortion.

This lack of abortion access in large swaths of the country poses significant barriers for pregnant people experiencing IPV who are seeking an abortion, particularly people who have low incomes and some communities of color, who, on average, have fewer resources to travel to obtain care (Pleasants et al., 2022; Rader et al, 2022). Many would need to travel out of state to obtain this essential service, which will likely be even more challenging during a PHE (Pleasants et al., 2022; Rader et al., 2022). Those seeking an abortion without a partner's knowledge have even more limited access after the *Dobbs* ruling.

Sexual Assault Nurse Examiners

Sexual Assault Nurse Examiners (SANEs) play an important role in providing care for individuals who have experienced IPV-related sexual assault. SANEs are trained to provide "comprehensive and compassionate specialty care to sexual assault survivors" (Hollender et al., 2023, p. 1). Sexual assault forensic medical examinations may be performed by clinicians who have not been trained to perform these exams (GAO, 2016). However, researchers have found that patients are more likely to accept services offered from SANEs, they report feeling more cared for, and are more likely to be offered pregnancy tests and emergency contraception (Chandramani et al., 2020; Hollender et al., 2023). A nationwide survey of

---

[22] *Dobbs, State Health Officer of the Mississippi Department of Health et al. v. Jackson Women's Health Organization et al.* 597 US_ (2022).

[23] *Jane Roe, et al., Appellants v. Henry Wade* 410 U.S. 113 (1973).

[24] *Planned Parenthood of Southeastern Pennsylvania, et al. v. Casey, Governor of Pennsylvania, et al.* 505 U.S. 833 (1992).

315 advocates from 119 sexual assault crisis centers across 44 states about emergency department preparedness to care for people who experience sexual assault found that the presence of a SANE was associated with an increased likelihood of availability of post-discharge resources (Chalmers et al., 2023). While data on the exact number of SANEs across the United States is limited, several studies conducted at the local and state level have highlighted a shortage of SANEs across the country, particularly in rural areas (GAO, 2016; Mitchell et al., 2022; Miyamoto et al., 2021; Morris et al., 2022; Thiede and Miyamoto, 2021). A 2016 Government Accountability Office (GAO) report noted that state officials from all six of the states included in their research reported that the number of SANEs in their respective states did not meet the need for exams (GAO, 2016). The GAO report said that several state officials offered examples to illustrate the SANE shortage in their respective states. For example, in rural western Colorado, someone who has been sexually assaulted may need to travel over an hour to reach a facility that has a SANE available, and in Nebraska they may need to drive 2 or more hours (GAO, 2016). This shortage represents a serious barrier to care access for women experiencing sexual IPV. The shortage of SANE workers was elevated in March 2022 when President Biden signed the *Supporting Access to Nurse Exams (SANE) Act* into law as part of the *Violence Against Women Reauthorization Act of 2022*[25] with the goal to increase access to SANE care. This law is intended to help address the SANE shortage by providing funding for SANE salaries in rural, tribal, and underserved communities, establish regional training centers, provide additional funding for pediatric SANEs, and provide funding for mobile SANE units (Hanson, 2023).

Mental Health Professionals

Women that experience IPV have substantial needs for mental health care, including behavioral health care such as substance abuse treatment. In 2023, there were 166 million people residing in areas classified as mental health provider shortage areas according to tracking by HRSA (HRSA, 2023c).[26] As illustrated in Figure 5-5, most of the United States has some degree of mental health professional shortage. With few exceptions, large metropolitan areas are less likely to have a shortage than rural areas. HRSA's national-level projections of supply adequacy for

---

[25] *Violence Against Women Reauthorization Act of 2022*, Public Law 117-103 Division W, 117th Congress (March 15, 2022).

[26] The providers included in HRSA's data for mental health providers include adult psychiatrists, addiction counselors, child psychiatrists, marriage and family therapists, mental health counselors, psychiatric nurse practitioners, psychiatric physician assistants, psychologists, school counselors, and social workers.

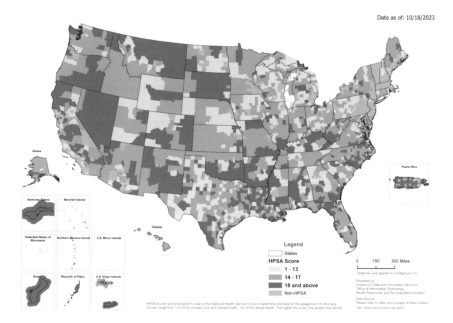

FIGURE 5-5 Health Resources and Services Administration (HRSA) Mental Health Professional Shortage Area Map.
SOURCE: HRSA (2023e).

mental health providers indicate likely shortages by 2035 of many of the professions that care for women who experience IPV, including adult psychiatry, child and adolescent psychiatry, psychologists, addiction counselors, mental health counselors, and under some scenarios, marriage and family therapists (HRSA, 2022). Prior to the COVID-19 pandemic, rural mental health and substance abuse treatment providers had begun efforts to use telehealth to increase access (Uscher-Pines et al., 2020; Vakkalanka et al., 2022). The COVID-19 pandemic and associated policy changes brought about a substantial increase in use of telehealth for mental health and substance abuse treatment. However, barriers associated with the digital divide, including lack of internet access and technological devices needed to access the internet (i.e., smartphones or laptop computers) have perpetuated mental health access barriers for people in both urban and rural settings (Summers-Gabr, 2020). In addition to shortages, a systematic review including 20 studies found that mental health providers lacked in-depth training on IPV and felt underprepared when working with someone who had experienced IPV (Sutton et al., 2021).

Adolescent Care Professionals

Accessibility to comprehensive adolescent care remains a major barrier for youth across the country, especially those who are immigrants, are uninsured, live in a rural area, or live in a neighborhood with a concentrated disadvantage. Even with federal and state insurance coverage for minors, including increases in receipt of care with the Patient Protection and Affordable Care Act (ACA), fewer than half of adolescents in the United States receive well visits (Adams et al., 2019).

POLICY AND REGULATORY CONSIDERATIONS

Referral and Financing

One challenge for providing the entire constellation of services that people experiencing IPV might need is financing and payment, which tends to be siloed between buckets of services. Most women are covered by private insurance or Medicaid, which has broad coverage for many medical care services but limited coverage for abortion services. The federal *Hyde Amendment*[27] blocks certain federal funds from being used to pay for abortion outside of the exceptions for rape, incest, or when the pregnancy is determined to endanger the pregnant person's life. This has resulted in severely limited coverage of abortion under Medicaid and other federal programs, including the Indian Health Service (IHS) and the federal employees' health benefits program (Liu and Shen, 2022). Under private insurance, several states also impose restrictions on the circumstances under which private insurance plans can cover abortion services (Guttmacher Institute, 2023).

Health insurance coverage is also limited for nonmedical support services, such as transportation and housing, which are essential for some people experiencing IPV. Some models may be promising for integrated coverage. The state of North Carolina's Medicaid program is operating the Healthy Opportunities pilot program, which allows for reimbursement of some non-medical services that address specific social needs and are linked to health or health outcomes, including safe housing, transportation, food, and interpersonal safety for state Medicaid enrollees that are considered high need (NCDHHS, n.d.).

---

[27] *Hyde Amendment* Public Law 94-439 § 209 94th Congress, September 30, 1976 (original). Most recently enacted version Public Law 117-103. Div. H, §§ 506–507, 117th Congress, March 15, 2022.

Confidentiality and Privacy Requirements

Privacy and confidentiality requirements present challenges for integrated service models in a steady state context. For example, medical–legal partnerships, which "address the health-harming social and legal needs of patients and communities by integrating the expertise of health care, public health, and legal professionals," face legal impediments to sharing data among members of interprofessional care teams (Mantel and Knake, 2018, p. 184). During a PHE, barriers to data sharing may be exacerbated by the displacement and disruption of access to mechanisms for secure communication. For example, during a hurricane, health care facilities may lose power, and communications systems may be affected (Horahan et al., 2014). At the same time, barriers to data sharing may be eased by orders suspending privacy regulations pursuant to federal or state declarations. During the federally declared PHE for COVID-19 under Section 319 of the *Public Health Services Act*,[28] the HHS Secretary exercised authority to waive sanctions and penalties against covered hospitals for failure to comply with specific provisions of the *Health Insurance Portability and Accountability Act* (HIPAA) Privacy Rule.[29]

Confidentiality and accessibility are critical for adolescent health services. Adolescents are generally amenable to having trusted adults, including parents and caregivers, involved in important health care decisions. However, the ability to seek care confidentially is a well-documented factor that increases the likelihood of an adolescent receiving needed health care, including preventive services and behavioral health treatment (Ford et al., 2004). Although great variability exists in laws governing consent for adolescent patients, some protections exist in all U.S. states for some provision of confidential care, generally in reproductive and sexual health and behavioral health.

Title X Regulations

Title X[30] regulations require participating clinics to provide pregnant clients with non-directive pregnancy options counseling. At the same time, it is prohibited to use Title X funds for the provision of abortion services. The program does allow for the co-location of family planning and abortion services. However, in 2019 regulations were revised to require Title X-funded clinicians to maintain strict physical and financial separation of abortion services. This resulted in a large decline in the network of Title X clinicians and in the number of clients served (Fowler et al., 2022). Those regulations were revoked, but an ongoing legal challenge seeks to reinstate the ban on

---

[28] *Public Health Service Act* 42 USC 247d §319.

[29] *Health Insurance Portability and Accountability Act of 1996 Privacy Rule* 45 CFR Part 160 and Subparts A and E of Part 164.

[30] *Title X of the Public Health Service Act* 42 USC § 300 to 300a-6.

abortion counseling and referral and disqualify family planning sites that provide abortion services (Frederiksen et al., 2021). This ongoing threat could eventually compromise the Title X network of clinicians and reduce access to clinicians with expertise in making family planning services available to people experiencing IPV.

Payment and Insurance Challenges

Access to essential health care services related to IPV depends in part on insurance coverage of those services, availability of in-network clinicians to deliver them, and laws ensuring or restricting access to certain services regardless of insurance coverage or prevailing clinical standards of care. These matters vary by insurance type, service type, and geographic jurisdiction.

Rates of Coverage and Enrollment Challenges

According to a KFF analysis of data from the 2021 American Community Survey, among nonelderly adult women ages 19–64, 60 percent were covered by private employer–sponsored group health plans; private nongroup plans covered 8 percent; 18 percent relied on Medicaid coverage; 3 percent relied on Medicare, military, or other public programs; and 11 percent were uninsured (as of 2021) (KFF, 2023c). This analysis found that coverage patterns were similar among women and teenage girls of reproductive age (15–49). In 2021, 58 percent were covered by employer-sponsored group health plans, one in five were covered by Medicaid (21 percent), and one in ten were uninsured (11 percent) (KFF, 2023c).

Experiencing IPV may qualify an individual to initiate or change type of health insurance, with associated changes in the network of clinicians from whom the individual may seek covered services. Under the ACA,[31] health insurers and self-insuring employers are prohibited from refusing to issue or renew coverage or charging higher premiums based on an applicant's history of conditions arising from experiencing domestic violence, pregnancy, and other health status–related factors.

In March 2020, at the outset of the COVID-19 pandemic, the *Families First Coronavirus Response Act*[32] was enacted into federal law. The law required that states keep people continuously enrolled in the Medicaid program through the end of the COVID-19 PHE in exchange for increased

---

[31] *Patient Protection and Affordable Care Act*, Public Law 118-148, 111th Congress (March 23, 2010).

[32] *Families First Coronavirus Response Act*, Public Law 116-127, 116th Congress (March 18, 2020).

federal funding. Research has found that Medicaid enrollment grew during the PHE partly because of this policy (Benitez and Dubay, 2022; Mandal et al., 2022). With the end of the COVID-19 PHE, many states have restarted administrative verifications of Medicaid eligibility, and many people have already been disenrolled from the program. Given the intense health needs of many people experiencing IPV, maintaining stable coverage is vital for connecting to and receiving health care services. States can employ policies and practices that facilitate access to coverage for people experiencing IPV, such as partnering with IPV service agencies for outreach and streamlining enrollment processes to minimize paperwork requirements (Wagner, 2021).

Restrictive provider networks may limit access to health care services for individuals enrolled in private insurance plans (group or nongroup) and those enrolled in privatized Medicaid managed care plans (which cover the majority of Medicaid recipients) or privatized Medicare plans (GAO, 2022). Health plans establish provider networks through contracts with clinicians and facilities. When enrollees seek care from out-of-network clinicians, their health plan may deny coverage or charge higher out-of-pocket costs. Health plan provider networks are often geographically limited (GAO, 2022). Therefore, it is reasonable to assume that displacement due to IPV or a PHE may hinder access to affordable health care services.

Access to Abortion Services

Access to abortion services varies by insurance type and jurisdiction. As previously noted, a federal restriction known as the *Hyde Amendment*[33] prohibits using certain federal funds to cover abortion services. This greatly limits access for individuals covered by Medicaid, Medicare, and IHS (Liu and Shen, 2022). Several states have restricted coverage of abortion services by private health plans. However, these restrictions on benefit design are preempted by the federal *Earned Retirement Income Security Act*[34] and therefore do not apply to health plans sponsored by employers who self-insure. Since the Supreme Court's 2022 ruling in *Dobbs v. Jackson Women's Health Organization*,[35] several states have also restricted the provision of abortion services regardless of insurance.

---

[33] *Hyde Amendment* Public Law 94-439 § 209 94th Congress, September 30, 1976 (original). Most recently enacted version Public Law 117-103. Div. H, §§ 506–507, 117th Congress, March 15, 2022.

[34] *Earned Retirement Income Security Act of 1974.* Public Law 93-406, amended through Public Law 117-328, 117th Congress, (December 29, 2022).

[35] *Dobbs, State Health Officer of the Mississippi Department of Health et al. v. Jackson Women's Health Organization et al.* 597 US_ (2022).

Required Coverage for Services

Federal and state governments ensure or restrict access to health care through various means. One approach is to require health plans to cover certain types of services, such as preventive care. Health plan benefits are regulated by overlapping federal and state laws, which vary by insurance type and service. In addition, government agencies may be required to ensure no-cost provision of certain services regardless of insurance status. Finally, states may restrict or prohibit the provision of certain types of services, such as abortion, even if the services are deemed essential under prevailing clinical standards of care.

Federal law requires most private health plans and some Medicaid plans to cover IPV screening. A provision in the ACA requires most private health plans to cover the total cost of certain preventive services, including those that receive an A or B rating from the USPSTF, which HRSA recommends via the Women's Preventive Services Initiative (WPSI).[36] WPSI recommends screening adolescents and women for interpersonal and domestic violence at least annually and, when needed, providing or referring for initial intervention services (including, but not limited to, counseling, education, harm reduction strategies, and referral to appropriate supportive services).[37] A separate provision in the ACA requires Medicaid Alternative Benefit Plans (which cover all Medicaid enrollees eligible as part of the ACA's expansion population and other enrollees in some states) to cover the same slate of preventive services as private plans. States may opt to cover these services in their traditional Medicaid plans with financial assistance from the federal government but are not required to do so.

In addition to screening for IPV, the preventive services recommended by USPSTF and WPSI include many important services for caring for women experiencing IPV. These include the full range of FDA-approved contraceptives for women, STI screenings, well-woman visits, screening for depression and anxiety, and a broad range of pregnancy-related tests and services.

---

[36] 42 USC § 300gg–13; see also https://www.kff.org/health-reform/report/preventive-services-tracker/ (accessed August 25, 2023). The same provision also requires most private health plans to cover services that receive an A or B rating from USPSTF, including IPV screening for women of reproductive age. In 2023 this requirement was vacated by a federal district court order applicable to all benefit design mandates triggered by USPSTF recommendations issued after 2010; however, the requirement to cover WPSI-recommended services is not currently affected by this ruling (see Braidwood Management Inc., et al. v. Xavier Becerra et al. 666 F.Supp.3d 613 [5th Cir. 2023]).

[37] WPSI defines *interpersonal and domestic violence* as including physical violence, sexual violence, stalking and psychological aggression (including coercion), reproductive coercion, neglect, and the threat of violence, abuse, or both.

Out-of-Pocket Expenses

While preventive services are covered without cost sharing, the health consequences of IPV can be severe, and many people who experience IPV have significant care needs beyond preventive services. As a result, many face substantial out-of-pocket expenses. According to data from the 2016–2017 NISVS, 35 percent of women had injuries from IPV during their lifetimes (Leemis et al., 2022). Common injuries include bruises, scratches, cuts, and black eyes. Furthermore, 28 percent reported mental or emotional harm related to IPV during their lifetime (Leemis et al., 2022). Analysis of 2016–2017 NISVS data found 13.9 percent of women reported needing medical care due to IPV related injuries during their lifetime (Leemis et al., 2022). This care can be costly. A 2007 study found that women who experienced IPV had higher utilization of primary care, specialty visits, and prescription medications (Rivara et al., 2007). Another analysis using 2014 costs estimated that a woman experiencing IPV would have an additional $65,165 in medical costs during her lifetime (Peterson et al., 2018).

In cases of sexual assault, the *Violence Against Women Act* (VAWA)[38] requires states, local governments, and IHS to ensure no-cost access to medical forensic exams, regardless of insurance status (Hanson, 2023). However, services ancillary to the evidence-gathering portion of the medical forensic exam—such as treatment for injuries, pregnancy testing, and emergency contraception—are not required under VAWA-mandated programs. The no-cost provision of these ancillary services is governed by state law, which varies from jurisdiction to jurisdiction (Ramaswamy et al., 2022). These services may be covered by insurance, possibly without cost-sharing, depending on how the services are classified and the type of insurance the individual has, as described above. In correspondence with the *New England Journal of Medicine*, researchers noted that many patients are still charged out-of-pocket fees when they seek care for sexual violence in emergency departments (Dickman et al., 2022).

Challenges with Confidentiality

Another challenge with insurance, particularly private insurance, is confidentiality. Private insurers typically send beneficiaries billing statements that enumerate the health services they received and the associated costs. For people experiencing IPV, this can be dangerous, particularly if the patient received services that the partner opposes, such as contraception

---

[38] *Violence Against Women Reauthorization Act of 2019*, H.R. 1585, 116th Cong., 1st Session (April 10, 2019), H. Rept. 116-21.

or abortion. HIPAA[39] does allow patients to request that explanation of benefits statements are kept confidential, but enforcement has been uneven (English and Lewis, 2016). Similarly, some states have added confidentiality protections, but these are limited and do not cover most people with private insurance (English ct al., 2012).

CHAPTER SUMMARY

Essential health care services related to IPV are those that address the most prevalent and serious physical health issues related to IPV, behavioral health issues related to IPV, and those that facilitate disclosure of IPV, protect the safety of the person experiencing IPV (and their children if needed), and meet these individuals' basic needs for food and shelter. They are delivered in a variety of settings within and outside of the traditional health care system. Community-based support services are an important component of care delivery for essential health care services related to IPV. Health care deserts, particularly for primary care, maternal and reproductive health care, adolescent care, and SANEs, create barriers to accessing essential health care services related to IPV. Additional barriers to accessing essential health care services related to IPV include state-level restrictions on reproductive health care, limitations on insurance coverage, and inadequate availability of culturally and linguistically appropriate care.

REFERENCES

Abramsky, T., K. M. Devries, L. Michau, J. Nakuti, T. Musuya, N. Kyegombe, and C. Watts. 2016. The impact of SASA!, a community mobilisation intervention, on women's experiences of intimate partner violence: Secondary findings from a cluster randomised trial in Kampala, Uganda. *Journal of Epidemiology and Community Health* 70(8):818-825.

Acharya, M., M. M. Ali, C. J. Hayes, C. A. Bogulski, E. F. Magann, and H. Eswaran. 2023. Trends in telehealth visits during pregnancy, 2018 to 2021. *JAMA Netw Open* 6(4):e236630.

ACOG (American College of Obstetricians and Gynecologists). 2012. ACOG committee opinion no. 518: Intimate partner violence. *Obstet Gynecol* 119(2 Pt 1):412-417.

Adams, E. N., H. M. Clark, M. M. Galano, S. F. Stein, A. Grogan-Kaylor, and S. Graham-Bermann. 2021. Predictors of housing instability in women who have experienced intimate partner violence. *J Interpers Violence* 36(7-8):3459-3481.

Adams, S. H., M. J. Park, L. Twietmeyer, C. D. Brindis, and C. E. Irwin, Jr. 2019. Young adult preventive healthcare: Changes in receipt of care pre- to post-affordable care act. *J Adolesc Health* 64(6):763-769.

---

[39] *Health Insurance Portability and Accountability Act of 1996*, Public Law 104-91, 104th Congress (August 21, 1996).

Adjognon, O. L., J. E. Brady, M. R. Gerber, M. E. Dichter, A. R. Grillo, A. B. Hamilton, S. W. Stirman, and K. M. Iverson. 2021. Getting routine intimate partner violence screening right: Implementation strategies used in Veterans Health Administration (VHA) primary care. *The Journal of the American Board of Family Medicine* 34(2):346-356.

Ahmad, F., S. Hogg-Johnson, D. E. Stewart, H. A. Skinner, R. H. Glazier, and W. Levinson. 2009. Computer-assisted screening for intimate partner violence and control: A randomized trial. *Ann Intern Med* 151(2):93-102.

Alhusen, J. L., E. Ray, P. Sharps, and L. Bullock. 2015. Intimate partner violence during pregnancy: Maternal and neonatal outcomes. *J Womens Health (Larchmont)* 24(1):100-106.

Anderson, C. A., and D. B. Arciniegas. 2010. Cognitive sequelae of hypoxic-ischemic brain injury: A review. *NeuroRehabilitation* 26(1):47-63.

Anderson, J. R., S. M. Stith, M. D. Johnson, M. M. Strachman-Miller, Y. Amanor-Boadu, and D. J. Linkh. 2013. Multi-couple group and self-directed prep formats enhance relationship satisfaction and improve anger management skills in Air Force couples. *American Journal of Family Therapy* 41(2):121-133.

Ard, K. L., and H. J. Makadon. 2011. Addressing intimate partner violence in lesbian, gay, bisexual, and transgender patients. *J Gen Intern Med* 26(8):930-933.

Ascione, F. R., C. V. Weber, T. M. Thompson, J. Heath, M. Maruyama, and K. Hayashi. 2007. Battered pets and domestic violence: Animal abuse reported by women experiencing intimate violence and by nonabused women. *Violence Against Women* 13(4):354-373.

Auger, N., N. Low, G. E. Lee, A. Ayoub, and T. M. Luu. 2022. Pregnancy outcomes of women hospitalized for physical assault, sexual assault, and intimate partner violence. *J Interpers Violence* 37(13-14):NP11135.

Bair-Merritt, M. H., A. Lewis-O'Connor, S. Goel, P. Amato, T. Ismailji, M. Jelley, P. Lenahan, and P. Cronholm. 2014. Primary care-based interventions for intimate partner violence: A systematic review. *Am J Prev Med* 46(2):188-194.

Barrett, B. J., A. Fitzgerald, R. Stevenson, and C. H. Cheung. 2020. Animal maltreatment as a risk marker of more frequent and severe forms of intimate partner violence. *J Interpers Violence* 35(23-24):5131-5156.

Basile, K. C., S. DeGue, K. Jones, K. Freire, J. Dills, S. G. Smith, and J. L. Raiford. 2016. *Stop SV: A technical package to prevent sexual violence.* National Center for Injury Prevention and Control (U.S.). Division of Violence Prevention.

Basile, K. C., S. G. Smith, Y. Liu, M. J. Kresnow, A. M. Fasula, L. Gilbert, and J. Chen. 2018. Rape-related pregnancy and association with reproductive coercion in the US. *American Journal of Preventive Medicine* 55(6):770-776.

Benitez, J. A., and L. Dubay. 2022. COVID-19-related Medicaid enrollment in Medicaid expansion and non-expansion states. *Health Services Research* 57(6):1321-1331.

Bent-Goodley, T. B. 2007. Health disparities and violence against women: Why and how cultural and societal influences matter. *Trauma Violence Abuse* 8(2):90-104.

Bergmann, J. N., and J. K. Stockman. 2015. How does intimate partner violence affect condom and oral contraceptive use in the United States?: A systematic review of the literature. *Contraception* 91(6):438-455.

BLS (Bureau of Labor Statistics). 2023. *Occupational outlook handbook.* https://www.bls.gov/ooh/healthcare/registered-nurses.htm (accessed September 13, 2023).

Braithwaite, S. R., and F. D. Fincham. 2014. Computer-based prevention of intimate partner violence in marriage. *Behaviour Research Therapy* 54:12-21.

Brigance, C., R. Lucas, E. Jones, A. Davis, K. Oinuma, K. Mishkin, and Z. Henderson. 2022. *Nowhere to go: Maternity care deserts across the U.S. 2022 report.* March of Dimes.

Britto, M. T., B. K. Klostermann, A. E. Bonny, S. A. Altum, and R. W. Hornung. 2001. Impact of a school-based intervention on access to healthcare for underserved youth. *J Adolesc Health* 29(2):116-124.

Brown, R. B., S. Miller-Walfish, S. Scott, A. Ali, A. Marjavi, E. Miller, and E. A. McGuier. 2023. Cross-sector collaboration in project catalyst: Creating state partnerships to address the health impact of intimate partner violence. *Prev Med Rep* 33:102204.

Burnett, C., J. Crowder, L. J. Bacchus, D. Schminkey, L. Bullock, P. Sharps, and J. Campbell. 2021. "It doesn't freak us out the way it used to": An evaluation of the domestic violence enhanced home visitation program to inform practice and policy screening for IPV. *Journal of Interpersonal Violence* 36(13-14):NP7488-NP7515.

Calton, J. M., L. B. Cattaneo, and K. T. Gebhard. 2016. Barriers to help seeking for lesbian, gay, bisexual, transgender, and queer survivors of intimate partner violence. *Trauma Violence Abuse* 17(5):585-600.

Campbell, J. C. 1986. Nursing assessment for risk of homicide with battered women. *Advances in Nursing Science* 8(4):36-51.

Campbell, J., and N. Glass. 2009. Safety planning, danger, and lethality assessment. In *Intimate partner violence: A health-based perspective*. New York, NY: Oxford University Press. Pp. 319-334.

Campbell, J. C., D. Webster, J. Koziol-McLain, C. Block, D. Campbell, M. A. Curry, F. Gary, N. Glass, J. McFarlane, C. Sachs, P. Sharps, Y. Ulrich, S. A. Wilt, J. Manganello, X. Xu, J. Schollenberger, V. Frye, and K. Laughon. 2003. Risk factors for femicide in abusive relationships: Results from a multisite case control study. *Am J Public Health* 93(7):1089-1097.

Campbell, J. C., D. W. Webster, and N. Glass. 2009. The danger assessment: Validation of a lethality risk assessment instrument for intimate partner femicide. *J Interpers Violence* 24(4):653-674.

Cantor, A. G., H. D. Nelson, M. Pappas, C. Atchison, B. Hatch, N. Huguet, B. Flynn, and M. McDonagh. 2023. Telehealth for women's preventive services for reproductive health and intimate partner violence: A comparative effectiveness review. *J Gen Intern Med* 38(7):1735-1743.

Center for Health Care Strategies. 2018. *Incorporating patients' voices at the women's HIV program: University of California, San Francisco*. https://www.traumainformedcare.chcs.org/incorporating-patients-voices-at-the-womens-hiv-program-university-of-california-san-francisco/ (accessed September 11, 2023).

Chalmers, K., M. Hollender, L. Spurr, R. Parameswaran, N. Dussault, J. Farnan, S. Oyola, and K. Carter. 2023. Emergency department preparedness to care for sexual assault survivors: A nationwide study. *West J Emerg Med* 24(3):629-636.

Chandramani, A., N. Dussault, R. Parameswaran, J. Rodriguez, J. Novack, J. Ahn, S. Oyola, and K. Carter. 2020. A needs assessment and educational intervention addressing the care of sexual assault patients in the emergency department. *J Forensic Nurs* 16(2):73-82.

Chang, J. C., P. A. Cluss, L. Ranieri, L. Hawker, R. Buranosky, D. Dado, M. McNeil, and S. H. Scholle. 2005. Health care interventions for intimate partner violence: What women want. *Womens Health Issues* 15(1):21-30.

Chisholm, C. A., L. Bullock, and J. E. J. Ferguson, 2nd. 2017. Intimate partner violence and pregnancy: Screening and intervention. *Am J Obstet Gynecol* 217(2):145-149.

Chouinard, A.-F., M. J. Troulis, and E. T. Lahey. 2016. The acute management of facial fractures. *Current Trauma Reports* 2:55-65.

Clayton, S., T. Chin, S. Blackburn, and C. Echeverria. 2010. Different setting, different care: Integrating prevention and clinical care in school-based health centers. *Am J Public Health* 100(9):1592-1596.

Coker, A. L., B. S. Fisher, H. M. Bush, S. C. Swan, C. M. Williams, E. R. Clear, and S. DeGue. 2015. Evaluation of the green dot bystander intervention to reduce interpersonal violence among college students across three campuses. *Violence Against Women* 21(12):1507-1527.

Coker, A. L., D. R. Follingstad, H. M. Bush, and B. S. Fisher. 2016. Are interpersonal violence rates higher among young women in college compared with those never attending college? *Journal of Interpersonal Violence* 31(8):1413-1429.

Collins, E. A., A. M. Cody, S. E. McDonald, N. Nicotera, F. R. Ascione, and J. H. Williams. 2018. A template analysis of intimate partner violence survivors' experiences of animal maltreatment: Implications for safety planning and intervention. *Violence Against Women* 24(4):452-476.

Condon, M. C., D. Charlot-Swilley, and T. Rahman. 2022. At the feet of storytellers: Equity in early relational health conversations. *Infant Ment Health J* 43(3):390-409.

Dawson-Rose, C., Y. P. Cuca, M. Shumway, K. Davis, and E. L. Machtinger. 2019. Providing primary care for HIV in the context of trauma: Experiences of the health care team. *Womens Health Issues* 29(5):385-391.

Dickman, S. L., G. Himmelstein, D. U. Himmelstein, K. Strandberg, A. McGregor, D. McCormick, and S. Woolhandler. 2022. Uncovered medical bills after sexual assault. *N Engl J Med* 387(11):1043-1044.

DOJ (Department of Justice). 2023. *A national protocol for intimate partner violence medical forensic examinations.* Washington, DC: US Department of Justice.

Duchesne, E., A. Nathoo, M. Walker, and S. A. Bartels. 2022. Patient and provider emergency care experiences related to intimate partner violence: A systematic review of the existing evidence. *Trauma Violence Abuse* 24(5):2901-2921. https://doi.org/10.1177/15248380221118962.

Dyer, A. M., and C. G. Abildso. 2019. Impact of an intimate partner violence training on home visitors' perceived knowledge, skills, and abilities to address intimate partner violence experienced by their clients. *Health Educ Behav* 46(1):72-78.

Echeburúa, E., J. Fernández-Montalvo, P. de Corral, and J. J. López-Goñi. 2009. Assessing risk markers in intimate partner femicide and severe violence: A new assessment instrument. *Journal of Interpersonal Violence* 24(6):925-939.

Edwards, K. M. 2015. Intimate partner violence and the rural-urban-suburban divide: Myth or reality? A critical review of the literature. *Trauma Violence Abuse* 16(3):359-373.

Ellis, T. W., S. Brownstein, K. Beitchman, and J. Lifshitz. 2019. Restoring more than smiles in broken homes: Dental and oral biomarkers of brain injury in domestic violence. *Journal of Aggression, Maltreatment & Trauma* 28(7):838-847.

English, A., and J. Lewis. 2016. Privacy protection in billing and health insurance communications. *AMA J Ethics* 18(3):279-287.

English, A. G., R. B. Gold, E. Nash, and J. Levine. 2012. *Confidentiality for individuals insured as dependents: A review of state laws and policies.* Guttmacher Institute.

Ezie, C. 2023. Dismantling the discrimination to incarceration pipeline for trans people of color. *University of St. Thomas Law Journal* 19.

Feder, G. S., M. Hutson, J. Ramsay, and A. R. Taket. 2006. Women exposed to intimate partner violence: Expectations and experiences when they encounter health care professionals: A meta-analysis of qualitative studies. *Arch Intern Med* 166(1):22-37.

Feltner, C., I. Wallace, N. Berkman, C. E. Kistler, J. C. Middleton, C. Barclay, L. Higginbotham, J. T. Green, and D. E. Jonas. 2018. Screening for intimate partner violence, elder abuse, and abuse of vulnerable adults: Evidence report and systematic review for the US preventive services task force. *JAMA* 320(16):1688-1701.

Finnie, R. K. C., D. L. Okasako-Schmucker, L. Buchanan, D. Carty, H. Wethington, S. L. Mercer, K. C. Basile, S. DeGue, P. H. Niolon, J. Bishop, T. Titus, S. Noursi, S. A. Dickerson, D. Whitaker, S. Swider, P. Remington, and Community Preventive Services Task Force. 2022. Intimate partner and sexual violence prevention among youth: A community guide systematic review. *Am J Prev Med* 62(1):e45-e55.

Ford, C., A. English, and G. Sigman. 2004. Confidential health care for adolescents: Position paper for the Society for Adolescent Medicine. *J Adolesc Health* 35(2):160-167.

Ford-Gilboe, M., C. Varcoe, K. Scott-Storey, N. Perrin, J. Wuest, C. N. Wathen, J. Case, and N. Glass. 2020. Longitudinal impacts of an online safety and health intervention for women experiencing intimate partner violence: Randomized controlled trial. *BMC Public Health* 20(1):260.

Foshee, V. A., K. E. Bauman, S. T. Ennett, G. F. Linder, T. Benefield, and C. Suchindran. 2004. Assessing the long-term effects of the safe dates program and a booster in preventing and reducing adolescent dating violence victimization and perpetration. *Am J Public Health* 94(4):619-624.

Fowler, C. I., J. Gable, and B. Lastaer. 2022. *Family planning annual report 2021 national summary*. Rockville, Maryland: Health and Human Services.

Frederiksen, B., I. Gomez, and A. Salganicoff. 2021. *Rebuilding Title X: New regulations for the federal family planning program*. https://www.kff.org/womens-health-policy/issue-brief/rebuilding-title-x-new-regulations-for-the-federal-family-planning-program/ (accessed July 26, 2023).

Frederiksen, B., U. Ranji, M. Long, K. Diep, and A. Salganicoff. 2022. Contraception in the United States: A closer look at experiences, preferences, and coverage. https://www.kff.org/womens-health-policy/report/contraception-in-the-united-states-a-closer-look-at-experiences-preferences-and-coverage/ (accessed September 13, 2023).

Futures Without Violence. n.d. *Telehealth, COVID-19, intimate partner violence, and human trafficking: Increasing safety for people surviving abuse*. Edited by Futures Without Violence: IPV Health Partners.

Galgano, M., G. Toshkezi, X. Qiu, T. Russell, L. Chin, and L. R. Zhao. 2017. Traumatic brain injury: Current treatment strategies and future endeavors. *Cell Transplant* 26(7):1118-1130.

GAO (Government Accountability Office). 2016. *Sexual assault: Information on training, funding, and the availability of forensic examiners*. Washington, DC: U.S. Government Accountability Office.

GAO. 2022. *Private health insurance: State and federal oversight of provider networks varies*. Washington, DC: U.S. Government Accountability Office.

Garcia-Vergara, E., N. Almeda, F. Fernández-Navarro, and D. Becerra-Alonso. 2022. Risk assessment instruments for intimate partner femicide: A systematic review. *Frontiers in Psychology* 13.

Gavin, L., K. Pazol, and K. Ahrens. 2017. Update: Providing quality family planning services - recommendations from CDC and the U.S. Office of Population Affairs, 2017. *MMWR Morb Mortal Wkly Rep* 66(50):1383-1385.

Gee, R. E., N. Mitra, F. Wan, D. E. Chavkin, and J. A. Long. 2009. Power over parity: Intimate partner violence and issues of fertility control. *Am J Obstet Gynecol* 201(2):148 e141-e147.

Gibson, E. J., J. S. Santelli, M. Minguez, A. Lord, and A. C. Schuyler. 2013. Measuring school health center impact on access to and quality of primary care. *J Adolesc Health* 53(6):699-705.

Giesbrecht, C. J. 2022. Animal safekeeping in situations of intimate partner violence: Experiences of human service and animal welfare professionals. *J Interpers Violence* 37(17-18):NP16931-NP16960.

Gilbert, L., S. A. Shaw, D. Goddard-Eckrich, M. Chang, J. Rowe, T. McCrimmon, M. Almonte, S. Goodwin, and M. Epperson. 2015. Project wings (women initiating new goals of safety): A randomised controlled trial of a screening, brief intervention and referral to treatment (SBIRT) service to identify and address intimate partner violence victimisation among substance-using women receiving community supervision. *Crim Behav Ment Health* 25(4):314-329.

Gilmore, A. K., A. E. Jaffe, C. K. Hahn, L. E. Ridings, K. Gill-Hopple, G. B. Lazenby, and J. C. Flanagan. 2021. Intimate partner violence and completion of post-sexual assault medical forensic examination follow-up screening. *J Interpers Violence* 36(13-14):5991-6004.

Gilmore, A. K., G. McKee, J. C. Flanagan, R. M. Leone, D. W. Oesterle, C. M. Kirby, N. Short, and K. Gill-Hopple. 2022. Medications at the emergency department after recent rape. *Journal of Interpersonal Violence* 37(15-16):NP12954-NP12972.

Gilroy, H., J. McFarlane, J. Maddoux, and C. Sullivan. 2016. Homelessness, housing instability, intimate partner violence, mental health, and functioning: A multi-year cohort study of IPV survivors and their children. *Journal of Social Distress and the Homeless* 25(2):86-94.

Glass, N. E., N. A. Perrin, G. C. Hanson, T. L. Bloom, J. T. Messing, A. S. Clough, J. C. Campbell, A. C. Gielen, J. Case, and K. B. Eden. 2017. The longitudinal impact of an internet safety decision aid for abused women. *Am J Prev Med* 52(5):606-615.

Glass, N. E., A. Clough, J. T. Messing, T. Bloom, M. L. Brown, K. B. Eden, J. C. Campbell, A. Gielen, K. Laughon, K. T. Grace, R. M. Turner, C. Alvarez, J. Case, J. Barnes-Hoyt, J. Alhusen, G. C. Hanson, and N. A. Perrin. 2022. Longitudinal impact of the myPlan app on health and safety among college women experiencing partner violence. *J Interpers Violence* 37(13-14):NP11436-NP11459.

Gonzalez-Guarda, R. M., A. L. Florom-Smith, and T. Thomas. 2011. A syndemic model of substance abuse, intimate partner violence, HIV infection, and mental health among Hispanics. *Public Health Nurs* 28(4):366-378.

Grace, K. T., and J. C. Anderson. 2018. Reproductive coercion: A systematic review. *Trauma Violence Abuse* 19(4):371-390.

Grace, K. T., M. R. Decker, C. N. Holliday, J. Talis, and E. Miller. 2023. Reproductive coercion in college health clinic patients: Risk factors, care seeking and perpetration. *J Adv Nurs* 79(4):1464-1475.

Gray, S., and K. M. R. Sizemore, Jonathon. 2023. Coping strategies as a moderator for the association between intimate partner violence and depression and anxiety symptoms among transgender women. *Int. J. Environ. Res. Public Health* 20(11).

Guadalupe-Diaz, X. L., and J. Jasinski. 2017. "I wasn't a priority, I wasn't a victim": Challenges in help seeking for transgender survivors of intimate partner violence. *Violence Against Women* 23(6):772-792.

Gupta, R. C., K. A. Randell, and M. D. Dowd. 2021. Addressing parental adverse childhood experiences in the pediatric setting. *Adv Pediatr* 68:71-88.

Guruge, S., and J. Humphreys. 2009. Barriers affecting access to and use of formal social supports among abused immigrant women. *Can J Nurs Res* 41(3):64-84.

Gutowski, E. R., S. Freitag, S. Zhang, M. P. Thompson, and N. J. Kaslow. 2023. Intimate partner violence, legal systems and barriers for African American women. *J Interpers Violence* 38(1-2):NP1279-NP1298.

Guttmacher Institute. 2023. *Regulating insurance coverage of abortion.* https://www.guttmacher.org/state-policy/explore/regulating-insurance-coverage-abortion (accessed August 16, 2023).

Gwinn, C., G. Strack, S. Adams, and R. Lovelace. 2007. The Family Justice Center Collaborative Model. *St. Louis University Public Law Review* 27(1):79-120.

Haag, H., D. Jones, T. Joseph, and A. Colantonio. 2022. Battered and brain injured: Traumatic brain injury among women survivors of intimate partner violence—a scoping review. *Trauma, Violence, & Abuse* 23(4):1270-1287.

Hageman, T. O. N., L. Langenderfer-Magruder, T. Greene, J. H. Williams, J. St. Mary, S. E. McDonald, and F. R. Ascione. 2018. Intimate partner violence survivors and pets: Exploring practitioners' experiences in addressing client needs. *Families in Society* 99(2):134-145.

Hahn, C. K., A. K. Gilmore, R. O. Aguayo, and A. A. Rheingold. 2018. Perinatal intimate partner violence. *Obstet Gynecol Clin North Am* 45(3):535-547.

Hamberger, L. K., B. Ambuel, C. E. Guse, M. B. Phelan, M. Melzer-Lange, and A. Kistner. 2014. Effects of a systems change model to respond to patients experiencing partner violence in primary care medical settings. *Journal of Family Violence* 29(6):581-594.

Hamby, S., D. Finkelhor, H. Turner, and R. Ormrod. 2011. *Children's exposure to intimate partner violence and other family violence*. Edited by U.S. Department of Justice. Office of Justice Programs.

Hanson, E. J. 2023. *The 2022 Violence Against Women Act Reauthorization, Congressional Research Service reports*. Washington, DC: Congressional Research Service.

Hegarty, K., L. Tarzia, J. Valpied, E. Murray, C. Humphreys, A. Taft, K. Novy, L. Gold, and N. Glass. 2019. An online healthy relationship tool and safety decision aid for women experiencing intimate partner violence (i-decide): A randomised controlled trial. *Lancet Public Health* 4(6):e301-e310.

Hellman, C. M., C. Gwinn, G. Strack, M. Burke, R. T. Munoz, S. R. Brady, N. Aguirre, and Y. Aceves. 2021. Nurturing hope and well-being among survivors of domestic violence within the family justice center model. *Violence and Victims* 36(5):651-666.

HHS (Department of Health and Human Services). 2021. Ensuring access to equitable affordable, client-centered, quality family planning services. *Federal Register* 86(192).

Hollender, M., E. Almirol, M. Meyer, H. Bearden, and K. Stanford. 2023. Sexual assault nurse examiners lead to improved uptake of services: A cross-sectional study. *Western Journal of Emergency Medicine* 24(5).

Horahan, K., H. Morchel, M. Raheem, and L. Stevens. 2014. Electronic health records access during a disaster. *Online J Public Health Inform* 5(3):232.

HRSA (Health Resources and Services Administration). 2022. Behavioral health workforce projections, 2020-2035. https://bhw.hrsa.gov/sites/default/files/bureau-health-workforce/Behavioral-Health-Workforce-Projections-Factsheet.pdf (accessed August 16, 2023).

HRSA. 2023a. *2023-2025 HRSA strategy to address intimate partner violence*. Rockville, Maryland: Health Resources and Services Administration.

HRSA. 2023b. *2022 health center data*. https://data.hrsa.gov/tools/data-reporting/program-data/national/table?tableName=Full&year=2022 (accessed September 11, 2023).

HRSA. 2023c. *Health workforce shortage areas*. https://data.hrsa.gov/topics/health-workforce/shortage-areas (accessed August 21, 2023).

HRSA. 2023d. *Workforce projections*. https://data.hrsa.gov/topics/health-workforce/workforce-projections (accessed September 13, 2023).

HRSA. 2023e. *Map gallery*. https://data.hrsa.gov/maps/map-gallery (accessed August 21, 2023).

Hung, P., C. E. Henning-Smith, M. M. Casey, and K. B. Kozhimannil. 2017. Access to obstetric services in rural counties still declining, with 9 percent losing services, 2004-14. *Health Aff (Millwood)* 36(9):1663-1671.

Iverson, K. M., O. Adjognon, A. R. Grillo, M. E. Dichter, C. A. Gutner, A. B. Hamilton, S. W. Stirman, and M. R. Gerber. 2019. Intimate partner violence screening programs in the Veterans Health Administration: Informing scale-up of successful practices. *J Gen Intern Med* 34(11):2435-2442.

Iverson, K. M., S. B. Danitz, D. R. Shayani, D. Vogt, S. W. Stirman, A. B. Hamilton, C. T. Mahoney, M. R. Gerber, and M. E. Dichter. 2021. Recovering from intimate partner violence through strengths and empowerment: Findings from a randomized clinical trial. *J Clin Psychiatry* 83(1).

Iverson, K. M., S. B. Danitz, S. K. Low, J. A. Knetig, K. W. Doyle, and L. E. Bruce. 2022. Recovering from Intimate Partner Violence through Strengths and Empowerment (RISE): Initial evaluation of the clinical effects of rise administered in routine care in the US Veterans Health Administration. *International Journal of Environmental Research and Public Health* 19(14).

James, S. E., J. L. Herman, S. Rankin, M. Keisling, L. Mottet, and M. Anafi. 2016. *The report of the 2015 U.S. Transgender Survey.*

Jock, B. W. I., G. Dana-Sacco, J. Arscott, M. E. Bagwell-Gray, E. Loerzel, T. Brockie, G. Packard, V. M. O'Keefe, C. E. McKinley, and J. Campbell. 2022. "We've already endured the trauma, who is going to either end that cycle or continue to feed it?": The influence of family and legal systems on Native American women's intimate partner violence experiences. *J Interpers Violence* 37(21-22):NP20602-NP20629.

Jose, A., S. A. Nagori, B. Agarwal, O. Bhutia, and A. Roychoudhury. 2016. Management of maxillofacial trauma in emergency: An update of challenges and controversies. *J Emerg Trauma Shock* 9(2):73-80.

Judge-Golden, C. P., K. J. Smith, M. K. Mor, and S. Borrero. 2019. Financial implications of 12-month dispensing of oral contraceptive pills in the veterans affairs health care system. *JAMA Intern Med* 179(9):1201-1208.

Juszczak, L., P. Melinkovich, and D. Kaplan. 2003. Use of health and mental health services by adolescents across multiple delivery sites. *J Adolesc Health* 32(6 Suppl):108-118.

Kapur, N. A., and D. M. Windish. 2011. Optimal methods to screen men and women for intimate partner violence: Results from an internal medicine residency continuity clinic. *J Interpers Violence* 26(12):2335-2352.

Kast, N. R., M. E. Eisenberg, and R. E. Sieving. 2016. The role of parent communication and connectedness in dating violence victimization among Latino adolescents. *J Interpers Violence* 31(10):1932-1955.

Kasturirangan, A. 2008. Empowerment and programs designed to address domestic violence. *Violence Against Women* 14(12):1465-1475.

Kazmerski, T., H. L. McCauley, K. Jones, S. Borrero, J. G. Silverman, M. R. Decker, D. Tancredi, and E. Miller. 2015. Use of reproductive and sexual health services among female family planning clinic clients exposed to partner violence and reproductive coercion. *Maternal and Child Health Journal* 19:1490-1496.

KFF (Kaiser Family Foundation). 2023a. *Abortion in the United States dashboard.* https://www.kff.org/womens-health-policy/dashboard/abortion-in-the-u-s-dashboard/ (accessed August 24, 2023).

KFF. 2023b. *The availability and use of medication abortion.* https://www.kff.org/womens-health-policy/fact-sheet/the-availability-and-use-of-medication-abortion/ (accessed August 24, 2023).

KFF. 2023c. *State profiles for women's health.* https://www.kff.org/interactive/womens-health-profiles/?activeState=United%20States&activeCategory=coverage (accessed August 25, 2023a).

Kishton, R., L. Sinko, R. Ortiz, M. N. Islam, A. Fredrickson, N. E. Sheils, J. Buresh, P. F. Cronholm, and M. Matone. 2022. Describing the health status of women experiencing violence or abuse: An observational study using claims data. *J Prim Care Community Health* 13:21501319221074121.

Klein, L. B., B. R. Chesworth, J. R. Howland-Myers, C. F. Rizo, and R. J. Macy. 2021. Housing interventions for intimate partner violence survivors: A systematic review. *Trauma Violence Abuse* 22(2):249-264.

Kourti, A., A. Stavridou, E. Panagouli, T. Psaltopoulou, C. Spiliopoulou, M. Tsolia, T. N. Sergentanis, and A. Tsitsika. 2023. Domestic violence during the COVID-19 pandemic: A systematic review. *Trauma Violence Abuse* 24(2):719-745.

Kozhimannil, K. B., J. D. Interrante, M. K. S. Tuttle, and C. Henning-Smith. 2020. Changes in hospital-based obstetric services in rural US counties, 2014-2018. *JAMA* 324(2):197-199.

Kozhimannil, K. B., V. A. Lewis, J. D. Interrante, P. L. Chastain, and L. Admon. 2023. Screening for and experiences of intimate partner violence in the United States before, during, and after pregnancy, 2016-2019. *American Journal of Public Health* 113(3):297-305.

Koziol-McLain, J., A. C. Vandal, D. Wilson, S. Nada-Raja, T. Dobbs, C. McLean, R. Sisk, K. B. Eden, and N. E. Glass. 2018. Efficacy of a web-based safety decision aid for women experiencing intimate partner violence: Randomized controlled trial. *J Med Internet Res* 19(12):e426.

Krishnamurti, T., A. L. Davis, B. Quinn, A. F. Castillo, K. L. Martin, and H. N. Simhan. 2021. Mobile remote monitoring of intimate partner violence among pregnant patients during the COVID-19 shelter-in-place order: Quality improvement pilot study. *Journal of Medical Internet Research* 23(2):e22790.

Kulkarni, S. 2018. Intersectional trauma-informed intimate partner violence (IPV) services: Narrowing the gap between IPV service delivery and survivor needs. *Journal of Family Violence* 34(1):55-64.

Kurdyla, V., A. M. Messinger, and M. Ramirez. 2021. Transgender intimate partner violence and help-seeking patterns. *Journal of Interpersonal Violence* 36(19-20):NP11046-NP11069.

Leemis, R. W., N. Friar, S. Khatiwada, M. S. Chen, M.-j. Kresnow, S. G. Smith, S. Caslin, and K. C. Basile. 2022. The National Intimate Partner and Sexual Violence Survey: 2016/2017 report on intimate partner violence. Atlanta, GA: Centers for Disease Control and Prevention.

Liu, E. C., and W. W. Shen. 2022. The Hyde Amendment: An overview. *Congressional Research Service Reports*.

Logue, T. C., N. C. Danford, E. C. Bixby, M. M. Levitsky, and M. P. Rosenwasser. 2021. Neck and back sprain and hand flexor tendon repair are more common in victims of domestic violence compared with patients who were not victims of domestic violence: A comparative study of 1,204,596 patients using the National Trauma Data Bank. *JAAOS Global Research & Reviews* 5(9).

López-Ossorio, J. J., J. L. González-Álvarez, I. Loinaz, A. Martínez-Martínez, and D. Pineda. 2020. Intimate partner homicide risk assessment by police in Spain: The dual protocol VPR5.0-H. *Psychosocial Intervention* 30(1):47-55. https://doi.org/10.5093/pi2020a16.

Love, H. E., J. Schlitt, S. Soleimanpour, N. Panchal, and C. Behr. 2019. Twenty years of school-based health care growth and expansion. *Health Aff (Millwood)* 38(5):755-764.

Machtinger, E. L., K. B. Davis, L. S. Kimberg, N. Khanna, Y. P. Cuca, C. Dawson-Rose, M. Shumway, J. Campbell, A. Lewis-O'Connor, M. Blake, A. Blanch, and B. McCaw. 2019. From treatment to healing: Inquiry and response to recent and past trauma in adult health care. *Womens Health Issues* 29(2):97-102.

MacMillan, H. L., C. N. Wathen, E. Jamieson, M. Boyle, L. A. McNutt, A. Worster, B. Lent, M. Webb, and McMaster Violence Against Women Research Group. 2006. Approaches to screening for intimate partner violence in health care settings: A randomized trial. *JAMA* 296(5):530-536.

Maleku, A., B. Subedi, Y. K. Kim, H. Haran, and S. Pyakurel. 2022. Toward healing-centered engagement to address mental well-being among young Bhutanese-Nepali refugee women in the United States: Findings from the cultural leadership project. *Journal of Ethnic & Cultural Diversity in Social Work*:1-19.

Mandal, B., N. Porto, D. E. Kiss, S. H. Cho, and L. S. Head. 2022. Health insurance coverage during the COVID-19 pandemic: The role of Medicaid expansion. *J Consum Aff* 57(1):296-319.

Mantel, J., and R. Knake. 2018. Legal and ethical impediments to data sharing and integration among medical legal partnership participants. *Annals of Health Law* 27(2):183-204.

Markman, H. J., M. J. Renick, F. J. Floyd, S. M. Stanley, and M. Clements. 1993. Preventing marital distress through communication and conflict management training: A 4- and 5-year follow-up. *J Consult Clin Psychol* 61(1):70-77.

Marshall, K. J., D. N. Fowler, M. L. Walters, and A. B. Doreson. 2018. Interventions that address intimate partner violence and HIV among women: A systematic review. *AIDS Behav* 22(10):3244-3263.

Mastrocinque, J. M., D. Thew, C. Cerulli, C. Raimondi, R. Q. Pollard, Jr., and N. P. Chin. 2017. Deaf victims' experiences with intimate partner violence: The need for integration and innovation. *J Interpers Violence* 32(24):3753-3777.

McBain, R. K., J. Cantor, M. F. Pera, J. Breslau, D. M. Bravata, and C. M. Whaley. 2023. Mental health service utilization rates among commercially insured adults in the US during the first year of the COVID-19 pandemic. *JAMA Health Forum* 4(1). https://doi.org/10.1001/jamahealthforum.2022.4936.

McFarlane, J., A. Malecha, J. Gist, K. Watson, E. Batten, I. Hall, and S. Smith. 2004. Increasing the safety-promoting behaviors of abused women: In this study, a telephone intervention for victims of intimate-partner violence showed efficacy for 18 months. *AJN The American Journal of Nursing* 104(3):40-50.

Mcintosh-Clarké, D. R., M. N. Zeman, H. A. Valand, and R. K. Tu. 2019. Incentivizing physician diversity in radiology. *Journal of the American College of Radiology* 16(4, Part B):624-630.

McKay, T. E., M. L. Kan, J. Landwehr, and E. Miller. 2021. When disclosure isn't the goal: Exploring responses to partner violence victimization screening and universal education among youth and adults. *Journal of Family Violence* 37(3):487-504.

McLennan, J. D., and H. L. MacMillan. 2016. Routine primary care screening for intimate partner violence and other adverse psychosocial exposures: What's the evidence? *BMC Family Practice* 17(1):103.

Messing, J. T., Y. Amanor-Boadu, C. E. Cavanaugh, N. E. Glass, and J. C. Campbell. 2013. Culturally competent intimate partner violence risk assessment: Adapting the danger assessment for immigrant women. *Social Work Research* 37(3):263-275.

Messing, J. T., J. Campbell, J. Sullivan Wilson, S. Brown, and B. Patchell. 2017. The lethality screen: The predictive validity of an intimate partner violence risk assessment for use by first responders. *Journal of Interpersonal Violence* 32(2):205-226.

Messing, J. T., J. Campbell, K. Dunne, and S. Dubus. 2020. Development and testing of the danger assessment for law enforcement (da-le). *Social Work Research* 44(3):143-156.

Meyer, J. P., S. A. Springer, and F. L. Altice. 2011. Substance abuse, violence, and HIV in women: A literature review of the syndemic. *J Womens Health (Larchmt)* 20(7):991-1006.

Miller, E., M. R. Decker, A. Raj, E. Reed, D. Marable, and J. G. Silverman. 2010. Intimate partner violence and health care-seeking patterns among female users of urban adolescent clinics. *Maternal and Child Health Journal* 14:910-917.

Miller, E., M. R. Decker, H. L. McCauley, D. J. Tancredi, R. R. Levenson, J. Waldman, P. Schoenwald, and J. G. Silverman. 2011. A family planning clinic partner violence intervention to reduce risk associated with reproductive coercion. *Contraception* 83(3):274-280.

Miller, E., D. J. Tancredi, H. L. McCauley, M. R. Decker, M. C. D. Virata, H. A. Anderson, B. O'Connor, and J. G. Silverman. 2013. One-year follow-up of a coach-delivered dating violence prevention program: A cluster randomized controlled trial. *Am J Prev Med* 45(1):108-112.

Miller, E., H. L. McCauley, D. J. Tancredi, M. R. Decker, H. Anderson, and J. G. Silverman. 2014. Recent reproductive coercion and unintended pregnancy among female family planning clients. *Contraception* 89(2):122-128.

Miller, E., S. Goldstein, H. L. McCauley, K. A. Jones, R. N. Dick, J. Jetton, J. G. Silverman, S. Blackburn, E. Monasterio, L. James, and D. J. Tancredi. 2015. A school health center intervention for abusive adolescent relationships: A cluster RCT. *Pediatrics* 135(1):76-85.

Miller, E., D. J. Tancredi, M. R. Decker, H. L. McCauley, K. A. Jones, H. Anderson, L. James, and J. G. Silverman. 2016. A family planning clinic-based intervention to address reproductive coercion: A cluster randomized controlled trial. *Contraception* 94(1):58-67.

Miller, E., H. L. McCauley, M. R. Decker, R. Levenson, S. Zelazny, K. A. Jones, H. Anderson, and J. G. Silverman. 2017. Implementation of a family planning clinic-based partner violence and reproductive coercion intervention: Provider and patient perspectives. *Perspect Sex Reprod Health* 49(2):85-93.

Miller, E., K. A. Jones, A. J. Culyba, T. Paglisotti, N. Dwarakanath, M. Massof, Z. Feinstein, K. A. Ports, D. Espelage, J. Pulerwitz, A. Garg, J. Kato-Wallace, and K. Z. Abebe. 2020. Effect of a community-based gender norms program on sexual violence perpetration by adolescent boys and young men: A cluster randomized clinical trial. *JAMA Network Open* 3(12):e2028499.

Miller, C. J., K. Stolzmann, M. E. Dichter, O. L. Adjognon, J. E. Brady, G. A. Portnoy, M. R. Gerber, S. Iqbal, and K. M. Iverson. 2022. Intimate partner violence screening for women in the Veterans Health Administration: Temporal trends from the early years of implementation 2014-2020. *J Aggress Maltreat Trauma* a:1-19.

Miller-Walfish, S., J. Kwon, C. Raible, A. Ali, J. H. Bell, L. James, and E. Miller. 2021. Promoting cross-sector collaborations to address intimate partner violence in health care delivery systems using a quality assessment tool. *J Womens Health (Larchmt)* 30(11):1660-1666.

Mitchell, S. A., L. A. Charles, and N. Downing. 2022. Increasing access to forensic nursing services in rural and underserved areas of Texas. *J Forensic Nurs* 18(1):21-29.

Miyamoto, S., E. Thiede, L. Dorn, D. F. Perkins, C. Bittner, and D. Scanlon. 2021. The Sexual Assault Forensic Examination Telehealth (SAFE-T) Center: A comprehensive, nurse-led telehealth model to address disparities in sexual assault care. *J Rural Health* 37(1):92-102.

Mogos, M. F., W. N. Araya, S. W. Masho, J. L. Salemi, C. Shieh, and H. M. Salihu. 2016. The feto-maternal health cost of intimate partner violence among delivery-related discharges in the United States, 2002-2009. *J Interpers Violence* 31(3):444-464.

Monterrosa, A. E. 2021. How race and gender stereotypes influence help-seeking for intimate partner violence. *J Interpers Violence* 36(17-18):NP9153-NP9174.

Morris, A., S. Goletz, and J. Friona. 2022. Indiana sexual assault nurse examiner training initiative: Positive impacts for medical forensic care. *J Forensic Nurs* 18(3):146-155.

Moynihan, M. M., V. L. Banyard, A. C. Cares, S. J. Potter, L. M. Williams, and J. G. Stapleton. 2015. Encouraging responses in sexual and relationship violence prevention: What program effects remain 1 year later? *J Interpers Violence* 30(1):110-132.

National Coalition Against Domestic Violence. n.d. *Resources.* https://ncadv.org/RESOURCES (accessed May 8, 2023).

Nelson, H. D., B. G. Darney, K. Ahrens, A. Burgess, R. M. Jungbauer, A. Cantor, C. Atchison, K. B. Eden, R. Goueth, and R. Fu. 2022. Associations of unintended pregnancy with maternal and infant health outcomes: A systematic review and meta-analysis. *JAMA* 328(17):1714-1729.

Niolon, P. H., M. C. Kearns, J. Dills, K. Rambo, S. M. Irving, T. L. Armstead, and L. K. Gilbert. 2017. *Preventing intimate partner violence across the lifespan: A technical package of programs, policies, and practices.* Atlanta, GA: National Center for Injury Prevention and Control, Centers for Disease Control and Prevention.

Niolon, P. H., A. M. Vivolo-Kantor, A. J. Tracy, N. E. Latzman, T. D. Little, S. DeGue, K. M. Lang, L. F. Estefan, S. R. Ghazarian, W. L. K. McIntosh, B. Taylor, L. L. Johnson, H. Kuoh, T. Burton, B. Fortson, E. A. Mumford, S. C. Nelson, H. Joseph, L. A. Valle, and A. T. Tharp. 2019. An RCT of dating matters: Effects on teen dating violence and relationship behaviors. *Am J Prev Med* 57(1):13-23.

North Carolina Department of Health and Human Services. *Healthy opportunities*. https://www.ncdhhs.gov/about/department-initiatives/healthy-opportunities (accessed August 25, 2023).

NYSDOH (New York State Department of Health). 2013. *Guidelines for integrating domestic violence screening into HIV counseling, testing, referral & partner notification*. https://www.health.ny.gov/diseases/aids/providers/regulations/domesticviolence/guide.htm (accessed May 8, 2023).

OASH (Office of the Assistant Secretary for Health). 2022. *Equitable long-term recovery and resilience*. https://health.gov/our-work/national-health-initiatives/equitable-long-term-recovery-and-resilience (accessed August 20, 2023).

O'Doherty, L., K. Hegarty, J. Ramsay, L. L. Davidson, G. Feder, and A. Taft. 2015. Screening women for intimate partner violence in healthcare settings. *Cochrane Database Syst Rev* 2015(7):CD007007.

Ogbe, E., S. Harmon, R. Van den Bergh, and O. Degomme. 2020. A systematic review of intimate partner violence interventions focused on improving social support and mental health outcomes of survivors. *PLoS ONE* 15(6):e0235177.

Olds, D., and E. Yost. 2020. Developing the nurse-family partnership. *Designing Evidence-Based Public Health and Prevention Programs*. London, UK: Routledge. Pp. 173-193.

Ollen, E. W., V. E. Ameral, K. Palm Reed, and D. A. Hines. 2017. Sexual minority college students' perceptions on dating violence and sexual assault. *J Counseling Psych* 64(1):112-119.

Ombayo, B., B. Black, and K. M. Preble. 2019. Adolescent–parent communication among youth who have and have not experienced dating violence. *Child and Adolescent Social Work Journal* 36(4):381-390.

Overstreet, N. M., and D. M. Quinn. 2013. The intimate partner violence stigmatization model and barriers to help-seeking. *Basic Applied Soc Psych* 35(1):109-122.

Pavao, J., J. Alvarez, N. Baumrind, M. Induni, and R. Kimerling. 2007. Intimate partner violence and housing instability. *Am J Prev Med* 32(2):143-146.

Pearce, M. E., K. Jongbloed, L. Demerais, H. MacDonald, W. M. Christian, R. Sharma, N. Pick, E. M. Yoshida, P. M. Spittal, and M. B. Klein. 2019. "Another thing to live for": Supporting HCV treatment and cure among indigenous people impacted by substance use in Canadian cities. *Int J Drug Policy* 74:52-61.

Peterson, C., M. C. Kearns, W. L. McIntosh, L. F. Estefan, C. Nicolaidis, K. E. McCollister, A. Gordon, and C. Florence. 2018. Lifetime economic burden of intimate partner violence among U.S. adults. *Am J Prev Med* 55(4):433-444.

Piolanti, A., and H. M. Foran. 2022. Efficacy of interventions to prevent physical and sexual dating violence among adolescents: A systematic review and meta-analysis. *JAMA Pediatr* 176(2):142-149.

Pleasants, E. A., A. F. Cartwright, and U. D. Upadhyay. 2022. Association between distance to an abortion facility and abortion or pregnancy outcome among a prospective cohort of people seeking abortion online. *JAMA Netw Open* 5(5):e2212065.

Ponce, A. N., M. S. Lawless, and M. Rowe. 2014. Homelessness, behavioral health disorders and intimate partner violence: Barriers to services for women. *Community Ment Health J* 50(7):831-840.

Porsch, L. M., M. Xu, C. B. Veldhuis, L. A. Bochicchio, S. S. Zollweg, and T. L. Hughes. 2022. Intimate partner violence among sexual minority women: A scoping review. *Trauma, Violence, & Abuse* 24(5):3014-3036. https://doi.org/10.1177/15248380221122815.

Pritchard, A. J., A. Reckdenwald, and C. Nordham. 2017. Nonfatal strangulation as part of domestic violence: A review of research. *Trauma, Violence, & Abuse* 18(4):407-424.

Rader, B., U. D. Upadhyay, N. K. R. Sehgal, B. Y. Reis, J. S. Brownstein, and Y. Hswen. 2022. Estimated travel time and spatial access to abortion facilities in the US before and after the *Dobbs v Jackson* women's health decision. *JAMA* 328(20):2041-2047.

Ragavan, M. I., and E. Miller. 2022. Healing-centered care for intimate partner violence survivors and their children. *Pediatrics* 149(6).

Ragavan, M. I., L. Risser, V. Duplessis, S. DeGue, A. Villaveces, T. P. Hurley, J. Chang, E. Miller, and K. A. Randell. 2022. The impact of the COVID-19 pandemic on the needs and lived experiences of intimate partner violence survivors in the United States: Advocate perspectives. *Violence Against Women* 28(12-13):3114 3134.

Ramaswamy, A., B. Frederiksen, M. Rae, U. Ranji, A. Salganicoff, and D. McDermott. 2022. *Rebuilding Title X: New regulations for the federal family planning program.* https://www.kff.org/womens-health-policy/issue-brief/out-of-pocket-charges-for-rape-kits-and-services-for-sexual-assault-survivors/ (accessed August 20, 2023).

Ravi, K. E., S. R. Robinson, and R. V. Schrag. 2022. Facilitators of formal help-seeking for adult survivors of IPV in the United States: A systematic review. *Trauma Violence Abuse* 23(5):1420-1436.

Reidy, D. E., K. M. Holland, K. Cortina, B. Ball, and B. Rosenbluth. 2017. Evaluation of the expect respect support group program: A violence prevention strategy for youth exposed to violence. *Prev Med* 100:235-242.

Rickert, V. I., C. M. Wiemann, S. D. Harrykissoon, A. B. Berenson, and E. Kolb. 2002. The relationship among demographics, reproductive characteristics, and intimate partner violence. *American Journal of Obstetrics and Gynecology* 187(4):1002-1007.

Rivara, F. P., M. L. Anderson, P. Fishman, A. E. Bonomi, R. J. Reid, D. Carrell, and R. S. Thompson. 2007. Healthcare utilization and costs for women with a history of intimate partner violence. *Am J Prev Med* 32(2):89-96.

Rivas, C., C. Vigurs, J. Cameron, and L. Yeo. 2019. A realist review of which advocacy interventions work for which abused women under what circumstances. *Cochrane Database of Systematic Reviews* 6.

Robinson, S. R., K. Ravi, and R. J. Voth Schrag. 2021. A systematic review of barriers to formal help seeking for adult survivors of IPV in the United States, 2005-2019. *Trauma Violence Abuse* 22(5):1279-1295.

Rodriguez, M., J. M. Valentine, J. B. Son, and M. Muhammad. 2009. Intimate partner violence and barriers to mental health care for ethnically diverse populations of women. *Trauma Violence Abuse* 10(4):358-374.

Rollins, C., N. E. Glass, N. A. Perrin, K. A. Billhardt, A. Clough, J. Barnes, G. C. Hanson, and T. L. Bloom. 2012. Housing instability is as strong a predictor of poor health outcomes as level of danger in an abusive relationship: Findings from the SHARE study. *J Interpers Violence* 27(4):623-643.

Rossi, F. S., M. Shankar, K. Buckholdt, Y. Bailey, S. T. Israni, and K. M. Iverson. 2020. Trying times and trying out solutions: Intimate partner violence screening and support for women veterans during covid-19. *J Gen Intern Med* 35(9):2728-2731.

Sabri, B., S. Tharmarajah, V. P. S. Njie-Carr, J. T. Messing, E. Loerzel, J. Arscott, and J. C. Campbell. 2021. Safety planning with marginalized survivors of intimate partner violence: Challenges of conducting safety planning intervention research with marginalized women. *Trauma, Violence, and Abuse* 23(5):1728-1751. https://doi.org/10.1177/15248380211013136.

Saftlas, A. F., K. K. Harland, A. B. Wallis, J. Cavanaugh, P. Dickey, and C. Peek-Asa. 2014. Motivational interviewing and intimate partner violence: A randomized trial. *Ann Epidemiol* 24(2):144-150.

Scheer, J. R., M. Lawlace, C. J. Cascalheira, M. E. Newcomb, and S. W. Whitton. 2023. Help-seeking for severe intimate partner violence among sexual and gender minority adolescents and young adults assigned female at birth: A latent class analysis. *J Interpers Violence* 38(9-10):6723-6750.

Scheer, J. R., A. Martin-Storey, and L. Baams. 2020. Help-seeking barriers among sexual and gender minority individuals who experience intimate partner violence victimization. In *Intimate partner violence and the LGBT+ community: Understanding power dynamics.* Edited by B. Russell. Cham: Springer International Publishing. Pp. 139-158.

Schmidt, M., S. K. Kedia, P. J. Dillon, and K. H. Howell. 2023. Challenges to help-seeking among women of color exposed to intimate partner violence. *J Interpers Violence* 38(13-14):8088-8113.

Schoenthaler, A., E. Montague, L. Baier Manwell, R. Brown, M. D. Schwartz, and M. Linzer. 2014. Patient–physician racial/ethnic concordance and blood pressure control: The role of trust and medication adherence. *Ethnicity & Health* 19(5):565-578.

Sharps, P. W., L. F. Bullock, J. C. Campbell, J. L. Alhusen, S. R. Ghazarian, S. S. Bhandari, and D. L. Schminkey. 2016. Domestic violence enhanced perinatal home visits: The DOVE randomized clinical trial. *J Womens Health (Larchmont)* 25(11):1129-1138.

Shorey, R. C., V. Tirone, and G. L. Stuart. 2014. Coordinated community response components for victims of intimate partner violence: A review of the literature. *Aggress Violent Behav* 19(4):363-371.

Smith, C. W., R. J. Kreitzer, K. A. Kane, and T. M. Saunders. 2022. Contraception deserts: The effects of Title X rule changes on access to reproductive health care resources. *Politics & Gender* 18(3):672-707.

Smith, E. J., B. A. Bailey, and A. Cascio. 2023. Sexual coercion, intimate partner violence, and homicide: A scoping literature review. *Trauma Violence Abuse* 25(1):341-353. https://doi.org/10.1177/15248380221150474.

Snyder, J. E., R. D. Upton, T. C. Hassett, H. Lee, Z. Nouri, and M. Dill. 2023. Black representation in the primary care physician workforce and its association with population life expectancy and mortality rates in the US. *JAMA Network Open* 6(4):e236687-e236687.

Sorenson, S. B. 2017. Guns in intimate partner violence: Comparing incidents by type of weapon. *J Womens Health (Larchmont)* 26(3):249-258.

Sorenson, S. B., and R. A. Schut. 2018. Nonfatal gun use in intimate partner violence: A systematic review of the literature. *Trauma Violence Abuse* 19(4):431-442.

Spencer, C. M., and S. M. Stith. 2020. Risk factors for male perpetration and female victimization of intimate partner homicide: A meta-analysis. *Trauma Violence Abuse* 21(3):527-540.

Sprague, S., K. Madden, S. Dosanjh, K. Godin, J. C. Goslings, E. H. Schemitsch, and M. Bhandari. 2013a. Intimate partner violence and musculoskeletal injury: Bridging the knowledge gap in orthopaedic fracture clinics. *BMC Musculoskelet Disord* 14(1):23.

Sprague, S., M. Bhandari, G. J. Della Rocca, J. C. Goslings, R. W. Poolman, K. Madden, N. Simunovic, S. Dosanjh, and E. H. Schemitsch. 2013b. Prevalence of abuse and intimate partner violence surgical evaluation (PRAISE) in orthopaedic fracture clinics: A multi-national prevalence study. *Lancet* 382(9895):866-876.

Stockman, J. K., M. B. Lucea, R. Bolyard, D. Bertand, G. B. Callwood, P. W. Sharps, D. W. Campbell, and J. C. Campbell. 2014. Intimate partner violence among African American and African Caribbean women: Prevalence, risk factors, and the influence of cultural attitudes. *Glob Health Action* 7:24772.

Stockman, J. K., H. Hayashi, and J. C. Campbell. 2015. Intimate partner violence and its health impact on ethnic minority women [corrected]. *J Womens Health (Larchmt)* 24(1):62-79.

Summers-Gabr, N. M. 2020. Rural-urban mental health disparities in the United States during COVID-19. *Psychol Trauma* 12(S1):S222-S224.

Sutherland, M. A., H. C. Fantasia, M. K. Hutchinson, and J. Katz. 2021. Individual and institutional predictors of IPV/SV screening in college health centers. *J Interpers Violence* 36(3-4):1330-1355.

Sutton, A., H. Beech, B. Ozturk, and D. Nelson-Gardell. 2021. Preparing mental health professionals to work with survivors of intimate partner violence: A comprehensive systematic review of the literature. *Affilia* 36(3):426-440.

Tarzia, L., M. A. Bohren, J. Cameron, C. Garcia-Moreno, L. O'Doherty, R. Fiolet, L. Hooker, M. Wellington, R. Parker, J. Koziol-Mclain, G. Feder, and K. Hegarty. 2020. Women's experiences and expectations after disclosure of intimate partner abuse to a healthcare provider: A qualitative meta-synthesis. *BMJ Open* 10(11):e041339.

Taylor, C. A., J. M. Bell, M. J. Breiding, and L. Xu. 2017. Traumatic brain injury-related emergency department visits, hospitalizations, and deaths - United States, 2007 and 2013. *MMWR Surveillance Summaries* 66(9):1-16.

Thackeray, J., N. Livingston, M. I. Ragavan, J. Schaechter, E. Sigel, Council on Child Abuse and Neglect, Council on Injury, Violence, and Poison Prevention. 2023. Intimate partner violence: Role of the pediatrician. *Pediatrics* 152(1).

Thiede, E., and S. Miyamoto. 2021. Rural availability of sexual assault nurse examiners (SANES). *J Rural Health* 37(1):81-91.

Turkstra, L. S., K. Salanki, E. MacIntyre, N. Kim, J. Jin, S. Sprague, T. Scott, and M. Bhandari. 2023. What is the prevalence of intimate partner violence and traumatic brain injury in fracture clinic patients? *Clin Orthop Relat Res* 481(1):132-142.

Uscher-Pines, L., J. Cantor, H. A. Huskamp, A. Mehrotra, A. Busch, and M. Barnett. 2020. Adoption of telemedicine services by substance abuse treatment facilities in the U.S. *J Subst Abuse Treat* 117:108060.

Uscher-Pines, L., C. M. McCullough, J. L. Sousa, S. D. Lee, A. J. Ober, D. Camacho, and K. A. Kapinos. 2023. Changes in in-person, audio-only, and video visits in California's federally qualified health centers, 2019-2022. *JAMA* 329(14):1219-1221.

USPSTF (U.S. Preventive Services Task Force), S. J. Curry, A. H. Krist, D. K. Owens, M. J. Barry, A. B. Caughey, K. W. Davidson, C. A. Doubeni, J. W. Epling, Jr., D. C. Grossman, A. R. Kemper, M. Kubik, A. Kurth, C. S. Landefeld, C. M. Mangione, M. Silverstein, M. A. Simon, C. W. Tseng, and J. B. Wong. 2018. Screening for intimate partner violence, elder abuse, and abuse of vulnerable adults: US Preventive Services Task Force final recommendation statement. *JAMA* 320(16):1678-1687.

Vakkalanka, J. P., M. M. Nataliansyah, K. A. S. Merchant, L. J. Mack, S. Parsons, N. M. Mohr, and M. M. Ward. 2022. Telepsychiatry services across an emergency department network: A mixed methods study of the implementation process. *American Journal of Emergency Medicine* 59:79-84.

Valera, E. M., J. C. Daugherty, O. C. Scott, and H. Berenbaum. 2022. Strangulation as an acquired brain injury in intimate-partner violence and its relationship to cognitive and psychological functioning: A preliminary study. *Journal of Head Trauma Rehabilitation* 37(1):15-23.

Vavala, G., Q. Wang, S. Jimenez, W. E. Ramos, M. A. Ocasio, A. Romero-Espinoza, R. Flynn, R. Bolan, M. I. Fernandez, P. Doan, E. M. Arnold, D. Swendeman, W. S. Comulada, and J. D. Klausner. 2022. Substance use, violence, and sexual risk among young cis-gender women placed at high-risk for human immunodeficiency virus infection. *AIDS Behav* 26(9):3008-3015.

Velonis, A. J., P. O'Campo, J. J. Rodrigues, and P. Buhariwala. 2019. Using implementation science to build intimate partner violence screening and referral capacity in a fracture clinic. *J Eval Clin Pract* 25(3):381-389.

Wadsworth, P., C. Kothari, G. Lubwama, C. L. Brown, and J. Frank Benton. 2018. Health and health care from the perspective of intimate partner violence adult female victims in shelters: Impact of IPV, unmet needs, barriers, experiences, and preferences. *Fam Community Health* 41(2):123-133.

Wagner, A. L., S. Sheinfeld Gorin, M. L. Boulton, B. A. Glover, and J. D. Morenoff. 2021. Effect of vaccine effectiveness and safety on COVID-19 vaccine acceptance in Detroit, Michigan, July 2020. *Hum Vaccin Immunother* 17(9):2940-2945.

Wallace, M., L. Dyer, E. Felker-Kantor, J. Benno, D. Vilda, E. Harville, and K. Theall. 2021. Maternity care deserts and pregnancy-associated mortality in Louisiana. *Womens Health Issues* 31(2):122-129.

Weigel, G., B. Frederiksen, U. Ranji, and A. Saiganicoff. 2021. Obgyns and the provision of sexual and reproductive health care: Key findings from a national survey. https://www.kff.org/womens-health-policy/report/obgyns-and-the-provision-of-sexual-and-reproductive-health-care-key-findings-from-a-national-survey/#:~:text=The%20vast%20majority%20of%20OBGYNs%20provided%20most%20forms%20of%20hormonal,and%20resources%20to%20address%20psychosocial (accessed September 13, 2023).

White House. 2013. *Addressing the intersection of HIV/AIDS, violence against women and girls, & gender–related health disparities.* https://obamawhitehouse.archives.gov/sites/default/files/docs/vaw-hiv_working_group_report_final_-_9-6--2013.pdf (accessed August 21, 2023).

White, K. O., and C. Westhoff. 2011. The effect of pack supply on oral contraceptive pill continuation: A randomized controlled trial. *Obstet Gynecol* 118(3):615-622.

Wiggins, B., K. Anastasiou, and D. N. Cox. 2021. A systematic review of key factors in the effectiveness of multisector alliances in the public health domain. *Am J Health Promot* 35(1):93-105.

Willie, T. C., L. Sharpless, M. Monger, T. S. Kershaw, W. B. Mahoney, and J. K. Stockman. 2022. Enhancing domestic violence advocates' ability to discuss HIV pre-exposure prophylaxis (PREP): Feasibility and acceptability of an educational intervention. *Womens Health (Lond)* 18:17455065211070548.

Wilson, K. S., M. R. Silberberg, A. J. Brown, and S. D. Yaggy. 2007. Health needs and barriers to healthcare of women who have experienced intimate partner violence. *Journal of Women's Health* 16(10):1485-1498.

WPSI (Women's Preventive Services Initiative). 2022. *Women's Preventive Services Initiative 2022 coding guide.* American College of Obstetricians and Gynecologists.

6

Sustaining Intimate Partner Violence Services During Public Health Emergencies

ESSENTIAL HEALTH CARE SERVICES DURING PUBLIC HEALTH EMERGENCIES

The World Health Organization (WHO) has described the process of prioritizing essential services during a public health emergency (PHE) as "context relevant." In its *Maintaining Essential Health Services: Operational Guidance for the COVID-19 Context (June 2020)*, WHO provided the following list of high-priority categories (WHO, 2020, p. 6):

- Essential prevention measures for communicable diseases, including immunizations;
- Services related to reproductive health, including during pregnancy and childbirth;
- Care for vulnerable populations, such as infants and older adults;
- Provision of medications and supplies to support the ongoing management of chronic diseases, including mental health conditions;
- Uninterrupted critical inpatient care;
- Management of emergency health conditions and common acute presentations that require time-sensitive intervention; and
- Auxiliary services, such as basic diagnostic imaging, laboratory, and blood bank services.

While intimate partner violence (IPV) is not specifically called out here, the committee found this guidance to be a helpful resource to identify priorities. A recent study on U.S. policy responses to maintain essential health services built off WHO's guidance and defined essential services in this way: "Essential health services—including services for human immunodeficiency virus (HIV) infection and/or acquired immunodeficiency syndrome (AIDS), tuberculosis, malaria, routine immunization, noncommunicable diseases, nutrition and reproductive, maternal, newborn, child and adolescent health—are foundational to primary health care and vital for protecting population health" (Gurley et al., 2022, p. 168). Disruption to these services was found to increase mortality and widen existing inequities in care (Gurley et al., 2022). This study highlights two important aspects of defining some health care services as *essential*. First, they are *essential* in relationship to their impact on human health, not based on situational pressure. For example, malaria care is essential regardless of whether there are COVID-19 based pressures on the health care system. Essential health care services related to IPV will similarly be based on the conditions and sequelae that co-occur with IPV. A discussion of the most common health conditions related to IPV, as well as their impact on human health, can be found in Chapter 4. Second, there are documented existing inequities in accessing this care (Wasserman et al., 2019). That is, just because services are designated as *essential* does not mean that they are currently broadly available in all locations even in steady state conditions, let alone during PHEs. The committee acknowledges these services are unevenly available throughout the United States. The committee also notes that essential health care services are determined by the health care needs of populations and not the ability to provide them. Therefore, essential health care services retain their designation of essential, regardless of a system's status in the disaster cycle.

The committee sought to address the balance between essential health care services and the service obstacles created within a PHE. This led them to draw on the Federal Emergency Management Agency's (FEMA's) Community Lifelines approach and its associated toolkits, detailed in the current National Response Framework (DHS, 2019; FEMA, 2023). This approach designates critical Lifelines that support community function which should be stabilized and recovered during a disaster. One such Lifeline is Health and Medical, with public health as a key component (FEMA, 2023). By providing subsequent objectives leading to final stabilization of a given Lifeline, this framework both delineates which services are essential and outlines an order for the recovery of those services, given the constraints of the PHE.

The Community Lifelines Implementation Toolkit notes that the primary objective of the Lifelines is to ensure delivery of services critical to addressing immediate threats to life and property (FEMA, 2023). Medical services meeting that mark would be the first recovered (FEMA, 2023). However, the framework also states that the "network of assets, services, and capabilities that provide Lifeline services are used day-to-day to support the recurring

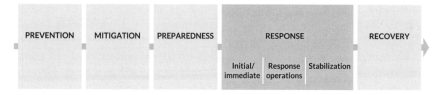

FIGURE 6-1 Five phases of emergency planning, with three phases of disaster response

needs of the community and enable all other aspects of society to function" (FEMA, 2023). This means that after life safety is established, the other services needed for the full function of the community should be reestablished as well. While these are not less essential for human well-being, they are less time sensitive based on immense resource constraints during PHEs.

RESTORING ESSENTIAL INTIMATE PARTNER VIOLENCE CARE IN PHASES

The committee identified the essential health care services related to IPV during steady state conditions in Chapter 4. The committee then defined three phases of disaster response, described below (also see Figure 6-1), and delineated which essential services to reestablish during each phase (Table 6-1).

The *initial* or *immediate response phase* occurs while the situation is unstable and unknown, before supplementary resources can be deployed to the affected area or resources within the community can be redirected. During this phase, disaster health responders' efforts are focused on saving and sustaining life using limited resources.[1] This is also the point at which initial requests for additional resources are made.

The *response operation phase* occurs once the health care system and associated jurisdictional authorities have assessed the incident and have stood up relevant incident coordination structures. During this phase, disaster health responders have begun to receive additional resources, such as supplies and staff to support temporary care delivery sites. At this point, while health care delivery capacity has increased beyond life-saving and -sustaining activities, resources are not adequate to support the full delivery of all essential health care services related to IPV for all individuals.

The *stabilization phase* occurs when basic lifeline services have been provided to PHE survivors, either by rapid reestablishment of those services

---

[1] For the purposes of this report, *disaster health responders* are the leaders and staff with expertise in public health and health care who are working and providing care in those settings during response to a PHE.

or through the employment of a contingency response solution. At this point all essential health care services related to IPV are available for all individuals.

The committee identified these phases of restoration not only to guide prioritization of specific essential health care services, but also to identify those services that, once they have been identified as part of public health preparedness planning, can be included as part of the process of identifying necessary supplies for emergency stockpiles and can, in some cases, be provided by a variety of clinical staff. As Table 6-1 depicts, the committee identified the services that need to be prioritized and what services could be restored once response operations and stabilization are occurring according to response plans. Chapter 4 details the evidence to support the services in Table 6-1. The table prioritizes services that require immediate access even during PHEs and ones that cannot be expected to be delivered when resources are severely restricted.

Recommendation: 5
Essential health care services related to intimate partner violence during steady state conditions remain essential during public health emergencies (PHEs), but health care systems should restore them in phases that consider the obstacles to delivering this care during different phases of the PHE response (see Table 6-1).

TABLE 6-1 Essential Health Care Services for Intimate Partner Violence During Public Health Emergencies—A Phased Return to Steady State

Essential Health Care Service	PHASE WHEN SERVICE SHOULD BE RESTORED		
	Initial	Response operations	Stabilization
Universal IPV screening/inquiry and education			
Safety planning			
Forensic medical exams			
Emergency medical care			
Treatment of physical injury			
Gynecologic and reproductive health care including pregnancy termination	Urgent	Non-urgent	
Obstetric care	Urgent	Non-urgent	
Perinatal home visits			
Contraception and emergency contraception	Contraceptives not requiring procedures or immediate follow-up	All types of contraceptives	
Screening and treatment of sexually transmitted infections and HIV	Treatment and rapid testing	Treatment and all screening	
Substance abuse treatment	Withdrawal mitigation	All treatment	
Pharmacy/medication management			
Primary and specialty care			
Mental health care	Urgent/Crisis	Non-urgent	
Dental care	Urgent treatment for acute injuries	Urgent treatment for acute injuries	
Support services including shelter, nutritional assistance, child care			

Restore services for all patients

Selectively restore services for acute needs or restore targeted services

Do not restore services during this phase

The committee integrated the Community Lifelines approach in the development of a phased approach to sustaining and restoring essential health care services related to IPV. It prioritized delivery of essential health care services related to IPV that are most integral to protecting life safety during the initial phase of PHE response. In some cases, specific components of an essential health care service are required to protect life. This is due to the severity and time-sensitive nature of certain IPV-related health conditions. In other cases, components are critical for averting serious or life-threatening outcomes in vulnerable patients, such as pregnant women. For example, during the initial phase of PHE response, a woman experiencing IPV with abnormal vaginal bleeding or discharge may have an urgent need for gynecologic care because these symptoms may indicate serious injury or infection that could rapidly progress to life-threatening hemorrhage or sepsis. In contrast, while timely preventive gynecologic care is essential for women's health, a *brief* delay during the initial phase of PHE response is unlikely to immediately lead to an acutely life-threatening condition. Additionally, as previously discussed, unintended pregnancy as well as IPV during pregnancy are associated with serious adverse health outcomes, including fetal death and intimate partner homicide. Thus, women who have experienced IPV-related rape or IPV-related unintended pregnancy that need to prevent or terminate a pregnancy have a time-sensitive need to access care. Emergency contraceptive methods generally need to be initiated within 3-5 days of the assault (Mazer-Amirshahi and Ye, 2023). During times of limited availability of providers and medical supplies, it is logical to engage medical interventions that have the least intensive needs for both. Medication-based protocols for pregnancy termination do not require special equipment and do not have the multiple and prolonged staff needs associated with surgical procedures. However, these medications need to be taken during the first 70 days of gestation (Beaman et al., 2020). Therefore, this care cannot be deferred.

The committee also considered PHE-induced constraints related to staff and supply availability during PHE response in the development of this phased approach. During the initial and response operations phases in particular, health care systems may reallocate staff and supplies in the short term to treat life-threatening injuries and conditions. This was exemplified on a large scale during the initial response to the COVID-19 pandemic. Many hospitals assigned clinicians who did not typically staff the intensive care unit (ICU) to their ICUs and cancelled elective surgeries so that both staff and supplies could be directed to caring for the surge of seriously ill patients (Mathews et al., 2022; Kerlin et al., 2021). The committee prioritized components of essential health care services that protect life safety and can be delivered safely and effectively using the least staff and supplies. For example, some forms of contraception, such as intrauterine devices or subdermal implants, require an office procedure and a specially trained clinician (Teal and Edelman, 2021). Such procedures usually require more than one staff member and additional supplies. Other forms of contraception can be delivered as an injection or pill (Teal and Edelman, 2021). Those forms of contraception require fewer staff members, less staff time, minimal supplies, and do not require a provider to be trained in a special procedure.

Universal education and screening are crucial for connecting women experiencing IPV to needed resources during PHEs, whether they seek care in traditional clinical settings or the various settings in which disaster health responders deliver care. However, the committee recognizes that during PHEs, health care delivery often occurs under substantial time constraints and levels of urgency, particularly during the initial phase of PHE response. As a result, universal IPV education in the form of substantial educational discussions may not be feasible. During this time, prominently displayed posters and easily accessed brochures can be used to make women aware of key IPV-related information and how to access resources. Posters can be displayed in a variety of places, including temporary health care facilities such as alternate care sites, vehicles used for transporting people affected by the PHE, and emergency shelters. Universal IPV screening can also be maintained throughout the PHE response phase but may need to be modified. For example, while most screening instruments involve several questions, screening during the initial phase of a PHE may need to be limited to one or two targeted questions due to the acute time constraints associated with caring for a high volume of people experiencing acutely life-threatening conditions. Disaster health responders will need to keep women's health, safety, and privacy in mind when asking such questions, just as providers do when screening during steady state conditions. The committee acknowledges that during the initial and response operations phases of PHE response, there are some circumstances and settings in which universal IPV screening and education are not appropriate. For example, the initial encounter with a woman in the moments after she has been extracted from a building that was destroyed by a tornado is not an appropriate time for IPV screening or education because the focus of care must be on ensuring that she is medically stable.

Crisis Standards of Care and Resource-Limited Conditions

Crisis standards of care (CSCs) were conceptualized as a means of guiding health care decision making during a disaster or PHE in times when a substantial change in the ability to deliver usual health care is experienced or expected (IOM, 2009). The goal of a CSC approach rests on a well known tenet of disaster management: do the greatest good for the greatest number of patients. The ethical challenges of implementing CSC guidelines were evident during the COVID-19 pandemic, when clinicians had to make difficult choices about resource allocation, such as reuse of PPE, identifying what surgeries must be performed and which should be delayed or canceled, and deciding who on the health care team was deemed essential. A lack of planning for women's health needs during PHEs potentially increases risks for those who have been experiencing IPV.

Thus, a CSC approach can be applied in IPV care to prioritize the allocation of resources for IPV survivors who are at the highest risk of harm, according to such criteria as severity of injuries, likelihood of survival, and potential to prevent further harm. In the context of IPV health care, a modification of the standards of care can mean providing more focused and streamlined services, such as prioritizing emergency medical care and safety planning over longer-term counseling or therapy.

CSCs emphasize the importance of collaboration and coordination among clinicians, emergency responders, and other stakeholders and could involve strengthening partnerships between clinicians and those community-based organizations that can provide additional resources and support (IOM, 2009). Clear communication and transparency about the allocation of resources and the decision-making process are central tenets of CSCs and are relevant to IPV care, as survivors may be hesitant to seek care or disclose their experiences because of fear of retaliation or stigma.

The COVID-19 pandemic served as a reminder that existing societal inequities are exacerbated during PHEs (Evans et al., 2020; Mishra et al., 2021). While CSCs rest on their ability to support unbiased and consistent health care decision making, unconscious biases and existing structural inequalities were clearly present in early pandemic health care (Evans et al., 2020; Hick et al., 2021; Mishra et al., 2021). For example, reports emerged describing how hospitals were not accepting or were delaying transfers based on the insurance status of patients (Evans et al., 2020). In IPV care during a PHE, ensuring equitable access to information, basic health care, testing, vaccinations, and early treatment is even more essential for individuals who may have pre-existing challenges in accessing health care (Evans et al., 2020; Hick et al., 2021). Incorporating CSC protocols with an equity focus is therefore essential in the development of IPV PHE protocols. While CSC protocols used for making urgent allocation decisions in a disaster are not expected to address structural inequity, they ought not worsen existing underlying disparities (Hick et al., 2021).

INTIMATE PARTNER VIOLENCE CARE DURING PUBLIC HEALTH EMERGENCIES IN GLOBAL CRISIS SETTINGS

There is much knowledge to be gained from the decades of advancements to support women and girls affected by gender-based violence (GBV) in global humanitarian crisis settings, which can inform federal plans. GBV is a broader term used to refer to acts of violence that disproportionately affect a group of people based on their gender. GBV includes IPV and other forms of abuse, such as child marriage, sexual harassment, and human trafficking (UN Women, 2022). Given the limited existing U.S.-based IPV and disaster protocols, this section first covers the available guidance on sheltering, followed by a discussion of standards for providing essential health care services from international guidance sources. These standards represent common agreement on what constitutes adequate quality and are developed to be universally relevant to all emergency settings, with the expectation that the guidance will be modified according to the specific context.

Inter-Agency Minimum Standards for Gender-Based Violence in Emergencies

The United Nations Population Fund's (UNFPA) Inter-Agency Minimum Standards for Gender-Based Violence in Emergencies[2] (GBVIMs) provides 16 minimum standards for GBV prevention and response programming in emergencies (UNFPA, 2019). The 16 minimum standards describe the capabilities needed to prevent and respond effectively to GBV across different sectors. Their objective is to establish a common understanding of what constitutes minimum prevention and response programming for GBV in emergencies. This guidance was useful to the committee during the process of identifying priorities for ensuring access to essential health care services related to IPV during PHEs in the United States.

In a U.S.-based IPV context, the GBVIMS can provide transferable guidance through four key mechanisms:

- **Developing policies and protocols** for screening, assessing, and treating patients who have experienced IPV (with contextualization, the guidelines can be used for mandatory reporting, particularly around supporting safety, confidentiality, and respect for self-determination);
- **Providing training and support** for training clinicians on identifying, responding to, and referring IPV survivors;
- **Strengthening partnerships and referral networks,** including collaboration and coordination among service providers, such as health care facilities, social service agencies, and law enforcement; and
- **Ensuring survivor-centered care** through guidance on responsive care that includes the needs and preferences of the IPV survivors, focusing on principles of dignity and respect.

---

[2] https://www.unfpa.org/minimum-standards (accessed August 25, 2023).

Individuals who experience IPV may be reluctant to disclose or ask for help if they do not encounter survivor-centered attitudes or if clinicians are not equipped to discuss or knowledgeable about IPV. Therefore, the GBVIMS guidance for survivor-centered care emphasizes the following actions for health care facilities:

- Having female staff present;
- Asking appropriate questions in a nonjudgmental manner;
- Having private spaces for consultation;
- Having protocols for provision of health care, essential medicines, and supplies to survivors;

BOX 6-1
Essential Actions to Support IPV Survivors During PHEs

- Pre-position supplies to ensure receipt of post-exposure prophylaxis for HIV and emergency contraception within 72 hours of potential exposure.
- Work with health care organizations through existing relationships (e.g., emergency management and Health Care Coalitions) to ensure immediate access to essential health care services at the onset of an emergency.
- Work with health care staff to ensure that survivors of IPV have access to high-quality, lifesaving health care.
- Work with health care entities to assess health care facility readiness and health care service provision and advocate to address gaps to ensure that an adequate health care response is in place and accessible to survivors.
- Enhance the capacity of the health care team, including nurses, to deliver quality care to survivors through training, support, and supervision, including training and education about IPV prevention and response and the clinical management of rape and IPV.
- Establish and maintain safe referral systems among health care and other services and among different levels of health care, particularly where life-threatening injuries or injuries necessitating surgical intervention require referral to a facility providing more complex care.

- Offering confidential mechanisms for documentation;
- Communicating clearly about the types of services that are available; and
- Communicating that any disclosure made will be approached with respect, sympathy, and confidentiality (UNFPA, 2019, p. 28).

See Box 6-1 for the GBVIMS standards, adapted slightly to fit the context of this report.

- Work with communities to develop safe access, including sheltering and transportation options for IPV survivors to obtain health services.
- Ensure that a consistent IPV point person is present in Health Care Coalition meetings and activities and that a non-clinical individual participates in IPV meetings.
- Train and support clinicians to guide medical and nonmedical personnel on the needs of IPV survivors and the importance of promoting survivor-centered, compassionate care that is appropriate to the survivor's age, gender, and developmental stage.
- Strengthen the capacity of community health providers and other community-based organizations, which are important entry points for referrals and basic support.
- Work with health care entities to ensure follow-up and referral for IPV cases.
- Work with clinicians and community leaders to inform the community about the urgency of, and the procedures for, referring survivors of IPV—if safe to do so.
- Disseminate information and engage communities on the health consequences of IPV—if PHE conditions allow.
- Reestablish comprehensive sexual and reproductive health care services and strengthen local health systems after the immediate emergency onset and during transition phases.

SOURCE: Adapted from the *Inter-Agency Minimum Standards for Gender-Based Violence in Emergencies* (2019, p. 27). https://www.unfpa.org/minimum-standards (accessed June 26, 2023).

Minimum Initial Services Package for Sexual and Reproductive Health

The Minimum Initial Services Package (MISP)[3] for Sexual and Reproductive Health is UNFPA's set of priority life-saving sexual and reproductive health services and activities designed to be implemented at the onset of all humanitarian emergencies (UNFPA, 2020). The goal of implementation of the MISP is to prevent or decrease sexual and reproductive health-related morbidity and mortality among the populations affected by the crisis (UNFPA, 2020).

The MISP and associated *Interagency Field Manual on Reproductive Health in Humanitarian Settings* provides guidance for clinical care in emergency settings for survivors of sexual violence, such as management of physical injuries and the provision of emergency contraception and prophylaxis for sexually transmitted infections and HIV as well as guidance on providing psychosocial support in emergencies, including counseling and other mental health services to support survivors (IAWG, 2018). Emergency triage is an important component of this guidance and involves quickly assessing the medical needs of survivors and prioritizing care based on the severity of their condition. Similar to the GBVIMS, key components include ensuring access to accurate and timely information about the patients' health and well-being and developing strong referral networks for connecting survivors with appropriate services and resources.

Essential Services Package

UNFPA's Essential Services Package (ESP) is designed to be applicable in any setting, although it was originally intended for stable settings where the response organizations have established communications and implementation processes. The ESP provides guidance for the identification of essential services needed for women and girls who have experienced GBV, with a focus on necessary services to be provided by health care, social services, police, and justice organizations (UNFPA, 2015).

The ESP, GBVIMS, and MISP each provide guidance about implementation, but they do so in different ways. While the GBVIMS and MISP were developed specifically for use in humanitarian emergencies and provide more targeted guidance on specific issues related to GBV and reproductive health services, the ESP provides a comprehensive set of guidelines for providing essential health care services. IPV care challenges that are not well defined in the United States (e.g., the triage of survivors in resource-limited settings, IPV toolkits for field triage, communications in resource-limited environments

---

[3] https://www.unfpa.org/resources/minimum-initial-service-package-misp-srh-crisis-situations (accessed August 25, 2023).

that allow for health care provider access, referral networks, procedures for just-in-time training, management of chronic and ongoing health conditions without causing further trauma) can be adapted from these international resources. This includes having well-established formal partnership agreements and protocols with health care centers in order to provide needed services, such as emergency contraception and related treatment under the direction of a licensed health professional.

ADDRESSING CHALLENGES IN SUSTAINING HEALTH CARE SERVICES

Training for Disaster Response Personnel

During the immediate response phase of a disaster, emergency health care may be delivered by local, state, or federal response teams or volunteer organizations active in disasters (VOADs), which come from diverse health care backgrounds, so IPV training may not be a requirement of their usual health care role (NVOAD, 2020). Scant evidence exists among federal disaster response entities, as well as among national VOADs, regarding protocols or guidance for IPV care in emergencies.

Ongoing capacity development for disaster health responders is imperative. This can be accomplished by dedicating time for participation in education and training focused on IPV identification and care in the context of PHEs. Incorporating IPV health care services will require the availability of clinicians qualified to perform such care. Licensing concerns may present an issue, as was seen in communities experiencing patient surges during the COVID-19 pandemic. Future planning will need to include consideration for "changes to licensing or certification requirements and suspension or modification of protocols, rules, or even certain laws may be necessary to coordinate the restoration of a health care system" (IOM, 2015, p. 176).

Access to Supplies and Community Resources

Protocols are needed to guide the allocation of resources, such as supplies and medications, when providing IPV care in austere or disrupted health care environments. Additionally, IPV resources outside of health care institutions are needed to ensure the safety, security, and community acceptability of the care setting (UNFPA, 2019). Long-term investments in local women's organizations can help ensure that IPV services are sustainable and viable both during and after PHEs. Investing resources—material, intellectual, and financial—in these groups can provide communities with effective IPV care during PHEs as well as sustainable services after an emergency. As evidenced in the MISP framework, input from women's rights activists, who have expertise on women's experiences, risks, and perspectives, can help guide decisions about resource allocation (UNFPA, 2020).

Challenges for Community-Based Organizations

During a PHE, community-based groups that help victims of IPV may face several unforeseen difficulties or challenges. These impediments can include a complete disruption in services, reduced and limited resources, an increase in demand for services, increased access for underserved populations, burnout, a lack of coordination, an increased risk of repetitive exposure to violence, and a myriad of mental health challenges. It is critical therefore to have established ongoing partnerships with essential community services providers before the emergency.

Restricted and Reduced Resources: PHEs may have a substantial impact on a region's economy, resulting in reduced financial resources available to community-based groups. Supply chains may also be disrupted, which limits access to supplies and equipment. This hampers these groups' ability to deliver care to people experiencing IPV (Garcia et al., 2022; Lauve-Moon and Ferreira, 2016; Sapire et al., 2022).

Disruption of Services: Disasters can result in infrastructure being destroyed, people being uprooted, and communication lines being disrupted, making it challenging for community-based groups to offer basic support services to women experiencing IPV. Virtual support might be limited as well, which could interrupt services such as telehealth (First et al., 2017; Lauve-Moon and Ferreira, 2016; Sapire et al., 2022).

Increased Demand for Services: Generally speaking, disasters cause stress levels to spike, and this increases vulnerability for those at risk for IPV. Community-based groups might be easier to access than traditional health care settings, but they lack sufficient capacity. During the COVID-19 pandemic, several services were deemed nonessential, resulting in a backlog of services for clients in need (First et al., 2017; Lauve-Moon and Ferreira, 2016; Sapire et al., 2022; Toccalino et al., 2022).

Burnout: During the COVID-19 pandemic, IPV and sexual assault workforces based at community-based organizations were on the front lines of the PHE, continuing to meet survivor needs (Garcia et al., 2022). Trauma associated with the PHE can combine with the trauma of caring for people experiencing IPV. As with other frontline workers (e.g., the medical workforce), IPV and sexual assault frontline workers experienced chronic burnout during the COVID-19 outbreak (Hu et al., 2020; Morgantini et al., 2020; Stogner et al., 2020). Community-based organizations that help IPV victims may lessen these difficulties by forming solid alliances with other groups, creating emergency plans, and boosting their capacity to deliver trauma-informed support services.

Protecting Confidentiality

Protecting the confidentiality of individuals experiencing IPV is essential to health and personal safety. During the immediate response period, when usual health care operations are disrupted or care is being provided in austere settings, such as a field hospital, the standard means of communicating and reporting protected health information may be altered. Furthermore, mandatory reporting (which varies among states, tribes, and territories) may be disrupted by limited communications, limited law enforcement availability, or when local law enforcement is being supported by federal resources, such as the National Guard.

The federal law, HIPAA[4] sets national standards for the privacy of individuals' *protected health information*, which includes medical records and other individually identifiable health information. The law's Privacy Rule requires that clinicians, health plans, and other health care clearinghouses put in place measures to ensure that patients' health information remains confidential. While the Privacy Rule cannot be suspended during a national or public health emergency, certain provisions may be waived during declared disasters that present specific safety risks to individuals experiencing IPV who are seeking health care.[5] Additionally, support service providers who receive funding under the *Violence Against Women Act*[6] must follow a stricter set of confidentiality laws.

Health care clinicians have an ethical responsibility to protect the safety of their patients, and as such, their focus should remain on the individual who is experiencing IPV, including offering ongoing and supportive access to those health care resources that are available, addressing safety issues, and ensuring that the patient is aware of all available options (Lizdas et al., 2019). At the same time, information sharing on the part of care teams during PHEs is still beneficial to the provision of essential health care services. To best support the delivery of safe and equitable health care, protocols that define standards of patient confidentiality during periods when HIPAA provisions are waived need to be developed, including procedures for communications

---

[4] *Health Insurance Portability and Accountability Act of 1996 Privacy Rule.* 45 CFR Part 160 and Subparts A and E of Part 164. (December 28, 2003).

[5] Privacy Act provisions that may be waived during declared disasters include the requirements to obtain a patient's agreement to speak with family members or friends involved in the patient's care (45 CFR 164.510[b]), the requirement to honor a request to opt out of the facility directory (45 CFR 164.510[a]), the requirement to distribute a notice of privacy practices (45 CFR 164.520), the patient's right to request privacy restrictions (45 CFR 164.522[a]), and the patient's right to request confidential communications (45 CFR 164.522[b]). See https://www.hhs.gov/hipaa/for-professionals/faq/1068/is-hipaa-suspended-during-a-national-or-public-health-emergency/index.htm (accessed June 26, 2023).

[6] *Violence Against Women Reauthorization Act of 2019*, H.R 1585, 116th Cong., 1st Session (April 10, 2019) H. Rept. 116-21

and contacts for mandatory reporting and safeguarding protected health information when electronic health record systems are not functional.

CHAPTER SUMMARY

Essential health care services are defined in terms of their impact on human health. The essential health care services related to IPV during steady state conditions remain essential during PHEs. The response to a PHE is marked by conditions such as infrastructure damage and resource restrictions that create barriers to care delivery that improve as resources are directed to the affected geographic area. Therefore, a phased restoration of essential health care services related to IPV is the most practical approach that also ensures care access to those who need it most. Planning for restoration of these services can be informed by current disaster management strategies, such as the equitable application of crisis standards of care, as well as guidance from international humanitarian organizations.

Barriers to restoring and sustaining essential services can be overcome with a variety of strategies. These include cooperation with community-based organizations, incorporating considerations for delivering IPV-related care in PHE planning, and adequate training for disaster responders. Importantly, the confidentiality of people experiencing IPV should be protected in all services.

REFERENCES

Beaman, J., C. Prifti, E. B. Schwarz, and M. Sobota. 2020. Medication to manage abortion and miscarriage. *J Gen Intern Med* 35(8):2398-2405.

DHS (Department of Homeland Security). 2019. *National response framework, fourth ed.* Washington, DC: US Department of Homeland Security.

Evans, Y. N., S. Golub, G. M. Sequeira, E. Eisenstein, and S. North. 2020. Using telemedicine to reach adolescents during the COVID-19 pandemic. *J Adolesc Health* 67(4):469-471.

Evans, M., A. Berzon, and D. Hernandez. 2020. *Some California hospitals refused COVID-19 transfers for financial reasons, state emails show.* https://www.wsj.com/articles/some-california-hospitals-refused-covid-19-transfers-for-financial-reasons-state-emails-show-11603108814 (accessed August 25, 2023).

FEMA (Federal Emergency Management Agency). 2023. *Community lifelines.* https://www.fema.gov/emergency-managers/practitioners/lifelines (accessed August 25, 2023).

First, J. M., N. L. First, and J. B. Houston. 2017. Intimate partner violence and disasters: A framework for empowering women experiencing violence in disaster settings. *Affilia* 32(3):390-403.

Garcia, R., C. Henderson, K. Randell, A. Villaveces, A. Katz, F. Abioye, S. DeGue, K. Premo, S. Miller-Wallfish, J. C. Chang, E. Miller, and M. I. Ragavan. 2022. The impact of the COVID-19 pandemic on intimate partner violence advocates and agencies. *J Fam Violence* 37(6):893-906.

Gurley, N., E. Ebeling, A. Bennett, J. K. Kashondo, V. A. Ogawa, C. Couteau, C. Felten, N. Gomanie, P. Irungu, K. D. Shelley, and J. C. Shearer. 2022. National policy responses to maintain essential health services during the COVID-19 pandemic. *Bull World Health Organ* 100(2):168-170.

Hick, J. L., D. Hanfling, M. K. Wynia, and E. Toner. 2021. Crisis standards of care and covid-19: What did we learn? How do we ensure equity? What should we do? *NAM Perspect* 2021.

Hu, D., Y. Kong, W. Li, Q. Han, X. Zhang, L. X. Zhu, S. W. Wan, Z. Liu, Q. Shen, J. Yang, H. G. He, and J. Zhu. 2020. Frontline nurses' burnout, anxiety, depression, and fear statuses and their associated factors during the COVID-19 outbreak in Wuhan, China: A large-scale cross-sectional study. *EClinicalMedicine* 24:100424.

IAWG (Inter-Agency Working Group on Reproductive Health in Crises). 2018. Inter-agency field manual on reproductive health in humanitarian settings.

IOM (Institute of Medicine). 2009. *Crisis standards of care: Summary of a workshop series.* Edited by C. Stroud, B. M. Altevogt, L. Nadig and M. Hougan. Washington, DC: The National Academies Press.

IOM. 2015. *Healthy, resilient, and sustainable communities after disasters: Strategies, opportunities, and planning for recovery.* Washington, DC: The National Academies Press.

Kerlin, M. P., D. K. Costa, B. S. Davis, A. J. Admon, K. C. Vranas, and J. M. Kahn. 2021. Actions taken by US hospitals to prepare for increased demand for intensive care during the first wave of COVID-19: A national survey. *Chest* 160(2):519-528.

Lauve-Moon, K., and R. J. Ferreira. 2017. An exploratory investigation: Post-disaster predictors of intimate partner violence. *Clinical Social Work Journal* 45(2):124-135.

Lizdas, K., A. O'Flaherty, N. Durborow, A. Marjavi, and A. Ali. 2019. *Compendium of state and us territory statutes and policies on domestic violence and health care.* Edited by F. W. Violence. 4th ed.

Mathews, K. S., K. P. Seitz, K. C. Vranas, A. Duggal, T. S. Valley, B. Zhao, S. Gundel, M. O. Harhay, S. Y. Chang, and C. L. Hough. 2021. Variation in initial U.S. hospital responses to the coronavirus disease 2019 pandemic. *Crit Care Med* 49(7):1038-1048.

Mazer-Amirshahi, M., and P. Ye. 2023. Emergency contraception in the emergency department. *Am J Emerg Med* 63:102-105.

Mishra, V., G. Seyedzenouzi, A. Almohtadi, T. Chowdhury, A. Khashkhusha, A. Axiaq, W. Y. E. Wong, and A. Harky. 2021. Health inequalities during COVID-19 and their effects on morbidity and mortality. *J Healthcare Leadership* 13:19-26.

Morgantini, L. A., U. Naha, H. Wang, S. Francavilla, O. Acar, J. M. Flores, S. Crivellaro, D. Moreira, M. Abern, M. Eklund, H. T. Vigneswaran, and S. M. Weine. 2020. Factors contributing to healthcare professional burnout during the COVID-19 pandemic: A rapid turnaround global survey. *PLoS ONE* 15(9):e0238217.

NVOAD (National Voluntary Organizations Active in Disaster). 2020. *Our work.* https://www.nvoad.org/ (accessed November 6, 2023).

Sapire, R., J. Ostrowski, M. Maier, G. Samari, C. Bencomo, and T. McGovern. 2022. COVID-19 and gender-based violence service provision in the United States. *PLoS ONE* 17(2):e0263970.

Stogner, J., B. L. Miller, and K. McLean. 2020. Police stress, mental health, and resiliency during the COVID-19 pandemic. *Am J Crim Justice* 45(4):718-730.

Teal, S., and A. Edelman. 2021. Contraception selection, effectiveness, and adverse effects: A review. *JAMA* 326(24):2507-2518.

Toccalino, D., H. L. Haag, M. J. Estrella, S. Cowle, P. Fuselli, M. J. Ellis, J. Gargaro, A. Colantonio, and the COVID TBI-IPV Consortium. 2022. The intersection of intimate partner violence and traumatic brain injury: Findings from an emergency summit addressing system-level changes to better support women survivors. *J Head Trauma Rehabil* 37(1):E20-E29.

UN Women. n.d. *UN women.* https://www.unwomen.org/en (accessed August 18, 2023).

UNFPA (United Nations Population Fund). 2015. *Essential services package for women and girls subject to violence.* https://www.unfpa.org/essential-services-package-women-and-girls-subject-violence (accessed August 25, 2023).

UNFPA. 2019. *The inter-agency minimum standards for gender based violence in emergencies programming.* https://www.unfpa.org/minimum-standards (accessed August 25, 2023).

UNFPA. 2020. *Minimum initial service package for sexual and reproductive health.* https://www.unfpa.org/resources/minimum-initial-service-package-misp-srh-crisis-situations (accessed August 25, 2023).

Wasserman, J., R. C. Palmer, M. M. Gomez, R. Berzon, S. A. Ibrahim, and J. Z. Ayanian. 2019. Advancing health services research to eliminate health care disparities. *Am J Public Health* 109(S1):S64-S69.

WHO (World Health Organization). 2020. *Maintaining essential health services: Operational guidance for the COVID-19 context: Interim guidance, 1 June 2020.* https://www.who.int/publications/i/item/WHO-2019-nCoV-essential_health_services-2020.2 (accessed August 25, 2023).

7

Planning and Operationalization of Intimate Partner Violence Essential Health Care Services During Public Health Emergencies

All-hazards protocols for intimate partner violence (IPV) care can draw from the past effective use of the *systems, supplies, staff, space* organizational approach to disaster preparedness and response (CDC, 2019; IOM, 2005). This approach describes four variables. Defined in terms of all-hazards IPV protocols, they are:

- Systems: The decision-making channels, logistical networks, and communication necessary for preparedness and response.
  - o Decision making for stocking supplies
  - o Coordination across disaster response agencies (both federal and state, local, tribal, and territorial) and other actors involved in IPV care
  - o Community-based organizations
  - o Identifying adaptations for how organizations can deliver care during disasters
- Supplies: The countermeasures, equipment, and basic necessities required to care for people experiencing IPV during an emergency.
  - o Tailored supply caches for IPV care
  - o Strategic National Stockpile resources
  - o Medications
  - o Guidance from the *Inter-Agency Emergency Reproductive Health Kits for Use in Humanitarian Settings* (UNFPA, 2019)
  - o Materials for standing up makeshift shelters sufficient for people at risk for experiencing IPV

- Staff: The deployment of disaster health responders as well as the training that responders will need to adequately care for people experiencing IPV.
  - On-call and telehealth IPV resources
  - Just-in-time training modules
  - Federal response specific training (Disaster Medical Assistance Teams, Veterans Health Administration, U.S. Public Health Service Public Health Emergency Response Strike Teams)
- Space: Considerations for the physical and built environment for providing adequate care for people experiencing IPV, as well as such factors that may prevent IPV during sheltering.
  - Sheltering[1]
    - Disaster shelters
    - IPV emergency shelters

Many of the examples above have been developed for use in general emergency preparedness. However, they largely have not been adapted for IPV care during an emergency. Developing protocols specific to IPV will help sustain essential health care services related to IPV during public health emergencies (PHEs). This chapter discusses these four factors and how they affect care for people experiencing IPV during emergencies.

SYSTEMS FOR INTIMATE PARTNER VIOLENCE CARE DURING PUBLIC HEALTH EMERGENCIES

Opportunities for Intimate Partner Violence Care within Existing Systems and Settings

Federal Medical Stations

Federal medical stations (FMSs) are deployable supply caches that can be rapidly deployed to convert a pre-identified building into a temporary medical facility to support health care systems anywhere in the United States (ASPR, n.d.-b). Each FMS has enough medical and pharmaceutical resources to serve up to 250 stable primary or critical care patients needing medical and nursing services for 3 days. Essentially a *hospital in a box*, FMSs are managed by the Strategic National Stockpile and can be deployed during disasters and

---

[1] Guidance about organizing emergency shelters to protect from IPV is found in this chapter. Guidance about the materials and processes needed to efficiently stand up emergency shelters in general can be found in the International Federation of the Red Cross and Red Crescent (IFRC) Shelter Kit Guidelines (https://www.ifrc.org/document/shelter-kit-guidelines) (accessed November 27, 2023).

PHEs (ASPR, n.d.-a). An FMS could be designed to have a women's health module that provides for IPV essential care and supplies.

Health Care Coalitions

Health Care Coalitions (HCCs), described in Chapter 3, coordinate and organize throughout the disaster management cycle. The role of HCCs in disseminating information and preparing health care organizations for PHEs may provide an opportunity to ensure the provision of IPV care. Moreover, HCCs provide a forum for communication and coordination between different actors (ASPR, 2016). By including IPV-related efforts in their preparedness tasks, HCCs can help sustain essential health care services related to IPV. However, HCCs often struggle with a lack of funding and resources, so they may be reluctant to take on additional roles (Barnett et al., 2022).

HCCs are uniquely positioned to locally implement promising practices and other evidence-based interventions. An example of this is training in trauma-informed care, which acknowledges a patient's life experiences (including IPV and other traumatic stressors) and is crucial for providing effective essential health care services related to IPV. In the context of a PHE, trauma-informed care recognizes the patient's past traumatic experiences and the immediate disaster incident when planning for and delivering care.

One example of an HCC incorporating trauma-informed care is the Los Angeles County Hospital Preparedness Program, which trains staff in hospitals and community clinics to provide trauma-informed health care during PHEs (Los Angeles County Health Services, 2007). Los Angeles County offers three such training modules, each designed for a specific set of end users: administrative, disaster planning, and disaster response staff; hospital and clinic staff, which includes clinical, non-clinical, and mental health staff; and Los Angeles County mental health staff. These trainings include level-setting with regard to key definitions and procedures as well as examples of how staff can plan for and implement trauma-informed care into disaster operations. Other trainings and planning documents offer more specific programmatic guidance, such as recommendations to include mental health professions in disaster planning, identifying mental health staff for hospital incident command roles, and including mental health in annual exercise programs (Shields, 2011). This program also employs the PsySTART Disaster Mental Health Triage system, which allows emergency medical and primary health care professionals to rapidly determine the risk for trauma-related stress disorders during a PHE, considering a patient's prior trauma history (Schreiber et. al., 2014). Los Angeles County has several training documents explaining PsySTART to health care professionals. Other HCCs that train staff for trauma-informed care include the North

Central Texas Trauma Regional Advisory Council and My Health My Resources of Tarrant County, Texas.

Alternate Care Sites

Alternate care sites (ACSs) are locations converted, usually temporarily, to provide health care services when existing facilities are either compromised by a hazard impact or when an expected volume of patients exceeds the available capacity and capability of the local health care system (ASPR, 2023). As part of the design process for an ACS, locations that are appropriate for the type of patient care intended to be delivered are selected. ACSs are sometimes situated inside of the health care systems they are intended to support, particularly when a specific type of care is needed. More commonly, ACSs are set up outside of the traditional health care setting. During the COVID-19 pandemic, ACSs existed in convention centers, athletic facilities, and former hospitals and clinics (Bell et al., 2021).

Although ACSs are generally thought of as providing acute or chronic care, they can be designed to meet the needs of the population affected by the PHE. For example, an ACS may be designed to provide women's health care services when these are lacking in the community. ACSs can support IPV care by intentional design choices or through post hoc changes depending on the community's specific needs.

ACS design needs to include the necessary amounts of staff and equipment in an appropriate setting so that patients can continue to receive the optimal quality of care and practitioners can provide care that does not compromise their safety (Bell et al., 2021). The development and implementation of ACS in multiple locations may pose challenges regarding staffing and supplies, especially during times of national or global emergency. The large number of ACSs that were rapidly scaled up across the country during the COVID-19 pandemic meant that essential supplies, most notably personal protective equipment but also including cots, linens, and privacy screens, were difficult or impossible to source, as supply chains were overwhelmed or limited because of global disruptions (Bell et al., 2021).

PROMISING MODELS FOR INTIMATE PARTNER VIOLENCE CARE IN PUBLIC HEALTH EMERGENCIES

Rapid Response Teams and Mobile Health Clinics

Some countries have developed models of IPV care delivery for use during humanitarian crises, in some cases through nongovernmental organizations. One such example is the Panzi Foundation, founded by 2018

Nobel Peace Prize winner, Dr. Denis Mukwege in the Democratic Republic of Congo (Panzi Foundation, 2021). While the contexts in which the Panzi Foundation serves may seem far removed from those of the United States, learning from this organization's approach and structure can help to advance IPV care during PHEs in the United States.

The Panzi Foundation has mobile care clinics and rapid response teams to address gender-based violence (Panzi Foundation, 2021). When reports of mass rape or other severe attacks on women and girls are received, the Panzi Foundation deploys rapid response teams composed of doctors, psychosocial assistants, and legal advocates urgently to provide on-the-ground care. Additionally, the Panzi Foundation's mobile health clinics include medical staff, psychosocial assistants, and lawyers who travel to remote locations to identify and provide health care to women and girls who have experienced severe gynecological trauma (Panzi Foundation, 2021). These health clinics are interdisciplinary and aim to provide holistic care to women and the affected community. Specifically, mobile health clinics provide communities with medications, supplies, and general medical care for the entire community. The Panzi Foundation partners with local health clinics to ensure they have a reliable stock of post-exposure prophylaxis medications and supplies (Panzi Foundation, 2021).

Mobile health clinics have been used in the United States as well. Some have been used specifically to deliver women's health care, including perinatal care (Edgerley et al., 2007). An analysis of 2007–2017 data from 811 mobile health clinics found that 55 percent of clients that used those clinics were women (Malone et al., 2020). As seen in overseas humanitarian crises, this model could be used to deliver IPV care during PHEs.

Integrating Intimate Partner Violence Care with Other Health Care

Primary care and other non-IPV health care units are settings in which clinicians may help ensure that their patients receive effective IPV health care and support services. Screening, universal education, and referral are three key tools that health care professionals can use in this context. However, some models have built out broader systems around these concepts. For example, the Pathways Program[2] at Chicago's Swedish Hospital[3] is a model designed to bridge the gap between health care services, support services, and social services for intimate partner violence, such as those offered

---

[2] See https://swedishcovenant.org/community/pathways-program (accessed September 15, 2023)

[3] The information about the Pathways Program in this paragraph and the next is based on a presentation to the committee by Maria Balata, *Gender-Based Violence Response in Health Care Settings*, Meeting 2, February 23, 2023.

BOX 7-1
Swedish Hospital Pathways Program

"The Pathways program is a program of Swedish, which is a community hospital located in an underserved area of Chicago—so we have one of those federal qualifications of a medically underserved area. And the program was founded in 2015 with the idea of helping bridge the gap between the services that already exist in the community through domestic violence agencies and other social service providers and our health care providers and what they were seeing here within the health care setting.

"So the thought is these services exist in the community. They're critical. They're necessary. But sometimes just giving a patient a phone number or a brochure isn't enough to actually give them the care that they need, especially if there is high acuity. And so what our program aims to do is to provide bedside crisis intervention to our patients."

- Maria Balata,
Director of Pathways,
Swedish Hospital

SOURCE: Balata, M. 2023. *Gender-Based Violence Response in Health Care Setting.* Presented at Sustaining Essential Health Care Services Related to Intimate Partner Violence During Public Health Emergencies Meeting 2, Irvine, CA.

---

by governmental domestic violence agencies and community organizations (see Box 7-1). Clinicians at Swedish Hospital identify patients who may be experiencing IPV via screening, universal education, or observation. Patients may be referred from the hospital's emergency department, inpatient units, labor and delivery unit, psychology unit, outpatient medical offices, and community partners. Once a patient is identified, the Pathways Program offers bedside crisis intervention and trauma-informed care.

Like many clinics, the Pathways Program makes connections and referrals to community organizations. However, it also takes an active role in providing care and resources to patients. Services provided include on-site mental health services, safety planning, transportation, and burner cellular phones.[4] These services are provided on a free and confidential basis in sev-

---

[4] A burner phone is a cellular phone that does not require registration with a cellular service provider and instead operates on prepaid service credits and is usually intended to be disposed of after use. See https://www.merriam-webster.com/dictionary/burner%20phone (accessed August 25, 2023).

eral languages. The Pathways Program serves people of all gender identities, sexual orientations, immigration statuses, and housing statuses. Because the health care setting is more discreet than going to a shelter or seeking counseling services elsewhere, it provides both cover and privacy for people experiencing IPV. Hospitals allow for more ambiguity, as routine treatments are provided there and allow for an easy explanation as to why someone might see a medical professional. However, mandatory reporting and clinician training may negatively affect patients' comfort with the program.

Clinics can also take a role beyond screening and referral. The PurpLE (Purpose, Listen and Engage) Health Foundation[5] has created a model designed to do so. PurpLE is a nonprofit organization intended to "advance health equity for women and girls and people across the gender spectrum who have experienced gender-based violence, no matter where they are in their survivorship journey" (see Box 7-2). PurpLE uses a trauma-informed care lens in a three-part care model that includes primary care, mental health services, and a survivor-led care navigation program. PurpLE stresses the importance of recognizing patients' social history and how lived experiences affect the type of care patients are comfortable with receiving. Integrating social histories as part of the patient intake process allows for strong care coordination and prescribing care that the patient is likely to follow through with. The PurpLE Health Foundation patient population consists of those currently experiencing IPV or trafficking, those who have recently left a relationship due to IPV, and those who are several years removed from an abusive relationship and still struggling to receive care.

PurpLE also emphasizes continuity of care for patients and aims to keep those services consistent regardless of the social service that referred the patient. PurpLE tracks barriers to care and works to mitigate the structures in place that keep patients from seeking care. PurpLE incorporates the following considerations and strategies in their IPV prevention framework:

- Considering ways to provide care for those currently experiencing IPV, e.g., contraception, safety planning, documentation, exit plan;
- Minimizing the risk for reentry into a dangerous situation or reexposure to trauma by removing financial barriers to accessing health care and assisting with housing, employment, incarceration prevention, child custody; and
- Identifying advocacy opportunities to address the systemic problems that created the need for the above care.

---

[5] See https://purplehealthfoundation.org/ (accessed September 15, 2023) The information about the PurpLE Health Foundation in this paragraph and the following paragraphs is based on a presentation to the committee by Anita Ravi, *PurpLE Health Foundation*, Meeting 3B, April 4, 2023.

BOX 7-2
PurpLE Health Foundation

"Our care model is threefold. So we do direct service care. We have an affiliated medical practice where we do primary care. We have mental health and therapy services. And then we have a survivor leader care navigation program . . .

"A big part of the work that we do and our impact [is] because every case that we see, whether it's from referral or from the process of whether or not someone was able to make it to an appointment, or decided to come back for care, or they could access the medications were recommended, we meticulously write down and we try to understand barriers to care—how we can change our own check-in process to improve care delivery."

- Anita Ravi,
Chief Executive Officer and Cofounder,
PurpLE Health Foundation

SOURCE: Ravi, A. 2023. *PurpLE Health Foundation.* Presented at Sustaining Essential Health Care Services Related to Intimate Partner Violence During Public Health Emergencies Meeting 3B, Washington, D.C.

A core component of the PurpLE organization is planning for long-term survivorship, and it is committed to helping IPV victims regardless of insurance coverage. The organization scaled up its model by educating clinicians. PurpLE has successfully trained 10,000 health care professionals across the country in trauma-informed care (Ravi, 2023).

Intimate Partner Violence Care for American Indian/Alaska Native Communities

IPV care is more effective when it is culturally relevant and salient for the people to whom it is delivered. Models of providing IPV care to American Indian/Alaska Native (AI/AN) communities demonstrate this. The Family Spirit Home Visiting Program[6] is a home visitation program

---

[6] See https://cih.jhu.edu/programs/family-spirit-home-visiting-program/ (accessed September 15, 2023). The information about the Family Spirit Program Foundation in this paragraph and the next is based on a presentation to the committee by Lisa Martin, *Family Spirit Home Visiting Program Connections and Impact on IPV during Public Health Emergencies*, Meeting 3A, March 29, 2023.

rooted in traditional Indigenous and cultural practices. Family Spirit was co-created by AI/AN communities and is centered on strength-based, culture-based, and evidence-based programming that promotes tribal sovereignty while demonstrating impact (see Box 7-3). The team at Family Spirit has developed 63 lessons across six modules. These curricula include lessons about goal setting, reproductive health, family planning, substance abuse, nutrition, budgeting, conflict resolution, and problem solving. Home visits begin during pregnancy and last through 3 years postpartum. Decision-making and assessment tools are in place to help home visitors navigate IPV in the household. If a family is in crisis, there is a structured process that home visitors are trained in to provide the best support necessary. The program was designed with the hope of having a multi-generational impact, by modeling healthy behaviors and cycles that will last beyond the nuclear family and onto the following generation.

BOX 7-3
Family Spirit Home Visiting Program

"Family Spirit is an evidence-based home visitation program taught by Native American home visitors generally. There are some communities that hire nonindigenous home visitors that they feel are part of their community and that they're trusted.

"The program is targeting and is tested with young mothers from pregnancy to age 3. So the research is spanning that age group and time period. It's designed for home-based outreach. However, as I'll mention in the presentation, it doesn't have to be home-based. We're meeting families where they're at. So we can meet in public spaces, we can meet wherever the family feels comfortable.

"It's supporting family involvement, but also connection to the community. We realize that as a home visitation program, we can't fix everything or do everything for families, but we can serve as a connection between services within the community that are available that a family might need."

- Lisa Martin,
Senior Research Associate,
Johns Hopkins Center for Indigenous Health

SOURCE: Martin, L. 2023. *Family Spirit Home Visiting Program Connections and Impact on IPV during Public Health Emergencies.* Presented at Sustaining Essential Health Care Services Related to Intimate Partner Violence During Public Health Emergencies Meeting 3A, Washington, D.C.

The Family Spirit program serves tribal communities by recognizing the specific strengths and barriers that are present in each community. Home visitor educators are thoroughly trained in the model, so they are well versed in the curriculum. The Family Spirit program has been delivered in 155 communities across 24 states. A key component in the success of the program is the strong relationships fostered with the families and the home visitors. The model works with small and large agencies. Working with different types of agencies allows for adaptation and flexibility for the program to be delivered to a variety of communities while meeting their specific needs.

Another unique challenge for providing IPV care for AI/AN women is the remoteness of many reservations. Amá Dóó Álchíní Bíghan (ADABI) Healing Shelter, Incorporated,[7] provides services to people experiencing intimate partner violence, domestic violence, sexual assault, and rape in the Chinle Agency of the Navajo Nation. It provides shelter, food, transportation, and support groups in a culturally relevant manner. ADABI refers clients to the Chinle Indian Health Service, which in turn refers clients to ADABI. This relationship has helped both organizations serve clients more effectively, such as by ensuring private spaces and safe exits for people experiencing gender-based violence.

ADABI staff have had to adapt to unique challenges, including the geography of the Navajo Nation (see Box 7-4). For example, the sparse, muddy terrain makes transportation more difficult, cell reception is sparse in many parts of the reservation, and there are not many stores, gas stations, or other support service providers from which survivors can seek help. Some families have many children, necessitating the use of several vehicles to transport them to the shelter. ADABI's 24-hour on-call line and network of shelters are designed to help overcome these challenges.

Telehealth and Other Technology-Delivered Interventions

Prioritizing access, privacy, and safety is critical for successfully implementing any technology-delivered platform during a PHE. Safety guidelines for addressing domestic violence during PHEs through technology have been released by various entities, including Futures Without Violence, the National Domestic Violence Hotline, the National Network to End Domestic Violence (NNEDV), the National Coalition Against Domestic Violence, the Center for Court Innovation, and the Sexual Violence Research Initiative (Emezue, 2020). IPV care providers, advocates, and clinicians can

---

[7] See https://www.adabihealingshelter.org/ (accessed September 15, 2023). The information on Amá Dóó Álchíní Bíghan in this paragraph and the next is based on a presentation to the committee by Lorena Halwood, *Amá Dóó Álchíní Bíghan Healing Shelter*, Meeting 3A, March 29, 2023.

BOX 7-4
Amá Dóó Álchíní Bíghan (ADABI) Healing Shelter

"We assist victims of domestic violence, sexual assault, rape victims, within the Chinle Agency of the Navajo Nation. Chinle Agency, we have 16 chapters in the Chinle Agency. So my staff, I have a staff of six. I have four advocates, one is part-time. They go from one end of the reservation to the other, seems like, and we are very remote, especially now with this bipolar weather, it's just been really hard, it's just too muddy with the snow melting right now, and even to our building here, it gets pretty muddy and we all mud bog to work in the morning or sometimes we walk over here, it's that muddy. So it's very challenging for victims to get to a highway, try to get help when they are stranded.

"And more so during the pandemic. I think it gave the batterers more tools, more chances, to abuse the victims and the children because they were quarantined with the batterer, they can't go anywhere. And a lot of our cell phones don't work in certain areas; just can you imagine a victim and six children, eight children, nowhere to go, especially if they live in a hogan, which is a round structure and everyone is in there and the victim cannot escape. Maybe sometimes she'll take her phone, hide her phone, and use it, and try to ask for help.

"We were one of the programs, we were the only two shelters, my shelter and another shelter in Kayenta, which is an hour away. We were the only two shelters that remained open during the pandemic, but it was still difficult for my staff because two of my staff, they got COVID three times, and we don't know when we pick up the victims at the emergency room or the police department if they're positive or not, and we can double mask, we can take all the precautions, but then when the family gets to a shelter, maybe a day later, another shelter, they'll call and say the person you brought, they're all COVID-positive. So that means now I have to quarantine all my staff again and we start all over again."

- Lorena Halwood,
Executive Director, ADABI

SOURCE: Halwood, L. 2023. *Amá Dóó Álchíní Bíghan (ADABI) Healing Shelter.* Presented at Sustaining Essential Health Care Services Related to Intimate Partner Violence During Public Health Emergencies Meeting 3A, Washington, D.C.

use these guidelines to gauge the applicability, usefulness and safety of different digital tools for those experiencing IPV (Emezue, 2020). NNEDV developed a PHE digital services toolkit, as part of the Safety Net Project, which outlines best practices for using various types of tools, including text, chat, and video, to communicate with people with experiences of IPV during a PHE (NNEDV, 2020). The toolkit also offers worksheets and recorded webinars focused on assessing capacity and choosing an appropriate delivery platform (NNEDV, 2020).

Many technology-based solutions were implemented during the COVID-19 pandemic, ranging from online- and phone-delivered support to conversion from in-person to digital services provided by an advocate or IPV care provider and mobile self-help apps (e.g., I-DECIDE) (Su et al., 2022). Expanding web-based services for those experiencing IPV, combined with 24-7 digitalized responses (e.g., domestic violence hotlines, telehealth services including counseling, and guidance on relevant mobile apps) have been highlighted as important resources during the COVID-19 stay-at-home orders (Emezue, 2020).

Digital Services Provided by Advocates and Clinicians

During PHEs, the physical delivery of social and support services may no longer be feasible. As a result, such services may need to be delivered digitally. For example, the Crystal Judson Family Justice Center in Pierce County, Washington, shifted to digital services during the COVID-19 pandemic (Moyer et al., 2022). They offered both traditional (e.g., domestic violence hotlines) and new services in a digital modality. Such new services included advocate follow-up to assess past-year clients' conditions and consider potential changes as well as mobile follow-up for IPV-related 911 calls to offer short- and long-term support.

Increased time investments may be needed for advocates, clinicians, and staff to provide trauma-informed care, create safety plans, and provide other sources of support (e.g., orders of protection) (Moyer et al., 2022). This time increase is partly due to the nature of the introductory content included in these interactions, which ensures ongoing safety and educates individuals about the risks of digital services. The unique safety issues associated with digital service means that IPV care providers also may need to educate clients on how to erase internet browser histories, use incognito browsers, and identify cookies as part of safety education (Schrag et al., 2022).

Mobile Applications

Novel mobile applications (apps) have been developed or modified and deployed during PHEs. Snapchat, a popular multimedia messaging app, partnered with NNEDV to include more resources for users affected by IPV and those who wanted to support a friend in such a situation (Fried, 2020). The resources were made available in subtitles for those who did not feel comfortable or safe viewing content with the sound on.

Another mobile app, Promoting Safety in Emergencies, or PROMiSE has been adapted from an individualized safety planning web app known as Pathways (O'Campo et al., 2021). PROMiSE allows women to assess the severity, danger, and potential lethality of violent behaviors in their relationship, identify safety priorities, and develop and maximize safety planning discreetly in the context of PHEs through decision-support tools (O'Campo et al., 2021). PROMiSE was developed with a disguise feature, wherein the app content is overlaid onto an innocuous webpage (e.g., Pinterest board for Home and Garden television channel) to account for women being near their partner during a PHE (O'Campo et al., 2021).

The VictimsVoice app, collaboratively designed with attorneys and law enforcement, guides users in collecting the evidence needed to inform an IPV criminal case while keeping all of the collected information (e.g., photos of injuries, physical exam details, doctor visit documentation) in one safe and secure place (Victims Voice, n.d.). All data are encrypted and stored off-device, and there is a safety exit button to ensure the site does not remain in the browser history. VictimsVoice is currently being used in all U.S. states (Victims Voice, n.d.)

The Digital Divide

Although telehealth and technology-delivered interventions designed to address IPV have advantages, several disadvantages and barriers need to be considered in the implementation process during a PHE. The key disadvantages or risks include compromising personal safety (e.g., video call software automatically storing call history), loss of privacy (e.g., disclosure of abuse via message threads intentionally or unintentionally viewed by someone else), and loss of confidentiality (e.g., personally identifying information on a mobile device used by advocates) (NNEDV, 2020). The digital divide—inequitable access to the internet and technology due to socioeconomic barriers, language barriers, low literacy levels, and limited access to technology-delivered interventions and services—affects the widespread uptake and continued IPV service provision to those in need (Ghidei et al., 2022; Storer and Nyerges, 2023). Some individuals from socially marginalized backgrounds (e.g., unhoused, AI/AN, and immigrant populations) do not have equitable access to technology-delivered IPV services.

Unstable or unavailable internet connectivity can contribute to inequities in delivering IPV services. In part, the residential or neighborhood context contributes to the inequity. One study found that even when an organization could provide clients with the equipment and technology they needed, their clients could not access a stable internet connection due to their geographical location (Ghidei et al., 2022).

As noted earlier, AI/AN people often reside in isolated and remote areas within tribal lands and reservations, which may lack health and public safety infrastructure to address IPV (Sabri et al., 2019). Within these tribal lands and reservations, individuals may reside in concentrated and dense housing with limited privacy and limited cell phone access. Even with access to cell phones, the service may not work due to connectivity issues. This issue was further complicated during the COVID-19 pandemic when court closures resulted in increased reliance on email for some court documents (see Box 7-5).

Additionally, women who are immigrants or refugees may reside in over-crowded households, limiting their ability to have privacy to engage in technology-delivered IPV interventions (Rai et al., 2020).

Individuals with disabilities also experience unique barriers to access-ing digital technologies, further exacerbating IPV-related disparities (Ghidei et al., 2022). For example, it may be difficult for members of the deaf community to access interpreters virtually or to receive services through video-based options because they rely on lip-reading (Ghidei et al., 2022). Currently, few telehealth platforms interface well with assistive technologies used by people with disabilities (Valdez, 2021).

BOX 7-5
American Indian and Alaska Native
Communities and the Digital Divide

"During the pandemic, [getting services] was even harder because the courts were closed. You either had to drop off the protection order outside the courthouse, then they had to wait until 24 hours to pick up the court papers. Or they had to email them, and with our remote areas, they don't have emails. Our cell phones don't even work."

- Lorena Halwood,
Executive Director, ADABI

SOURCE: Halwood, L. 2023. *Amá Dóó Álchíní Bíghan (ADABI) Healing Shelter.* Presented at Sustaining Essential Health Care Services Related to Intimate Partner Violence During Public Health Emergencies Meeting 3A, Washington, D.C.

Advocating for youth and young adults in communities with limited access to the internet, computers, and cameras is critical for reducing inequities in health care delivery. The available models include providing telemedicine in schools and other community settings, partnering with community organizations to reach unstably housed youth or those involved in the juvenile justice system, and expanding connections to specialty adolescent care in rural settings (Evans et al., 2020).

Challenges in the virtual delivery of IPV services emerge differently for IPV care providers. Qualitative studies of the transition to virtual delivery during the COVID-19 pandemic revealed that it was difficult for many IPV care providers accustomed to in-person settings to develop authentic emotional connections, thus making it challenging in these virtual environments to build solid therapeutic relationships (Ragavan et al., 2022; Voth Schrag et al., 2023). Other challenges included the inability to contact clients, difficulties with technology once contact had been made with a client, and the inability to engage in important aspects of their job virtually (e.g., safety assessments with children, fear that others in the home or other environment were listening into a session or tracking a client's movements electronically) (Voth Schrag et al., 2023; Williams et al., 2021).

The digital divide remains a substantial barrier to accessing IPV care. This barrier can be reduced through greater and more equitable access to internet-capable devices and the internet, language equity in digital IPV resource development, accessible digital resources for people with disabilities, and strategies to build computer literacy.

Disaster Case Management

During an emergency, access to basic necessities such as food, water, and shelter is often disrupted. These harms can be exacerbated for people experiencing IPV. Services uniquely for people experiencing IPV can also be disrupted. For example, IPV shelter operations may be interrupted during an emergency, leaving shelter clients unable to secure housing away from the person engaging in IPV. Disaster case management (DCM) is one way to connect people experiencing IPV to the services and resources they may need.

DCM is a time-limited partnership between a trained case manager and a disaster survivor that entails the development of a disaster recovery plan and a shared effort to meet the unmet needs caused by the disaster that are outlined in the recovery plan (FEMA, 2023). This disaster recovery plan aids in assessing and addressing disaster survivors' unmet needs. The plan includes resources, decision-making priorities, direction, and tools to assist the disaster survivor with an effective recovery (FEMA, 2023). DCM planning could be contextualized to fit the needs of people experiencing IPV.

Additionally, disaster case managers may be some of the first disaster health responders with whom a disaster survivor interacts. Training disaster case managers in recognizing the signs and symptoms of IPV, universal education and screening, and how to connect clients to relevant support services can help connect those experiencing IPV to vital resources.

Community-Based Intimate Partner Violence Programs

State, local, tribal, and territorial (SLTT) governments can help ensure that people experiencing IPV have the resources they need by linking them to key social and support services. For instance, Miami-Dade County's Violence Prevention and Intervention Division[8] provides several community-based resources to community members experiencing IPV (see Box 7-6). These programs include emergency shelters, long-term residential housing options, access to legal services and advocates, a one-stop center that houses many community partners, and a program that partners with the state authority on child abuse to provide resources to those experiencing domestic violence. Ensuring confidentiality within all programs is a crucial component to the safety of the survivors and the success of their programs (see Box 7-6). All programs within the Violence Prevention and Intervention Division are certified in using the Danger Assessment tool and use that alongside other needs assessments to help determine the best safety plan for their community members.

Operating community-based programs can present a variety of challenges. Some of the challenges that the Miami programs have encountered include tension with police officers who may not understand the confidentiality requirements of the different programs, families wanting to track their family members, navigating a co-ed emergency shelter space, providing additional protections to undocumented clients and residents, and a need for further education about survivorship for those working in the long-term residential housing units. The COVID-19 pandemic presented several issues for emergency shelters and residences due to room shortages and social distancing. Following the COVID-19 outbreak, programs began to integrate the use of updated technology practices into their programs, leading to further efficiency of intake and support services. Technology is something that will continue to be used throughout these programs as they continue to grow and develop.

---

[8] The information about Miami-Dade County's Violence Prevention and Intervention Division in this section is based on a presentation to the committee by Ivon Mesa, *Miami-Dade County Violence Prevention and Intervention Division*, Meeting 2, February 23, 2023.

BOX 7-6
Miami-Dade County
Violence Prevention and Intervention Division

"[W]e have statutory protections that allow employees across the division to have confidentiality and communication privileges. And definitely the confidentiality of programs is definitely a source of safety for our clients, but at the same time it becomes an issue particularly as it relates to confidential conversations and communication privileges.

"And the reason why I think this is very important, for safety purposes obviously, but it also creates certain barriers for our clients and for the services that we provide. For example, when we need to make a referral, when we need to transfer a client into a permanent housing setting for example, one of the challenges that we currently have is that most of our service providers here would like to see what has happened for that survivor, how has that survivor improved, what she or he has accomplished, so on and so forth, they like for us to share information, and statutorily we would not be able to share any information, not even with the police department.

"So if a police officer shows up at one of our facilities and they demand to speak to so and so, we will not be able to confirm or deny that that individual is there. That is very challenging because very often do I end up speaking to the chief of the police because police officers are not well trained and they don't understand the privileges and the benefits of this type of setting, so that's very upsetting to a lot of people, not being able to get any information, not being able to basically share information. But again, we are protected under the statute Florida 741.30 that provides that type of confidentiality provisions and that type of confidential communication and privileges as well."

- Ivon Mesa,
Citizen Director,
Miami-Dade County Community Action
and Human Services Department

SOURCE: Mesa, I. 2023. *Miami-Dade County Violence Prevention and Intervention Division.* Presented at Sustaining Essential Health Care Services Related to Intimate Partner Violence During Public Health Emergencies Meeting 2, Irvine, CA.

---

[a] *Florida Statutes Title XLIII. Domestic Relations* §741.30.

Multi-Sector Collaboration

Some IPV care providers have engaged in collaborative efforts to address certain adverse health effects of intimate partner violence. One example is the CACTIS Foundation,[9] a community-based organization that conducts continuing medical education, supports research-focused preclinical and clinical programs, and supports clinical trials. Currently the foundation focuses on traumatic brain injuries (TBIs) in several populations, including people experiencing IPV. Much of their work in this area has focused on improving the epidemiological measurement of concussion incidence among people experiencing IPV (see Box 7-7).

The CACTIS Foundation has developed a number of brief questionnaires and point-of-incident concussion assessments tailored for use by frontline workers and IPV care providers to assess people who have experienced IPV. CACTIS has partnered with and trained police departments, social workers, and domestic violence shelters to screen for concussions. This training also helps these frontline workers to recognize behaviors that are symptoms of concussions that they may have overlooked or attributed to other things, such as drug use (see Box 7-7). The organization is collaborating with the University of Arizona's rural pharmacy program to pilot an IPV and concussion education program in community pharmacies in rural Arizona.

Role of the Hyperlocal Response

Hyperlocal responses build on the strengths and collective impact of communities. In many cases, communities have already developed avenues for meeting their needs, which can be used during a PHE to address health care needs. For example, hyperlocal responses to COVID-19 testing and vaccinations were critical for increasing access to these public health interventions during the pandemic, especially among historically marginalized populations (Thoumi et al., 2021). A report describing hyperlocal response during the COVID-19 pandemic described three guiding principles for hyperlocal response (Thoumi et al., 2021):

- Tailoring the approach to address the unique barriers to uptake that are experienced by the community;
- Delivering services with attention to linguistic and cultural needs and preferences and Americans with Disabilities Act accessibility; and
- Using partnerships and community-engaged decision making.

---

[9] The information about the CACTIS Foundation in this section is based on a presentation to the committee by Hirsch Handmaker, *Sustaining Essential Health Care Services Related to Intimate Partner Violence During Public Health Emergencies,* Meeting 3B, April 4, 2023.

BOX 7-7
The CACTIS Foundation

"We reached out to the police departments in Mesa, a community of 400,000 people, and Tempe, to talk to them about whether their officers at the call when they were called out to a scene, would they be willing to assess a quick history like we talked about in the form I provided, and take with them their social workers. The advocates and navigators do ride-alongs, and this CARE7 group has been instrumental in us learning about victims' willingness to talk to someone about whether the event occurred because of intimate partner violence . . .

"[W]hen the officers talk to them it raises their suspicion that if they're wearing sunglasses it's not because they're a druggy or hiding something, it's because they have photophobia from the concussion. It may be that they can't fill out a form because of their double vision. It may be that the story they tell on the initial event will be different than what they tell at the end of the event, an hour later, and then worse, in terms of a deposition with regard to prosecuting the abuser, the story may be different.

"They're not lying, it is like Steve Young in the Super Bowl that he won: didn't remember a day later the names of the wide receivers who received the touchdown passes. So it is not reasonable to think that the story is going to be consistent if a victim has sustained a concussion."

- Hirsch Handmaker,
Chief executive officer and chairman,
CACTIS Foundation

SOURCE: Handmaker, H. 2023. *Sustaining Essential Health Care Services Related to Intimate Partner Violence During Public Health Emergencies.* Presented at Sustaining Essential Health Care Services Related to Intimate Partner Violence During Public Health Emergencies Meeting 3B, Irvine, CA.

Many communities that provide services to women experiencing IPV have adopted a Coordinated Community Response (CCR) approach that could be used during a PHE as part of a hyperlocal response. The CCR approach involves coordinating a combination of services made available to women who experience IPV, such as shelters, advocacy, and legal protection (Shorey et al., 2014). This approach was initially developed to address the needs of individuals engaging in IPV and was adapted to coordinate services for those experiencing IPV (Gamache, 2012). Coordination councils are a cornerstone of the CCR approach. A coordination council representing different agencies and sectors involved in addressing IPV (e.g., advocates, police, IPV care providers, the court system, and faith and community organizations) works to ensure that the person experiencing IPV can access services across systems, helping to navigate these multiple systems and increasing awareness of and access to services (e.g., plenary orders of protection), and minimizing the burden on the person experiencing IPV (Allen et al., 2013; Gamache, 2012; Javdani and Allen, 2011). These central bodies for coordination can be embedded in emergency planning and management teams.

Cross-sector collaborations can be bolstered through continued investment in implementing and nurturing partnerships and policies that explicitly promote collaboration. In particular, disaster health responders should partner more deeply with social service providers and IPV-related community-based organizations. These partnerships would allow for improved coordination and sustainment of strategies for enhancing collaboration including formal partnership agreements, clear protocols that facilitate bidirectional referrals, and opportunities for cross-training health care and agency staff (Gmelin et al., 2018; IPV Health Partners, 2017). Health centers and support services agencies' organizational readiness can be assessed using checklists to assist sites in reviewing protocols and practices relevant to care for IPV survivors, staff support and training, clinical workflows, accessibility of educational materials, inclusion of diverse populations, and data collection (IPV Health Partners, 2017). Supporting the implementation of incremental changes within health systems and support services agencies can be accomplished through collaborations that promote quality improvement (Miller-Walfish et al., 2021). Agencies can also be trained to integrate health services into their intake procedures and workflow (Gmelin et al., 2018).

SUPPLIES FOR INTIMATE PARTNER VIOLENCE CARE IN PUBLIC HEALTH EMERGENCIES

Several federal systems exist to supply disaster health responders during emergencies. These include:

- the Strategic National Stockpile (SNS), which maintains a supply of key medical supplies and countermeasures;
- the medical supplies deployed with Disaster Medical Assistance Teams (DMATs), which are intended to provide basic and life-saving health care for roughly 72 hours; and
- the resources included as part of a Federal Medical Station's (FMS's) deployment kit.

While these caches are typically supplemented by supplies maintained by private and SLTT actors, kits meant for acute deployment (such as DMAT and FMS kits) are pre-packaged and standardized. They are designed to help responders provide care in austere settings where the supplies they bring are the only health care supplies available. Therefore, such caches include necessary equipment and supplies to address essential health care—including the needs of IPV survivors during the initial response period.

The global humanitarian crisis response field has generated evidence for the types of supplies that can be cached to address IPV care needs. The United Nations Population Fund (UNFPA) maintains guidelines, the *Inter-Agency Emergency Reproductive Health Kits for Use in Humanitarian Settings*, most recently updated in 2019, that comprehensively describe necessary supplies and their use across a variety of women's health needs (UNFPA, 2019). Inter-Agency Emergency Reproductive Health (IARH) kits are designed for use in the initial response phase of a PHE and are tailored to the knowledge, competencies, and qualifications required to use each of the supplies in the kit. Different kits exist for different types of care. Examples include a post-rape treatment kit, oral and injectable contraception kit, and sexually transmitted infection kit (UNFPA, 2019). It is important to note that certain settings in the United States may encounter challenges with procuring specific and vital supplies for IPV care, such as emergency contraception. Even so, cached supplies need to be rapidly deployable in any type of PHE. An IARH-like approach of breaking down supply lists by function may be useful for training and checklist development.

TRAINING STAFF FOR INTIMATE PARTNER VIOLENCE CARE IN EMERGENCIES

Those who provide health care services during PHEs have diverse needs, and the contexts they serve vary greatly. This section addresses the need to train disaster health responders and IPV care providers in IPV identification and care and strategies to manage stress and reduce the likelihood of burnout. Also discussed is the Health Resources and Services Administration's (HRSA's) training strategy, which emphasizes cross-collaboration between health care systems and agencies serving those who have experienced IPV (HRSA, 2023).

Training Disaster Health Responders

Health care professionals, emergency medical services, police officers, and community health workers may all be considered disaster health responders in a PHE. Disaster health responders, both in health care and community settings, need to be able to recognize the signs and symptoms of IPV and feel confident in addressing IPV. Critical education and training needs for IPV care providers and disaster health responders in a PHE are summarized below.

Training in trauma-informed approaches to addressing IPV is critical for disaster health responders. The Centers for Disease Control and Prevention's Office of Readiness and Response collaborated with the Substance Abuse and Mental Health Service Administration National Center for Trauma-Informed Care to develop training for disaster health responders in PHEs that can be used for addressing IPV (CDC, 2020b). The training identified six principles that guide a trauma-informed approach (CDC, 2020b):

- safety;
- trustworthiness and transparency;
- peer support;
- collaboration and mutuality;
- empowerment and choice; and
- cultural, historical, and gender issues.

Given the intersectional identities of women experiencing IPV, the syndemic context of IPV (i.e., co-occurrence with other traumas, behavioral health issues such as substance abuse, and health conditions such as HIV), and the disproportionate burden experienced by historically marginalized groups, such as racially and ethnically minoritized women and lesbian, bisexual, transgender, and queer (LGBTQ+) populations, practitioners have encouraged an intersectional and culturally responsive approach to training in trauma-informed IPV care (Kulkarni, 2018). Training needs to engage the populations served in the development and evaluation process to ensure responsiveness to identities, context, and culture.

Just-in-Time Training

Despite preparedness planning, disaster health responders may need additional preparation for the setting and type of care needs of the PHE community, underscoring the need for just-in-time training (Weiner and Rosman, 2019). Just-in-time disaster health care training is an opportunity—perhaps the only opportunity—to reinforce prior disaster knowledge and convey other vital information about the PHE, including:

- the response setting,
- the current operational status and capacity of local health care facilities,
- other health care disaster response capacity on hand,
- local condition-specific health care practices,
- the disaster team and individual roles,

- unique vulnerabilities of the population,
- the types of patient care expected due to the PHE, and
- the environment and duration over which patients are likely to present (Weiner and Rosman, 2019).

Just-in-time disaster training, delivered as close to deployment as possible that includes local knowledge of the community and the hazard, is critical to providing effective and safe care (Weiner and Rosman, 2019). Such training is crucial for health care professionals needing more expertise or experience in PHEs and austere settings or in the care needs specific to the community. Just-in-time training can be tailored to the needs of the PHE and the community. It represents a unique opportunity to provide IPV-specific education and training.

Training Health Care Professionals

Many training options for health care professionals to respond to IPV can be used during PHEs. The National Resource Center on Domestic Violence has created a collection of educational materials related to IPV care and disaster planning (VAWnet, 2021). However, most of this guidance is targeted at IPV and domestic violence programs. The collection does include one educational item for personnel involved in disaster preparedness and response (VAWnet, 2021). However, systematic reviews of IPV training have found that although these educational strategies may positively affect health care professionals' attitudes toward individuals experiencing IPV, there is limited evidence about how these affect the identification of IPV and safety planning (Kalra et al., 2021). To increase its effectiveness, clinician education needs to be part of an ongoing process integrated with a comprehensive approach (Ambikile et al., 2022). A literature review of studies about training programs for health care providers suggested that existing programs could be enhanced by conducting initial and ongoing training to increase clinician self-efficacy in screening for and addressing IPV, building institutional support and promoting institutional champions, implementing screening protocols, and providing immediate access to advocacy and other support services (Ambikile et al., 2022). Although these principles have been evaluated in a health care context, they can be expanded to different contexts and clinicians, such as community health workers during a PHE, when health care professionals may be less accessible (Saboori et al., 2022).

Training about evidence-based protocols and promising practices to address IPV needs to be tailored to clinician type and context. Examples include:

- evidence-based prevention curriculum offered in schools and other settings that address dating violence (e.g., Dating Matters; see Niolon et al., 2019);
- universal screening for IPV among women of reproductive age in health care settings that involves validated screening tools and referral to ongoing support services (USPSTF, 2018);
- cross-sector collaboration and referral protocols between health centers and service agencies (Brown et al., 2023; Miller-Walfish, 2021; Scott et al., 2023);
- dangerousness assessment and safety planning, such as the Lethality Assessment Program for police officers, which involves screening and immediate connection to a domestic violence advocate (Messing et al., 2015);
- the Coordinated Community Response Council for hyperlocal responses (Shorey et al., 2014);
- emerging interventions based on information and communications technologies (El Morr and Layal, 2020);
- empowerment-based advocacy (Trabold et al., 2020); and
- treatment for psychological and somatic symptoms of trauma survivors, such as cognitive–behavioral therapy (Arroyo et al., 2017; Trabold et al., 2020).

A recent Cochrane review assessed the effectiveness of training programs that sought to improve health care professionals' identification of and response to IPV against women, compared with no intervention, waitlist, placebo, or training as usual (Kalra et al., 2021). Within 12 months post-intervention, the evidence suggests that IPV training may improve IPV care providers' attitudes toward IPV survivors, their self-perceived readiness to respond to IPV survivors, and their knowledge of IPV (Kalra et al., 2021). Additional research is needed to determine the longer-term effectiveness of the training, as well as the impact of the training on the health and well-being of abused women.

Project Catalyst is a demonstration project focused on developing statewide leadership teams to promote health center and IPV agency collaborations and disseminate healing-centered approaches to care for survivors of IPV seeking care in community health centers (Brown et al., 2023; Scott et al., 2023). This emphasis on cross-sector collaboration is evident in the updated HRSA IPV Strategy, and research-informed materials, including training guides and evaluation tools. These tools are available from the National Training and Technical Assistance Program called the Health Partners on IPV and Exploitation (Futures Without Violence, 2023).

Wellness and Anti-Burnout Training

IPV care providers and disaster health responders experience secondary traumatic stress, burnout, and compassion fatigue, which are exacerbated in a PHE (Benincasa et al., 2022; Ragavan et al., 2022; Vagni et al., 2022). All clinicians and stakeholders need training for addressing potential burnout and compassion fatigue as well as supportive environments that do not contribute to burnout. Mindfulness-based interventions are an evidence-based approach to reducing stress and improving well-being among health care providers that could be beneficial for IPV care providers (Lomas et al., 2018). However, these strategies need to be couched within a systems-based approach that identifies and targets known external factors driving burnout while simultaneously including clinician and patient feedback (NASEM, 2019).

HRSA Training Strategy

Training IPV care providers and implementing system-level policies and protocols are essential components of ensuring the preparedness of health systems to address IPV and related health consequences. The *2023–2025 HRSA Strategy to Address Intimate Partner Violence* focuses on coordinating efforts to strengthen infrastructure and workforce capacity. It emphasizes that training is essential to promote culturally informed and trauma-informed care practices as well as improve skills and knowledge (HRSA, 2023). The strategy recommends integrating training for IPV care into existing programs and providing training and technical assistance specific to IPV to the health care workforce. The National Training and Technical Assistance Program, called Health Partners on IPV + Exploitation,[10] provides training on trauma-informed services, education, and tools for building partnerships, policy development, and integration of processes to promote prevention and increase referrals to services for individuals at risk for and experiencing IPV as well as exploitation (including human trafficking). Specifically, this training program works to implement and strengthen collaborations between health centers and agencies serving those who have experienced IPV.

Care Setting–Specific Protocols and Training

The limited existing protocols and training programs specific to essential health care services for IPV in PHEs underscores the need to develop such interventions. In keeping with an all-hazards framework, programming is needed that is rapidly deployable, that can be harmonized across

---

[10] https://healthpartnersipve.org/ (accessed September 4, 2023).

different care settings, and that can provide relevant and applicable but broad guidance.

The development of protocols needs to take an all-hazards approach. However, no one form of guidance will suit all situations. Tailoring protocols to address the contextual needs of populations and organizations will be beneficial, particularly for ensuring the equitable implementation of care practices (Brownson et al., 2021; Powell et al., 2017). Tailoring protocols to specific areas such as medically underserved areas, health care professional shortage areas, mental health professional shortage areas, areas served by Indian Health Services, community health centers, Federally Qualified Health Centers, the National Disaster Medical System, and HRSA need to be considered.

Training for Equitable, Culturally Aligned, and Linguistically Aligned Services

Some populations experience inequities in the consequences of IPV as well as systemic barriers to accessible health care related to IPV. These include minoritized racial/ethnic populations, immigrants, individuals with limited English proficiency (LEP), and individuals with disabilities.

Federal civil rights laws require federally funded emergency response and recovery services to provide language access to individuals with LEP as well as accommodations for individuals with disabilities[11] (DHS, 2019). The Department of Health and Human Services has provided a checklist with guidance for how to ensure language access and effective communication strategies during a PHE, which can be applied when designing and implementing essential IPV services (HHS, 2018). This includes:

- determining language and dialects spoken by individuals with LEP, who are hard of hearing, or have another disability requiring communication support in the community where services are being rendered;
- partnering with local community groups and organizations that are already serving these populations;
- coordinating with media to develop tailored messages for these groups related to the PHE; and
- providing language assistance, including access to interpreters using effective practices.

---

[11] See *Public Health Service* Act, Public Law 78-410, 78th Congress (July 1, 1944); *Robert T. Stafford Disaster Relief and Emergency Assistance Act*, Public Law 100-707, 100th Congress (May 22, 1974); *Post-Katrina Emergency Management Reform Act*, Public Law 109-295, 109th Congress (October 4, 2006); Executive Order 13166, August 11, 2000.

IPV care providers can provide culturally aligned social and health care services in PHEs. One way to ensure the delivery of culturally aligned services is to hire and train staff to develop expertise in culturally relevant care. Some services may not be culturally acceptable to specific populations, so new models of service with additional options may be needed. For example, protecting the family's reputation and stigma related to divorce have been shown to serve as barriers to Hispanic, Asian, and African immigrants seeking traditional IPV services in the United States (Hulley et al., 2023; Keller and Brennan, 2007). When designing interventions for diverse populations, it is essential to understand the varying sociocultural views concerning abusive relationships, expectations for leaving these relationships, the process in which women seek and obtain help, and perceptions of what would be helpful and safe (Barrios et al., 2021). Additionally, a more representative physician workforce can increase trust that patients have in the medical system and in their personal physician, leading to improved health outcomes (Gomez & Bernet, 2019; Jetty et al., 2022; Snyder et al., 2023).

Health care systems can ensure that services are culturally aligned by engaging racially, ethnically, and culturally diverse IPV care providers in the design and delivery of these services. A diverse health care workforce is a key strategy to addressing health inequities. Research has found that racially and ethnically minoritized clinicians are more likely to provide services to underserved communities, improve cultural and language concordance and effective communication, foster trust in clinicians and health care systems, and advocate for the needs of the populations they represent (HRSA, 2006).

Similarly, it is important to ensure that the IPV services being provided are salient to the cultural preferences of diverse groups of women during a PHE. Research has suggested that the designs of IPV services such as shelter and advocacy programs are not always inclusive for minoritized populations, which can lead to myriad barriers to help-seeking and engagement in services for historically marginalized and unserved populations (Kattari et al., 2017). The cultural tailoring of existing services could help enhance access and the effectiveness of these services. For example, in a recent evaluation of two IPV screening and prevention programs for Black women under community supervision in New York, researchers found that the protocol that included a culturally aligned navigator resulted in a 14-fold increase in engagement in IPV-related services (Goddard-Eckrich et al., 2022).

Expanding the Role of Nursing in Intimate Partner Violence Disaster Response

Nurses represent the largest health care workforce in the United States, making it imperative that the nursing workforce fully engage in disaster management (Smiley et al., 2023; Veenema et al., 2016). In health care settings where IPV survivors may present, nurses are often the first point of contact. They most frequently conduct initial triage and intake, and they generally spend more time with the patient than other health care team members.

In health care settings affected by disasters, nurses are critical at all phases of the disaster management cycle. Evidence from nurses during the COVID-19 pandemic, such as a national survey conducted by the American Nurses Association early in the pandemic, reported a lack of access to personal protective equipment; inadequate knowledge and skills related to pandemic response; a lack of decision rights as pertaining to workflow design, staffing decisions, and allocation of scarce resources; and a fundamental disconnect between frontline nurses and nurse executives and hospital administrators (ANA, 2020; Veenema et al., 2020). Longstanding efforts for nursing education in disaster preparedness and response have been sporadic, limited, and often focused on training activities related to specific disasters rather than being instilled as a standard and ongoing aspect of nursing education (Veenema et al., 2016). The recent National Academies of Sciences, Engineering, and Medicine consensus study report, *The Future of Nursing 2020–2030: Charting a Path to Achieve Health Equity,* specifically emphasizes that strengthening nurses' capacity to support disaster preparedness and PHE response is a pathway "to enhance nursing's role in addressing SDOH [social determinants of health] and improving health and health care equity" (NASEM, 2021, p. 248).

One innovative solution for increasing the availability of IPV care providers is implementing a protocol for an on-call, telehealth Sexual Assault Nurse Examiner (SANE). This could be especially relevant for federal response teams, who operate under a federal health care license and therefore would not have the same state licensure challenges as would SLTT teams or volunteers (HHS, 2017). Alternatively, state-level on-call SANE teams could be established that also cover overwhelmed emergency departments during non-disaster times. Additionally, Disaster Medical Assistance Teams could develop and offer IPV training through online modules accessible to all team members.

SPACE AND SHELTERING IN PUBLIC HEALTH EMERGENCIES

Guidance on Sheltering

The U.S. government and international organizations have developed standards for providing safe, equitable, and dignified shelter for populations affected by a disaster. While only some of these documents offer specific guidance for ensuring the safety of women and girls, many of the standards provided can help prevent IPV during sheltering.

At the federal level, the U.S. government has typically preferred that emergency sheltering for disaster survivors occur in facilities with large open spaces, such as schools, churches, and community centers (FEMA, 2021). Privacy for individuals and families is particularly challenging in these congregate spaces, also known as communal shelters in some literature. The risk of assault, abuse, and other forms of violence may increase in communal shelters, particularly at night (IASC, 2017). One review of international literature suggested that this may be due to the lack of physical divisions or boundaries, which remove the safety that some may associate with having a home (Aryanti and Muhlis, 2020). International standards have generally recommended that shelters provide adequate privacy between families (IASC, 2017; Sphere Association, 2018). At the same time, some level of openness in a shelter may allow for natural and communal defenses against violence, including IPV (Aryanti and Muhlis, 2020).

Federal disaster authorities have been flexible in allowing for noncongregate sheltering in appropriate situations. Most notably, the Federal Emergency Management Agency (FEMA) expanded public assistance funding for state and local governments' sheltering efforts to include noncongregate sheltering during the COVID-19 PHE (FEMA, 2021). Other federal policies and practices that can be extended to emergency shelters include respecting and providing services to sheltering individuals based on their gender identity; the development of clear procedures for sheltering individuals to report threats, violence, and other safety concerns; and reducing financial barriers to shelter access. These have been recommended as part of the Department of Housing and Urban Development's (HUD) *Emerging Practices to Enhance Safety at Congregate Shelters* (HUD, 2022). These guidelines were originally created for shelters for people experiencing homelessness, but they could apply to protecting the safety of people experiencing IPV who go to disaster shelters. Similar efforts to apply these HUD and FEMA policies may allow state and local governments flexibility and guidance for protecting people experiencing IPV during emergency sheltering.

International organizations have offered more specific guidance on how to ensure the safety of women and girls during sheltering. Many of these are specifically aimed at preventing IPV and other gender-based violence (IASC, 2017; Sphere Association, 2018). These include

- siting the shelter far from any violence or conflict that may put women and girls at risk;
- allowing for adequate privacy, particularly during bathing, changing, laundry, and menstrual hygiene management;
- ensuring that the shelter is well lit in all areas at all times, especially near toilets and chore areas; and

- avoiding overcrowding, which may increase the risk of IPV in the shelter.

The United Nations Inter-Agency Standing Committee developed a checklist for assessing gender equality in site selection, design, construction, and shelter allocation (IASC, 2017). While much of the language in the checklist is gender-binary, it is important to ensure that the experiences of transgender and gender-diverse people are considered in shelter planning.

CHALLENGES ASSOCIATED WITH SHELTERING

The guiding principles and recommendations for domestic violence shelters can be combined with those for PHE shelters to meet sheltering needs for those experiencing IPV during a PHE. The common characteristics between domestic violence and PHE shelters include having a welcoming space, accepting all those in need, (e.g., regardless of COVID-19 vaccination status or immigration status), and offering a safe setting (CDC, 2021; WSCADV, 2016). Screening protocols need to account for children and pets, the accessibility of the shelter (physical, linguistic, and cultural), the individual's health history (medical and substance use), and potential cultural, religious, and dietary needs, as well as transportation and safety concerns (WSCADV, 2016). Screening for IPV and safety concerns can still be prioritized if a shelter is open to the general population (e.g., not a domestic violence shelter) (Jenkins and Phillips, 2008).

The COVID-19 pandemic demonstrated that shelters can adapt steady state guidelines to the PHE context. This may involve screening for infection and trauma exposure, setting additional guidelines, supplementing communal shelters with non-congregate shelters such as hotels to provide social distancing, and making personal protective equipment accessible to clinicians and residents (CDC, 2021). The Centers for Disease Control and Prevention (CDC) Shelter Assessment Tool can be used to conduct an environmental health assessment, which addresses areas ranging from basic individual needs for food and water to wellness needs, such as pet companions (CDC, 2020a). When combined with tools for domestic violence, the CDC tool could address the intersecting needs of IPV and PHE survivors.

CHAPTER SUMMARY

The *systems, supplies, staff, space* organizing approach for disaster response seeks to ensure that service providers have the systems, supplies, staff, and space necessary to carry out their operations. IPV care during PHEs can be organized through this approach as well. Systems and settings that currently exist to support disaster response can be adapted to serve people experiencing IPV. For example, federal medical stations, Health Care Coalitions, and alternative care sites can all be designed for IPV care. Health care settings and community-based organizations have also developed models to treat IPV during PHEs such as the COVID-19 pandemic. These examples offer guidance for planning, operationalizing, and sustaining essential health services for IPV during PHEs.

REFERENCES

Allen, N. E., N. R. Todd, C. J. Anderson, S. M. Davis, S. Javdani, V. Bruehler, and H. Dorsey. 2013. Council-based approaches to intimate partner violence: Evidence for distal change in the system response. *Am J Community Psychol* 52(1-2):1-12.

Ambikile, J. S., S. Leshabari, and M. Ohnishi. 2022. Curricular limitations and recommendations for training health care providers to respond to intimate partner violence: An integrative literature review. *Trauma Violence Abuse* 23(4):1262-1269.

ANA (American Nurses Association). 2020. *COVID-19 survey March 20-April 10.* https://www.nursingworld.org/practice-policy/work-environment/health-safety/disaster-preparedness/coronavirus/what-you-need-to-know/covid-19-survey-results/ (accessed August 18, 2023).

Arroyo, K., B. Lundahl, R. Butters, M. Vanderloo, and D. S. Wood. 2017. Short-term interventions for survivors of intimate partner violence: A systematic review and meta-analysis. *Trauma Violence Abuse* 18(2):155-171.

Aryanti, T., and A. Muhlis. 2020. Disaster, gender, and space: Spatial vulnerability in post-disaster shelters. *IOP Conference Series: Earth and Environmental Science* 447:012012.

ASPR (Administration for Strategic Preparedness and Response). n.d.-a. *Products: Strategic national stockpile.* https://aspr.hhs.gov/SNS/Pages/Products.aspx (accessed August 18, 2023).

ASPR. n.d.-b. *Federal medical stations.* https://aspr.hhs.gov/SNS/Pages/Federal-Medical-Stations.aspx (accessed August 25, 2023).

ASPR. 2016. *2017-2022 health care preparedness and response capabilities.* Rockville, Maryland: U.S. Department of Health and Human Services.

ASPR. 2023. *Topic collection: Alternate care sites (including shelter medical care).* https://asprtracie.hhs.gov/technical-resources/48/alternate-care-sites-including-shelter-medical-care/47 (accessed September 15, 2023).

Barnett, D. J., L. Knieser, N. A. Errett, A. J. Rosenblum, M. Seshamani, and T. D. Kirsch. 2022. Reexamining health-care coalitions in light of COVID-19. *Disaster Med Public Health Prep* 16(3):859-863.

Barrios, V. R., L. B. L. Khaw, A. Bermea, and J. L. Hardesty. 2021. Future directions in intimate partner violence research: An intersectionality framework for analyzing women's processes of leaving abusive relationships. *J Interpers Violence* 36(23-24):NP12600-NP12625.

Bell, S. A., L. Krienke, and K. Quanstrom. 2021. Alternative care sites during the covid-19 pandemic: Policy implications for pandemic surge planning. *Disaster Med Public Health Prep* 1-3.

Benincasa, V., M. Passannante, F. Perrini, L. Carpinelli, G. Moccia, T. Marinaci, M. Capunzo, C. Pironti, A. Genovese, G. Savarese, F. De Caro, and O. Motta. 2022. Burnout and psychological vulnerability in first responders: Monitoring depersonalization and phobic anxiety during the COVID-19 pandemic. *International Journal of Environmental Research and Public Health* 19(5):2794.

Brown, R. B., S. Miller-Walfish, S. Scott, A. Ali, A. Marjavi, E. Miller, and E. A. McGuier. 2023. Cross-sector collaboration in project catalyst: Creating state partnerships to address the health impact of intimate partner violence. *Preventive Medicine Reports* 33:102204.

Brownson, R. C., S. K. Kumanyika, M. W. Kreuter, and D. Haire-Joshu. 2021. Implementation science should give higher priority to health equity. *Implement Sci* 16(1):28.

CDC (Centers for Disease Control and Prevention). 2019. *Space, staff, stuff - identifying your community's resources.* U.S. Department of Health and Human Services, Centers for Disease Control and Prevention.

CDC. 2020a. *Environmental health assessment for disaster shelters during COVID-19.* https://emergency.cdc.gov/shelterassessment/#:~:text=CDC%20Disaster%20Shelter%20Assessment&text=The%20tool%20is%20an%20assessment,tool%20to%20meet%20local%20needs (accessed August 25, 2023).

CDC. 2020b. *Infographic: 6 guiding principles to a trauma-informed approach.* https://www.cdc.gov/orr/infographics/6_principles_trauma_info.htm (accessed August 18, 2023).

CDC. 2021. *Guidance for general population disaster shelters during the COVID-19 pandemic.* https://www.cdc.gov/disasters/general-population-shelters-guidance.html?CDC_AA_refVal=https%3A%2F%2Fwww.cdc.gov%2Fcoronavirus%2F2019-ncov%2Fphp%2Feh-practitioners%2Fgeneral-population-disaster-shelters.html (accessed August 18, 2023).

DHS (Department of Homeland Security). 2019. *National response framework.* 4th ed. Washington, DC: Federal Emergency Management Agency.

Edgerley, L. P., Y. Y. El-Sayed, M. L. Druzin, M. Kiernan, and K. I. Daniels. 2007. Use of a community mobile health van to increase early access to prenatal care. *Matern Child Health J* 11(3):235-239.

El Morr, C., and M. Layal. 2020. Effectiveness of ICT-based intimate partner violence interventions: A systematic review. *BMC Public Health* 20(1):1372.

Emezue, C. 2020. Digital or digitally delivered responses to domestic and intimate partner violence during COVID-19. *JMIR Public Health and Surveillance* 6(3):e19831.

Evans, Y. N., S. Golub, G. M. Sequeira, E. Eisenstein, and S. North. 2020. Using telemedicine to reach adolescents during the COVID-19 pandemic. *J Adolesc Health* 67(4):469-471.

FEMA (Federal Emergency Management Agency). 2021. *FEMA emergency non-congregate sheltering during the covid-19 public health emergency: Policy 104-009-18.* Washington, DC: Department of Homeland Security.

FEMA. 2023. *Programs to support disaster survivors.* https://www.fema.gov/assistance/individual/disaster-survivors#case (accessed August 25, 2023).

Fried, I. 2020. *Exclusive: Snapchat to offer in-app domestic violence support.* https://www.axios.com/2020/05/11/exclusive-snapchat-to-offer-in-app-domestic-violence-support (accessed August 25, 2023).

Futures Without Violence. 2023. *Project catalyst: Statewide transformation on health, IPV, and human trafficking.* http://www.futureswithoutviolence.org/health/project-catalyst/ (accessed August 18, 2023).

Gamache, D. 2012. From victim safety to victim engagement: Comments on "the impact of victim-focused outreach on criminal legal system outcomes following police-reported intimate partner abuse." *Violence Against Women* 18(8):882-888.

Ghidei, W., S. Montesanti, L. Wells, and P. H. Silverstone. 2022. Perspectives on delivering safe and equitable trauma-focused intimate partner violence interventions via virtual means: A qualitative study during COVID-19 pandemic. *BMC Public Health* 22(1):1852.

Gmelin, T., C. A. Raible, R. Dick, S. Kukke, and E. Miller. 2018. Integrating reproductive health services into intimate partner and sexual violence victim service programs. *Violence Against Women* 24(13):1557-1569.

Goddard-Eckrich, D., B. F. Henry, S. Sardana, B. V. Thomas, A. Richer, T. Hunt, M. Chang, K. Johnson, and L. Gilbert. 2022. Evidence of help-seeking behaviors among Black women under community supervision in New York City: A plea for culturally tailored intimate partner violence interventions. *Women's Health Reports* 3(1):867-876.

Gomez, L. E., and P. Bernet. 2019. Diversity improves performance and outcomes. *Journal of the National Medical Association* 111(4):383-392.

Halwood, L. 2023. Amá Dóó Álchíní Bíghan (ADABI) Healing Shelter. Paper presented at Sustaining Essential Health Care Services Related to Intimate Partner Violence During Public Health Emergencies Meeting 3A, Washington, D.C.

Handmaker, H. 2023. Sustaining essential health care services related to intimate partner violence during public health emergencies. Paper presented at Presented at Sustaining Essential Health Care Services Related to Intimate Partner Violence During Public Health Emergencies Meeting 3B, Irvine, CA.

HHS (U.S. Department of Health and Human Services). 2017. *Calling on NDMS.* https://www.phe.gov/Preparedness/responders/ndms/Pages/calling-ndms.aspx (accessed August 18, 2023).

HHS. 2018. *Ensuring language access and effective communication during response and recovery: A checklist for emergency responders.* Department of Health and Human Services.

HRSA (Health Resources and Services Administration). 2006. *The rationale for diversity in the health professions: A review of the evidence.* Rockville, MD: U.S. Department of Health and Human Services.

HRSA. 2023. *2023-2025 HRSA strategy to address intimate partner violence.* Office of Women's Health. https://www.hrsa.gov/office-womens-health/addressing-intimate-partner-violence (accessed August 25, 2023).

HUD (U.S. Department of Housing and Urban Development). 2022. *Emerging practices to enhance safety at congregate shelters.* U.S. Department of Housing and Urban Development.

Hulley, J., L. Bailey, G. Kirkman, G. R. Gibbs, T. Gomersall, A. Latif, and A. Jones. 2023. Intimate partner violence and barriers to help-seeking among Black, Asian, minority ethnic and immigrant women: A qualitative metasynthesis of global research. *Trauma, Violence, & Abuse* 24(2):1001-1015.

IASC (Inter-Agency Standing Committee). 2017. *The gender handbook for humanitarian action.* https://interagencystandingcommittee.org/sites/default/files/migrated/2019-02/2018-iasc_gender_handbook_for_humanitarian_action_eng_0.pdf (accessed August 23, 2023).

IOM (Institute of Medicine) and NRC (National Research Council). 2005. *Public health risks of disasters.* Edited by W. H. Hooke and P. G. Rogers. Washington, DC: The National Academies Press.

IPV Health Partners. 2017. Prevent, assess, and respond: A domestic violence and human trafficking toolkit for health centers & domestic violence programs. https://ipvhealthpartners.org/wp-content/uploads/2020/10/Health-Partners-Toolkit_Oct-2020_final.pdf (accessed August 18, 2023).

Javdani, S., and N. E. Allen. 2011. Councils as empowering contexts: Mobilizing the front line to foster systems change in the response to intimate partner violence. *American Journal of Community Psychology* 48(3-4):208-221.

Jenkins, P., and B. Phillips. 2008. Battered women, catastrophe, and the context of safety after Hurricane Katrina. *NWSA Journal* 20(3):49-68.

Jetty, A., Y. Jabbarpour, J. Pollack, R. Huerto, S. Woo, and S. Petterson. 2022. Patient-physician racial concordance associated with improved healthcare use and lower healthcare expenditures in minority populations. *Journal of Racial and Ethnic Health Disparities* 9(1):68-81.

Kalra, N., L. Hooker, S. Reisenhofer, G. L. Di Tanna, and C. Garcia-Moreno. 2021. Training healthcare providers to respond to intimate partner violence against women. *Cochrane Database of Systematic Reviews* 5(5):CD012423.

Kattari, S. K., N. E. Walls, D. L. Whitfield, and L. Langenderfer Magruder. 2017. Racial and ethnic differences in experiences of discrimination in accessing social services among transgender/gender-nonconforming people. *Journal of Ethnic and Cultural Diversity in Social Work* 26(3):217-235.

Keller, E. M., and P. K. Brennan. 2007. Cultural considerations and challenges to service delivery for Sudanese victims of domestic violence: Insights from service providers and actors in the criminal justice system. *International Review of Victimology* 14(1):115-141.

Kulkarni, S. 2018. Intersectional trauma-informed intimate partner violence (IPV) services: Narrowing the gap between IPV service delivery and survivor needs. *Journal of Family Violence* 34(1):55-64.

Lomas, T., J. C. Medina, I. Ivtzan, S. Rupprecht, and F. J. Eiroa-Orosa. 2018. A systematic review of the impact of mindfulness on the well-being of healthcare professionals. *J Clin Psychol* 74(3):319-355.

Los Angeles County Health Services. 2007. *Disaster programs training index.* https://dhs.lacounty.gov/emergency-medical-services-agency/home/disaster-programs/disaster-programs-training-index/ (accessed August 11, 2023).

Malone, N. C., M. M. Williams, M. C. Smith Fawzi, J. Bennet, C. Hill, J. N. Katz, and N. E. Oriol. 2020. Mobile health clinics in the United States. *Int J Equity Health* 19(1):40.

Martin, L. 2023. Family spirit home visiting program connections and impact on IPV during public health emergencies. Paper presented at Sustaining Essential Health Care Services Related to Intimate Partner Violence During Public Health Emergencies Meeting 3A, Washington, D.C.

Mesa, I. 2023. Miami-Dade County violence prevention and intervention division. Paper presented at Sustaining Essential Health Care Services Related to Intimate Partner Violence During Public Health Emergencies Meeting 2, Irvine, CA.

Messing, J. T., J. Campbell, D. W. Webster, S. Brown, B. Patchell, and J. S. Wilson. 2015. The Oklahoma lethality assessment study: A quasi-experimental evaluation of the lethality assessment program. *Social Service Review* 89(3):499-530.

Miller-Walfish, S., J. Kwon, C. Raible, A. Ali, J. H. Bell, L. James, and E. Miller. 2021. Promoting cross-sector collaborations to address intimate partner violence in health care delivery systems using a quality assessment tool. *J Womens Health (Larchmont)* 30(11):1660-1666.

Moyer, R. A., C. J. Beck, N. Van Atter, and A. McLane. 2022. Advocacy services for survivors of intimate partner violence: Pivots and lessons learned during the COVID-19 quarantine in Tacoma, Washington. *Family Court Review* 60(2):288-302.

NASEM (National Academies of Sciences, Engineering, and Medicine). 2019. *Taking action against clinician burnout: A systems approach to professional well-being.* Washington, DC: The National Academies Press.

NASEM. 2021. *The future of nursing 2020-2030: Charting a path to achieve health equity.* Edited by M. K. Wakefield, D. R. Williams, S. Le Menestrel and J. L. Flaubert. Washington, DC: The National Academies Press.

Niolon, P. H., A. M. Vivolo-Kantor, A. J. Tracy, N. E. Latzman, T. D. Little, S. DeGue, K. M. Lang, L. F. Estefan, S. R. Ghazarian, W. L. K. McIntosh, B. Taylor, L. L. Johnson, H. Kuoh, T. Burton, B. Fortson, E. A. Mumford, S. C. Nelson, H. Joseph, L. A. Valle, and A. T. Tharp. 2019. An RCT of dating matters: Effects on teen dating violence and relationship behaviors. *Am J Prev Med* 57(1):13-23.

NNEDV (National Network to End Domestic Violence). 2020. *Safety net project.* https://www.techsafety.org/digital-services-during-public-health-crises (accessed August 18, 2023).

O'Campo, P., A. Velonis, P. Buhariwala, J. Kamalanathan, M. A. Hassan, and N. Metheny. 2021. Design and development of a suite of intimate partner violence screening and safety planning web apps: User-centered approach. *J Medical Internet Research* 23(12):e24114.

Panzi Foundation. 2021. *Reaching survivors at the last mile*. https://panzifoundation.org/mobile-clinics-and-rapid-response-missions/ (accessed August 18, 2023).

Powell, B. J., R. S. Beidas, C. C. Lewis, G. A. Aarons, J. C. McMillen, E. K. Proctor, and D. S. Mandell. 2017. Methods to improve the selection and tailoring of implementation strategies. *J Behavioral Health Services Research* 44(2):177-194.

Ragavan, M. I., L. Risser, V. Duplessis, S. DeGue, A. Villaveces, T. P. Hurley, J. Chang, E. Miller, and K. A. Randell. 2022. The impact of the COVID-19 pandemic on the needs and lived experiences of intimate partner violence survivors in the United States: Advocate perspectives. *Violence Against Women* 28(12-13):3114-3134.

Rai, A., S. Grossman, and N. Perkins. 2020. The effects of COVID-19 on domestic violence and immigrant families. *Greenwich Social Work Review* 2(1).

Ravi, A. 2023. PurpLE Health Foundation. Paper presented at Sustaining Essential Health Care Services Related to Intimate Partner Violence During Public Health Emergencies Meeting 3B, Washington, D.C.

Saboori, Z., R. S. Gold, K. M. Green, and M. Q. Wang. 2022. Community health worker knowledge, attitudes, practices and readiness to manage intimate partner violence. *J Community Health* 47(1):17-27.

Sabri, B., V. P. S. Njie-Carr, J. T. Messing, N. Glass, T. Brockie, G. Hanson, J. Case, and J. C. Campbell. 2019. The weWomen and ourCircle randomized controlled trial protocol: A web-based intervention for immigrant, refugee and indigenous women with intimate partner violence experiences. *Contemporary Clinical Trials* 76:79-84.

Schrag, R. V., S. Leat, and L. Wood. 2022. "Everyone is living in the same storm, but our boats are all different": Safety and safety planning for survivors of intimate partner and sexual violence during the COVID-19 pandemic. *J Interpers Violence* 37(23-24):NP21775-NP21799.

Schreiber, M. D., R. Yin, M. Omaish, and J. E. Broderick. 2014. Snapshot from Superstorm Sandy: American Red Cross mental health risk surveillance in lower New York State. *Ann Emerg Med* Jul;64(1):59-65. https://doi.org/10.1016/j.annemergmed.2013.11.009.

Scott, S. E., L. Risser, S. Miller-Walfish, A. Marjavi, A. Ali, J. Segebrecht, T. Branch, S. Dawson, and E. Miller. 2023. Policy and systems change in intimate partner violence and human trafficking: Evaluation of a federal cross-sector initiative. *J Womens Health (Larchmont)* 32(7):779-786.

Shields, S. 2011. *The LA County EMS agency programs for psychological consequences of disasters*. https://www.orau.gov/rsb/bridgingthegaps2011/presentations/PlanningPsychosocialBehavioralHealthinaRadiationEmergency-Shields.pdf (accessed August 18, 2023).

Shorey, R. C., V. Tirone, and G. L. Stuart. 2014. Coordinated community response components for victims of intimate partner violence: A review of the literature. *Aggression and Violent Behavior* 19(4):363-371.

Smiley, R. A., R. L. Allgeyer, Y. Shobo, K. C. Lyons, R. Letourneau, E. Zhong, N. Kaminski-Ozturk, and M. Alexander. 2023. The 2022 national nursing workforce survey. *Journal of Nursing Regulation* 14(1):S1-S90.

Snyder, J. E., R. D. Upton, T. C. Hassett, H. Lee, Z. Nouri, and M. Dill. 2023. Black representation in the primary care physician workforce and its association with population life expectancy and mortality rates in the US. *JAMA Network Open* 6(4):e236687-e236687.

Sphere Association. 2018. *The sphere handbook: Humanitarian charter and minimum standards in humanitarian response*. 4th edition. Geneva, Switzerland: Publisher Sphere Association.

Storer, H. L., and E. X. Nyerges. 2023. The rapid uptake of digital technologies at domestic violence and sexual assault organizations during the COVID-19 pandemic. *Violence Against Women* 29(5):1085-1096.

Su, Z., A. Cheshmehzangi, D. McDonnell, H. Chen, J. Ahmad, S. Segalo, and C. P. da Veiga. 2022. Technology-based mental health interventions for domestic violence victims amid COVID-19. *International Journal of Environmental Research and Public Health* 19(7).

Thoumi, A., K. Kaalund, C. Silcox, K. Greene, N. Chaudhry, J. Jacobs, K. Williamson, and M. McClellan. 2021. *Hyperlocal COVID-19 testing and vaccination strategies to reach communities with low vaccine uptake: Considerations for states and localities.* Washington, DC: Duke-Margolis Center for Health Policy.

Trabold, N., J. McMahon, S. Alsobrooks, S. Whitney, and M. Mittal. 2020. A systematic review of intimate partner violence interventions: State of the field and implications for practitioners. *Trauma Violence Abuse* 21(2):311-325.

UNFPA (United Nations Population Fund). 2019. *Inter-agency emergency reproductive health kits for use in humanitarian settings.* https://www.unfpa.org/minimum-standards (accessed August 25, 2023).

USPSTF (United States Preventive Services Task Force). 2018. Intimate partner violence, elder abuse, and abuse of vulnerable adults: Screening. *JAMA* 320(16):1678-1687.

Vagni, M., T. Maiorano, V. Giostra, D. Pajardi, and P. Bartone. 2022. Emergency stress, hardiness, coping strategies and burnout in health care and emergency response workers during the COVID-19 pandemic. *Front Psychol* 13:918788.

Valdez, R. S., C. C. Rogers, H. Claypool, L. Trieshmann, O. Frye, C. Wellbeloved-Stone, and P. Kushalnagar. 2021. Ensuring full participation of people with disabilities in an era of telehealth. *J Am Med Inform Assoc* 28(2):389-392.

VAWnet. 2021. *Disaster and emergency preparedness and response.* https://vawnet.org/sc/response (accessed August 18, 2023).

Veenema, T. G., A. Griffin, A. R. Gable, L. MacIntyre, R. N. Simons, M. P. Couig, J. J. Walsh Jr, R. P. Lavin, A. Dobalian, and E. Larson. 2016. Nurses as leaders in disaster preparedness and response—a call to action. *Journal of Nursing Scholarship* 48(2):187-200.

Veenema, T. G., D. Meyer, S. A. Bell, M. P. Couig, C. R. Friese, R. Lavin, J. Stanley, E. Martin, M. Montague, E. Toner, M. Schoch-Spana, A. Cicero, and T. Inglesby. 2020. *Recommendations for improving national nurse preparedness for pandemic response: Early lessons from COVID-19.* Johns Hopkins Bloomburg School of Public Health Center for Health Security.

Victims Voice. n.d. *Victims voice.* https://victimsvoice.app/ (accessed August 18, 2023).

Voth Schrag, R. J., S. Leat, B. Backes, S. Childress, and L. Wood. 2023. "So many extra safety layers:" Virtual service provision and implementing social distancing in interpersonal violence service agencies during COVID-19. *J Fam Violence* 38(2):227-239.

Weiner, D., and S. Rosman. 2019. Just-in-time training for disaster response in the austere environment. *Clinical Pediatric Emergency Medicine* 20(2):95-110.

Williams, E. E., K. R. Arant, V. P. Leifer, M. C. Balcom, N. C. Levy-Carrick, A. Lewis-O'Connor, and J. N. Katz. 2021. Provider perspectives on the provision of safe, equitable, trauma-informed care for intimate partner violence survivors during the COVID-19 pandemic: A qualitative study. *BMC Women's Health* 21(1):315.

WSCADV (Washington State Coalition Against Domestic Violence). 2016. *Screening and intake forms for domestic violence emergency shelters.* https://wscadv.org/resources/screening-intake-forms-guidelines/ (accessed August 25, 2023).

8

Recommendations[1]

The Committee on Sustaining Essential Health Care Services Related to Intimate Partner Violence During Public Health Emergencies carefully reviewed the available evidence about intimate partner violence (IPV) and public health emergency (PHE) planning and response, leading to the committee's eleven recommendations for Health Resources and Services Administration (HRSA) consideration. Following its thoughtful review and debate of compelling evidence, the committee recommends the following actions.

Essential Health Care Services

The committee used the Social Ecological Model to guide their understanding of the health care needs of women experiencing IPV and to identify the essential health care services related to IPV. That process was also informed by the Care Coordination Model's guidance that high-quality referrals and transitions to resources outside of the traditional health care system are a key component of effective health care delivery. This led the committee to conclude that the health consequences of IPV often require care that extends beyond the traditional health care system.

In order to identify the essential health care services related to IPV, the committee's review of evidence included several literature searches; recommendations from the U.S. Preventive Services Task Force (USPSTF), the Women's Preventive Services Initiative (WPSI), and the World Health

---

[1] This chapter does not include references. Evidence and citations to support the text and recommendations herein are provided in the body of the report.

Organization (WHO); and insight gleaned from presentations to the committee and a commissioned paper by experts in IPV-related care. This analysis identified numerous serious and high prevalence adverse health effects associated with experiencing IPV. Those adverse health outcomes fall in the following categories: acute physical injuries, gynecologic and reproductive health issues, perinatal and obstetric health issues, behavioral health issues (including mental health and substance use), and other chronic health issues that are either exacerbated by acute IPV or related to experiencing long-term IPV. A discussion of these conditions can be found in Chapter 4 as well as in Appendix B. The committee concluded that the essential health care services related to IPV were those that addressed the most common and most serious health conditions associated with experiencing IPV and those that facilitate disclosure and protect the safety of those experiencing IPV and their children, if needed. Recommendation 1 outlines the committee's recommendation as to what health care services related to IPV are essential. A detailed discussion of these services can be found in Chapter 5. The committee concluded that given the prevalence of IPV, it is likely that all U.S. health care systems provide care for women experiencing IPV. Therefore, the committee designated all U.S. health care systems as the responsible entities in this recommendation.

> Recommendation 1: The committee recommends that the Health Resources and Services Administration and all U.S. health care systems classify the following as essential health care services related to intimate partner violence (IPV):
> - Universal IPV screening and inquiry
> - Universal IPV education
> - Safety planning
> - Forensic medical examinations
> - Emergency medical care
> - Treatment of physical injuries
> - Gynecologic and reproductive health care, including all forms of Food and Drug Administration-approved contraception and pregnancy termination
> - Screening and treatment of sexually transmitted infections and HIV
> - Treatment for substance use disorders and addiction care
> - Pharmacy and medication management
> - Obstetric care, including perinatal home visits
> - Primary and specialty care
> - Mental health care
> - Support services, including shelter, nutritional assistance, and child care
> - Dental care

IPV disclosure is frequently the first step in accessing IPV-related health care services. Universal IPV screening is meant to facilitate that disclosure. However, women who are not aware of available resources or who feel that their clinician does not have time or is disinterested in addressing IPV are less likely to disclose. Universal IPV education that is either active (such as conversations about healthy relationships) or passive (such as prominently displayed posters and brochures) can reduce those perceptions. Additional discussion of the barriers to IPV disclosure can be found in Chapter 2 and additional discussion of universal IPV screening and education can be found in Chapter 5. Notably, both the USPSTF and WPSI recommendations for universal IPV screening include a recommendation to provide or refer a woman who screens positive for IPV to care and support services. Women who experience IPV are at high risk for traumatic brain injuries and mental health disorders, which make it difficult for them to navigate the often complex processes of accessing needed health care services. Warm referrals, in which a clinician directly connects an individual to referred services instead of simply providing a phone number or the address of a web site, are critical to facilitating access to essential health care services related to IPV during steady state conditions and PHEs.

> **Recommendation 2: Health care providers should consistently pair intimate partner violence (IPV) screening with universal IPV education and, for women who disclose IPV, provide warm referrals for health care and support services during both steady state conditions and public health emergencies.**

Reducing Health Inequities

Many of the populations that experience health inequities also report a greater prevalence of IPV. This includes minoritized racial and ethnic populations, those living in historically under-resourced communities (both rural and urban), people with low incomes, and sexual and gender minority populations. A more detailed discussion of populations disproportionately affected by IPV can be found in Chapter 2. This interaction exacerbates the negative health consequences of experiencing IPV. Women from these populations face substantial barriers to accessing essential health care services related to IPV. These barriers are discussed in detail in Chapter 5. The committee concluded that just as all U.S. health care systems are likely to care for people experiencing IPV, all U.S. health care systems have a responsibility to ensure that they deliver IPV-related health care services that are consistent with the needs of the populations they serve.

Recommendation 3: In order to reduce health inequities related to intimate partner violence (IPV), health care systems should:
- Ensure that individuals from historically marginalized communities and other communities adversely affected by health inequities are included in IPV care program development and planning.
- Provide culturally and linguistically specific resources for IPV care.
- Evaluate and monitor the reach of their IPV care programs' efforts to ensure equitable access to those programs.

Prevention for Adolescents

Many adults report that they first experienced IPV as an adolescent. Sadly, IPV is a common experience for adolescents. This is discussed further in Chapter 2. Adolescence is a period of complex biologic, cognitive, and social–emotional development, which makes it an important period for prevention strategies that can disrupt the developmental pathways toward IPV. The Centers for Disease Control and Prevention (CDC) developed guidance that includes specific prevention strategies for adolescents. While adolescents experience IPV in forms similar to those experienced by adults, the approach to their IPV care requires unique considerations. Confidentiality is especially important for adolescents. The presence of a trusted adult can support disclosure. School- and youth-based settings offer unique opportunities for disclosure and connection to care. Tailored IPV services for adolescents are critical to ensuring that this vulnerable population has access to appropriate, confidential care.

Recommendation 4: The Health Resources and Services Administration should disseminate best practices for ensuring that multi-sector, confidential services are available for adolescents experiencing intimate partner violence, including prevention services.

Essential Health Care Services Related to Intimate Partner Violence in Public Health Emergencies

The committee was tasked with identifying the essential health care services related to IPV during PHEs and strategies to ensure access to those health care services during PHEs. The committee began this process by asking "Does the list of essential health care services related to IPV during steady state conditions change during PHEs?" The committee considered evidence from U.S. policy and WHO guidance regarding essential health care services during the COVID-19 pandemic, and the adverse health effects related to experiencing IPV. This is discussed further in Chapter 6. The committee concluded that a health care service is essential due to its impact on health, not situational pressure. Therefore, the same health care services related to IPV that are essential during steady state conditions are essential during PHEs. However, health care systems face substantial obstacles to care delivery during PHEs. The committee sought to balance the need to deliver these essential health care services related to IPV with the reality of PHE-induced obstacles to care delivery. The committee drew on the Federal Emergency Management Agency's (FEMA's) Community Lifelines approach to develop a phased approach to delivery of essential health care services related to IPV during PHEs. This approach prioritizes those services that are essential for protecting life safety for immediate access, with other services that are essential but less time sensitive restored throughout PHE response as resources become more available. A discussion of the committee's application of the Community Lifelines approach can be found in Chapter 6. The committee defined three phases of PHE response for the purpose of this report, which organize this phased approach. These phases are defined below:

- The *initial or immediate-response phase* occurs while the situation is unstable and unknown before supplementary resources can be deployed to the affected area or resources within the community can be redirected. During this phase, the disaster health responders'[2] efforts are focused on saving and sustaining life using limited resources. This is also the point at which initial requests for additional resources are made.
- The *response operations phase* occurs once the health care system and associated jurisdictional authorities have assessed the incident and have stood up relevant incident coordination structures. During this phase, disaster health responders have begun to receive additional resources such as supplies and staff to support temporary care delivery sites. At this point, while health care delivery capacity has increased beyond life-saving and -sustaining activities, resources are not adequate to support full delivery of all essential health care services related to IPV for all individuals.
- The *stabilization phase* occurs when basic lifeline services have been provided to PHE survivors, either by rapid reestablishment of those services or through the employment of a contingency response solution. At this point all essential health care services related to IPV are available for all individuals.

---

[2] For the purposes of this report, disaster health responders are the leaders and staff with expertise in public health and health care who are working and providing care in those settings during response to a PHE.

The committee prioritized delivery of essential health care services related to IPV that are most integral to protecting life safety during the initial phase of PHE response. In some cases, specific components of an essential health care service are essential for protecting life due to the severity and time sensitive nature of certain IPV-related health conditions or are critical for women from groups that have an elevated risk for life threatening outcomes, such as pregnant women. Then, as health care staff and supplies become more available, the full essential health care service can be delivered more broadly. However, the committee emphasizes that all of these services are essential to IPV care regardless of the phase in which they recommend it be restored. These services are discussed in Chapter 5, and the phased model for restoration of services is discussed in Chapter 6. The phased model outlined in Recommendation 5 and the accompanying table (Table 8-1) are designed to balance the restoration of these essential services with the delivery challenges posed by PHEs.

Recommendation 5: Essential health care services related to intimate partner violence (IPV) during steady state conditions remain essential during public health emergencies (PHEs), but health care systems should restore them in phases that consider the obstacles to delivering this care during different phases of the PHE response (see Table 8-1).

TABLE 8-1 Essential Health Care Services for IPV During Public Health Emergencies—A Phased Return to Steady State

Essential Health Care Service	PHASE WHEN SERVICE SHOULD BE RESTORED		
	Initial	Response operations	Stabilization
Universal IPV screening/inquiry and education			
Safety planning			
Forensic medical exams			
Emergency medical care			
Treatment of physical injury			
Gynecologic and reproductive health care including pregnancy termination	Urgent	Non-urgent	
Obstetric care	Urgent	Non-urgent	
Perinatal home visits			
Contraception and emergency contraception	Contraceptives not requiring procedures or immediate follow-up	All types of contraceptives	
Screening and treatment of sexually transmitted infections and HIV	Treatment and rapid testing	Treatment and all screening	
Substance abuse treatment	Withdrawal mitigation	All treatment	
Pharmacy/medication management			
Primary and specialty care			
Mental health care	Urgent/Crisis	Non-urgent	
Dental care	Urgent treatment for acute injuries	Urgent treatment for acute injuries	
Support services including shelter, nutritional assistance, child care			

Restore services for all patients

Selectively restore services for acute needs or restore targeted services

Do not restore services during this phase

Planning and Operationalization of Intimate Partner Violence Care During Public Health Emergencies

The professionals who serve as disaster health responders during PHEs are expected to effectively deliver care in high stress and often unpredictable conditions. Given the increased prevalence and severity of IPV associated with PHEs, they are likely to encounter women who have experienced physical and psychological trauma related to IPV that may be compounded by trauma related to the PHE. Disaster health responders must be provided with adequate resources in the form of knowledge and skills, protocols, and supplies to ensure that they can effectively care for women experiencing IPV during PHEs. These resources are crucial for sustaining delivery of essential health care services related to IPV.

The committee took a pragmatic approach to developing recommendations targeted at facilitating delivery of essential health care services related to IPV during PHEs. The committee was intentional in their identification of the entity responsible for carrying out those recommendations. For example, the committee recognized that not all state, local, tribal, and territorial (SLTT) jurisdictions are organized in the same manner, with varying structures and titles for those agencies and offices responsible for emergency planning. Therefore, the committee concluded that naming specific agencies or offices at the SLTT level in recommendations for those entities could lead to confusion and contribute to a delay or failure of a jurisdiction to act on those recommendations. The recommendations in this section were developed to address key gaps that the committee identified in PHE preparedness and associated protocols related to IPV care that negatively affect both access to care for women experiencing IPV during PHEs and disaster health responders' ability to provide that care. A discussion of these gaps can be found in Chapter 7. These gaps include:

- standard guidance and best practices for the development of IPV care protocols for disaster health responders,
- public-facing PHE response plans that specifically address IPV care and formal coordination with community-based IPV care providers,
- training specifically focused on IPV for disaster health responders that is easy to find and access, and
- protocols to ensure medical supply caches for use in PHE response include all necessary items for delivery of the essential health care services related to IPV.

Disaster health responders come from diverse health care backgrounds, and some professions may not include IPV identification or care as part of their training. Additionally, they may not regularly care for women experiencing IPV in their steady state roles. Given that PHEs are associated with increases in IPV prevalence and severity, disaster health responders are likely to encounter women who have experienced IPV and need care. Adequate training provides disaster health responders with the knowledge they need to recognize that a woman is experiencing IPV and provide or connect her to the care she needs. Chapter 7 highlights opportunities for drawing on existing training mechanisms and structures to incorporate training about IPV for disaster health responders. The committee concluded that the Administration for Strategic Preparedness and Response (ASPR) and HRSA were well suited to develop and disseminate training and guidance for IPV care during PHEs in light of each entity's experience and existing structures that could support such efforts.

> **Recommendation 6: The Health Resources and Services Administration should partner with the Administration for Strategic Preparedness and Response to add an open access training hub on intimate partner violence (IPV) for disaster health responders and other personnel in health care and community settings that includes education about:**
> - **recognizing the signs and symptoms of IPV during public health emergencies;**
> - **appropriate use of supplies and care protocols unique to IPV-related health care services, including those related to reproductive health and forensic medical examinations; and**
> - **best practices for providing care and connections to support services for individuals experiencing IPV.**

Well-designed protocols are necessary to guide an effective PHE response. The existing guidance for development of IPV care protocols for disaster health responders is limited in nature and scattered across different documents from different entities. However, the committee identified international guidance, such as that developed by WHO and the United Nations Population Fund (UNFPA) that can inform development of guidance for domestic protocols. Chapter 3 discusses the committee's findings pertaining to protocols for IPV care during PHEs. It was common for existing U.S. guidance to discuss IPV as part of domestic violence or to only discuss domestic violence, framing IPV in the context of families with children and relationships with both partners living in the same home. This can lead planners and disaster health responders to overlook the possibility of IPV in families who do not have children, couples who do not live together, or former intimate partners. As previously noted, disaster health responders may not regularly provide care for women experiencing IPV in their steady state roles. They also may be reallocated to provide care in settings and geographic locations that differ from where they work during steady state conditions. This makes protocols for IPV care during PHEs that are based on standardized guidance an important tool for ensuring disaster health responders can effectively deliver essential health care services related to IPV.

> **Recommendation 7: The Health Resources and Services Administration should partner with the Administration for Strategic Preparedness and Response to develop and disseminate standardized guidance for developing protocols for intimate partner violence care for disaster health responders as well as the essential supplies required for delivering that care.**

Protocols for sustaining essential health care services related to IPV need to be incorporated into PHE planning at the federal and SLTT levels. Emergency Support Function 8 (ESF 8) of the National Response Framework, particularly the Public Health and Medical Service Annex of ESF 8, create a uniform structure with associated responsibilities at the federal level. Additional information about federal structures to guide PHE response planning can be found in Chapter 3 and Appendix A. However, SLTT jurisdictions vary in their organizational structure and allocate emergency planning responsibilities differently. The committee concluded that given the increased prevalence and severity of IPV associated with PHEs and the unique needs of women experiencing IPV during PHEs, emergency planning entities at all jurisdictional levels need to incorporate expertise in IPV care delivery. Additionally, community-based organizations are also frequently involved in responding to PHEs. Their staff are often trusted members of the community who have unique and critical knowledge about and credibility in their community. These groups are also frequently involved in providing IPV-related care. Representatives from these organizations can bring an important perspective to PHE response planning bodies. Their involvement can also increase community trust in those planning bodies.

> **Recommendation 8: Federal and state, local, tribal, and territorial government emergency response leaders should ensure that coordinated planning and response protocols for sustaining essential health care services related to intimate partner violence (IPV) during public health emergencies (PHEs) are in place before PHEs occur. Key steps in the planning process include:**
> - **At the federal level, the Department of Health and Human Services should ensure that protocols for IPV care are integrated into the planning and execution of all of the core competencies of the Emergency Support Function 8 Public Health and Medical Services Annex.**

- At the state, local, tribal, and territorial government level, IPV care planning and coordination should be assigned to a specific office or division that is part of the emergency planning or emergency management team.
- At all levels, jurisdictional emergency planning teams should include representation from social service providers and IPV-related community-based organizations to ensure that strong partnerships exist between disaster health responders and the organizations providing care for IPV survivors.

There are several federal sources of emergency medical supply caches. These are discussed in Chapters 3 and 7. While these caches are typically supplemented by supplies maintained by private and SLTT actors, kits meant for acute deployment are pre-packaged and standardized. Many of the essential health care services related to IPV during PHEs are the same as those for individuals not experiencing IPV. However, there are some unique and critical supply considerations, particularly related to caring for a woman who has experienced IPV-related sexual assault or rape. The committee found that standard protocols to guide the allocation of resources, such as supplies and medications, specific to providing IPV care in austere settings or in disrupted health care environments during PHEs are not currently widely available in the United States. However, international guidance, particularly the guidelines included in the UNFPA *Inter-Agency Emergency Reproductive Health Kits for Use in Humanitarian Settings* can inform domestic supply plans. This international guidance is discussed in Chapter 7. The committee acknowledges that those located in certain geographic areas in the United States may encounter challenges procuring specific and vital supplies for IPV care, such as emergency contraception or supplies needed for pregnancy termination. However, the committee emphasizes that emergency medical caches should include all of the necessary supplies to support delivery of all essential health care services related to IPV, regardless of geographic location.

> **Recommendation 9: Federal, state, local, tribal, and territorial governments' planning should take the following actions to ensure the availability of necessary supplies to deliver essential health care services for intimate partner violence (IPV) during public health emergencies (PHEs):**
> - Conduct an annual review of disaster response caches to ensure that appropriate supplies related to IPV are included.
> - Establish logistics and procurement plans for needed supplies for all entities that will be responsible for delivering that care, including disaster health responders, emergency shelter staff, and community-based support service providers engaged in IPV care.

Intimate Partner Violence Research

Early in the committee's deliberations, it was evident that data for the prevalence of IPV in the U.S. population has key limitations that negatively affect evidence-based care and prevention as well as evidence-based policy making related to IPV. Population-based surveys and clinic-based studies use varied terminology and reporting items when collecting IPV data. The variations in terminology and reporting items are discussed further in Chapter 2. This substantially limits the nation's ability to estimate the prevalence of IPV and restricts comparisons between datasets. It also creates barriers for data sharing. Inconsistent terminology across studies leads to substantial differences in what information is represented in each study's data and data categories. That precludes aggregation of shared data from across studies into common categories that would inform accurate analysis. These inconsistencies in terminology also limit the ability to compare outcomes across intervention studies. CDC sought to address these inconsistencies when it released its first version of *Intimate Partner Violence Surveillance: Uniform Definitions and Recommended Data Elements* in 1999 and an updated version in 2015. However, the guidance in this document has not been widely adopted.

Accurate and comparable prevalence data are critical for identifying populations that need additional targeted support and for tracking the effects of that additional support. Inconsistent and inadequately designed approaches to collection of demographic information have led to underrepresentation and erasure of some historically minoritized populations in data analyses, such as American Indian and Alaska Native women and Pacific Islanders. This is discussed further in Chapter 2. Standardized data reporting rules, including requiring the use of standard definitions for types of IPV and the collection of accurate demographic data, would greatly improve the accuracy of prevalence estimates for IPV. Standardized data reporting rules would also allow for the development of a more robust literature on promising models and practices for IPV care.

> **Recommendation 10: In order to improve consistency in intimate partner violence (IPV)-related terminology used in both the research and clinical setting, the Health Resources and Services Administration (HRSA) and all U.S. health care systems should adopt the IPV-related terminology defined in the Centers for Disease Control and Prevention *Intimate Partner Violence Surveillance: Uniform Definitions and Recommended Data Elements*. HRSA and other federally funded health care agencies can further support better alignment of clinical and survey data in IPV research by requiring the use of the recommended data elements in their funded projects.**

The committee identified several key gaps and limitations in the IPV-related research literature specific to this study's statement of task. These include:

- population-based studies of individual IPV intervention outcomes and the effectiveness of those interventions during steady state and PHE conditions;
- comparative effectiveness studies of adequate size to inform development of best practices for IPV identification and care in the health care setting during steady state and PHE conditions;
- population-based studies of the effects of different types of PHEs on IPV severity and prevalence;
- large population-based studies of IPV in populations that experience health disparities; and
- studies that clarify the occurrence and nature of harms associated with IPV screening and, if any harms are identified, best practices for reducing or avoiding those harms.

Numerous programs exist to help women experiencing IPV. However, beyond small-scale studies, there have been few efforts to evaluate the effectiveness of individual interventions. There are unique challenges associated with conducting IPV research that likely contribute to the relatively small study populations of many IPV-related studies. These unique challenges are discussed further in Chapter 1. Unfortunately, small populations limit the representativeness of the data. It is difficult to develop an understanding of IPV among minoritized populations without data that include adequate representation of those populations. While some in the fields of IPV care and advocacy have voiced concern about the potential harms associated with IPV screening, there is limited research available that clarifies the link between IPV screening and these harms or that elucidates the best practices to mitigate them. A more robust body of evidence about the degree to which such harms exist and effective strategies to reduce or prevent those harms can inform IPV screening and education protocols and reduce provider hesitancy around screening. Additionally, studies investigating the interaction between PHEs and IPV are limited and primarily focused on the recent COVID-19 pandemic. PHEs vary greatly. While the all-hazards[3] approach is generally the standard for planning and preparation, it is applied with the

---

[3] An all-hazards approach is an integrated approach to emergency preparedness planning that focuses on capacities and capabilities that are critical to prepare for, respond to, and recover from the full spectrum of emergencies or disasters, whether human-made or natural. The committee notes that their application of an all-hazards approach acknowledges that not all disasters and emergencies are identical, nor are their effects on different populations and communities.

understanding that different types of PHEs will require some differences in response activities. For example, response to an infectious disease outbreak may require the affected community to shelter-in-place and limit interactions with people from outside their homes for a period of time. However, response to a wildfire usually requires people to evacuate their homes, often to congregate shelters and unfamiliar locations. The different responses needed to address different types of PHEs affect communities differently. A greater understanding of whether and how different types of PHEs (infectious disease outbreaks, wildfires, oil spills, hurricanes, etc.) interact differently with IPV can provide important insight for all involved in IPV care and PHE planning. Strengthening the data and research infrastructure is core to developing a better understanding of how to reduce the incidence of IPV and how to best care for women who experience IPV. The committee concluded that HRSA is well-positioned to support efforts to address these gaps and build a more robust evidence base.

> **Recommendation 11: The Health Resources and Services Administration should fund research efforts that address:**
> - **Best practices for identifying and managing intimate partner violence (IPV) in routine clinical practice and during public health emergencies (PHEs);**
> - **The effectiveness of IPV interventions in improving physical and mental health outcomes in steady state conditions and PHEs;**
> - **The potential harms of IPV identification and management in steady state and PHEs and strategies to prevent or reduce those harms;**
> - **The prevalence and characteristics of IPV among specific populations, particularly those populations experiencing adverse effects of health disparities; and**
> - **The effect of PHEs on IPV frequency and severity.**

FINAL THOUGHTS

The committee's recommendations address gaps in knowledge about the essential health care needs related to IPV as well as its prevalence, effects, and effective interventions. They also build on HRSA's strategy to address IPV. Further, these recommendations offer specific guidance for incorporating IPV care into PHE planning for emergency planners and health care systems and ways to increase access to quality IPV-related health care services across all populations. If adopted, these recommendations will facilitate improvements in the health and well-being of women experiencing IPV, support disaster health responders to care for those women, and contribute to reducing health disparities in the United States.

Appendix A

Emergency Declarations and Federal Frameworks

Chapter 3 of this report provides an overview of public health emergencies (PHEs), including the role of federal and state governments in preparing for and responding to these disasters. This appendix provides additional background information about the government's role, specifically pertaining to emergency declarations at both federal and state levels and national frameworks for disaster planning and response.

FEDERAL AND STATE EMERGENCY DECLARATIONS

Although emergency and disaster management laws vary, the primary function of declarations is to trigger predetermined delegations of authority from the legislative branch to specified executive branch officials and agencies. Under the principle of separation of powers enshrined in the federal and state constitutions, executive branch agencies and officials are limited to exercising authority that is delegated to them by the constitution directly or (more commonly) by the legislative branch through statutes (Jaeger-Fine, 2020). Legislatures, recognizing that they are not well suited to implement swift responses or nimble adjustments, typically adopt emergency and disaster statutes that specify the conditions under which a declaration may be issued and the authority that will be automatically delegated to specific officials and agencies while that declaration is in effect (Wiley et al., 2021). Officials and agencies may use this delegated authority to make government expenditures and execute government contracts, to suspend or alter regulations that might otherwise impede an effective response, and to issue mandates or restrictions to facilitate the response—all without waiting for the legislative branch to act in response to a rapidly evolving situation (Wiley et al., 2021).

Although the federal role in PHE preparedness and response has grown in recent decades, state and local governments continue to bear primary responsibility. Most state and territorial legislatures have adopted civil defense, emergency, and disaster statutes to guide state, tribal, territorial, and local officials in responding to a PHE (Roberts, 2013). In many cases, these statutes were drafted with civil unrest and natural disasters in mind, but they are usually broad enough to encompass disease outbreaks as well. Civil defense statutes centered around ensuring the public's safety may similarly be interpreted to encompass measures to secure the public's health during an emergency (Wiley et al., 2021). State legislatures adopting civil defense, emergency, and disaster statutes during the mid-20th century generally left previous public health statutes in place that granted public health officials powers relevant to controlling the spread of infectious diseases (Wiley et al., 2021).

State emergency and disaster management statutes typically empower the governor to enact reasonable and necessary measures to "protect life and property or to bring the emergency situation within the affected area under control."[1] Powers delegated by many state statutes specifically authorize governors to control movement into, out of, and within an affected area.[2] A few state legislatures have delegated the entirety of the state's police powers (the broad authority to take actions to protect for the general welfare) to state executives during emergencies and disasters (Wiley et al., 2021). For example, California's Emergency Services Act grants the governor "complete authority over all agencies of the state government and the right to exercise within the area designated *all police power vested in the state* by the Constitution and laws of the State of California in order to effectuate the purposes of [emergency mitigation and protection of health and safety]."[3] The state's public health statute also authorizes public health officials to "take *any preventive measure* that may be necessary to protect and preserve the public health from any public health hazard during any 'state of war emergency,' 'state of emergency,' or 'local emergency' . . . within his

---

[1] See, e.g., Mich. C.L. 10.31(1). When Governor Whitmer relied on this provision to extend her authority to issue coronavirus emergency orders in 2020, the state supreme court determined that the statute violated the nondelegation doctrine enshrined in the state constitution. See Certified Questions from United States Dist. Court, W. Dist. of Michigan, S. Div., No. 161492, 2020 WL 5877599, at *24 (Mich. Oct. 2, 2020).

[2] Certified Questions from United States Dist. Court, W. Dist. of Michigan, S. Div., No. 161492, 2020 WL 5877599, at *24 (Mich. Oct. 2, 2020).

[3] CAL. GOV. CODE § 8627 (emphasis added).

or her jurisdiction."[4] Oregon's laws are similar; one emergency response law grants the state's governor "all police powers vested in the state by the Oregon Constitution in order to effectuate the purposes of [the statute]."[5] Examples of specific powers can be found in one of Oregon's public health statues, which provides more specific authorities to close facilities, regulate goods and services, and control "entry into, exit from, movement within, and occupancy of premises in any public area subject to or threatened by a public health emergency." This is subject to a 28-day limit on these expanded gubernatorial authorities.[6]

Most U.S. crisis response efforts are governed by the *Robert T. Stafford Disaster Relief and Emergency Assistance Act (Stafford Act)*,[7] passed in 1988 and last amended in 2021. It covers two types of incidents—more minor emergencies and larger major disasters—and provides both public assistance and individual assistance during disasters (Lee and Lindsay, 2021). The *Stafford Act* was rarely used for biologically driven public health disasters before it was employed for the West Nile Virus in New York and New Jersey in 2000 (Lee and Lindsay, 2021). The Section 501b clause of the *Stafford Act* was engaged to declare the COVID-19 pandemic a nationwide emergency in 2020 (Lee and Lindsay, 2021). This was the first time the *Stafford Act* had been used to declare a nationwide emergency. The declaration invited governors and territorial leaders to request major disaster declarations, which they all subsequently did. This also marked the first time the major disaster clause had been used for any infectious disease agent (Lee and Lindsay, 2021).

Separately, Section 319 of the *Public Health Service Act*[8] gives the federal Secretary of the Department of Health and Human Services (HHS) the authority to declare a PHE when:

- A disease or disorder presents a PHE; or
- A PHE, including significant outbreaks of infectious disease or bioterrorist attacks, otherwise exists.

Some definitions of a *public health emergency* are fairly limited in scope. For example, the World Health Organizations' International Health Regulations constrains PHEs of international concern within the "international spread of disease" (WHO, 2019). However, the *Public Health*

---

[4] Cal. Health & Saf. C. § 101040 (local health officers); § 101475 (city health officers) (emphasis added).

[5] Or. Rev. Stat. § 401.168(1).

[6] Or. Rev. Stat. § 433.441(4).

[7] *Robert T. Stafford Disaster Relief and Emergency Assistance Act*, Public Law 100-707, 100th Congress (May 22, 1974) (November 23, 1988).

[8] *Public Health Service Act* 42 USC 247d §319.

Service Act, which has been amended by pandemic preparedness measures several times, has been applied more broadly to disasters (Elsea et al., 2020). The federal government has declared PHEs for hurricanes including Katrina, Sandy, and Maria, as well as for infectious disease outbreaks, including H1N1 influenza, Zika virus, and SARS-CoV-2 (the virus that causes COVID-19), as well as for the United States' opioid crisis (ASPR, 2023a).

Federally, the declaration of a PHE under Section 319 of the *Public Health Service Act*[9] gives the Secretary of the Department of Health and Human Services (HHS) the ability to waive certain Medicaid and Medicare requirements, adjust grant deadlines, deploy personnel, and provide direct funding to impacted areas. CDC has developed a crisis-funding vehicle that is tied to these declarations and can be used to rapidly send money to impacted jurisdictions outside of the federal appropriations process (ASPR, 2023b). During the COVID-19 pandemic, the PHE designation helped to ensure insurance coverage for COVID-19 services and testing, allowed and surged telehealth use, and provided billions of dollars in aid to states and localities for their public health efforts (Lister et al., 2020).

Federal officials may issue several distinct declarations in response to a PHE:

- The President may issue a national emergency declaration under Section 201 of the *National Emergencies Act*[10] (NEA). An NEA declaration authorizes federal agencies to waive or suspend requirements and obligations under federal law. An NEA declaration lasts for 1 year and may be renewed for additional periods of up to 1 year unless it is terminated by the President or by a joint resolution of Congress.
- The Secretary of HHS may issue an Emergency Use Authorization (EUA) declaration under Section 564 of the *Federal Food, Drug, and Cosmetic Act*.[11] An EUA declaration authorizes the Food and Drug Administration (FDA) to issue EUAs for medical countermeasures, including personal protective equipment, diagnostics, therapeutics, and vaccines. A Section 564 declaration remains in effect indefinitely until terminated by the HHS Secretary.

---

[9] *Public Health Service Act* 42 USC 247d §319. See also https://aspr.hhs.gov/legal/PHE/Pages/Public-Health-Emergency-Declaration.aspx (accessed November 13, 2023).

[10] *National Emergencies Act*, Public Law 94-412, 94th Congress (September 14, 1976).

[11] *Federal Food, Drug, and Cosmetic Act* Section 564 21 USC § 360bbb-3.

- The HHS secretary may also issue a *Public Readiness and Emergency Preparedness (PREP) Act*[12] declaration under Section 319F-3 of the *Public Health Service Act*, which provides immunity from liability for specified activities related to medical countermeasures covered by the declaration.

FEDERAL FRAMEWORKS OVERVIEW

After the 2007 Homeland Security Strategy was established, the federal government issued national frameworks that covered both the response and recovery phases for disasters and emergencies. Both frameworks are meant to be aligned and to link up to the broader Department of Homeland Security strategy and the national preparedness systems.

Today, the National Response Framework (NRF)[13] and National Incident Management System (NIMS)[14] provide organizational structures and preparedness guidance for federal agencies. Whereas the NRF is explicitly designed for federal agency use, the principles within NIMS are meant to support all levels of government as well as nongovernment groups, such as nonprofit and private-sector organizations (FEMA, 2017). This means that most organizations that have structured emergency response apparatus use NIMS in some form—especially the Incident Command System (ICS), a flexible set of organization structures meant to encompass the entirety of a disaster or PHE response (FEMA, 2017).

The NRF implements NIMS within federal emergency operations centers through the Emergency Support Functions (ESFs) (DHS, 2019). The 15 ESFs cover a broad array of functions (e.g., Transportation, Search and Rescue) and provide the mechanism for coordination between federal agencies, which often have multiple overlapping responsibilities within various ESFs. For example, ESF 8, Public Health and Medical Services, is coordinated by HHS and includes such partners as the Departments of Energy, Labor, and Defense; the U.S. Postal Service; and the American Red Cross. Many of these agencies also have lead or supporting roles in other ESFs (DHS, 2019).

The National Disaster Recovery Framework (NDRF) provides guidance for coordinating the authorities and missions of federal agencies under a wide range of federal laws, including the Stafford Act, the Public Health

---

[12] *Department of Defense, Emergency Supplemental Appropriations to Address Hurricanes in the Gulf of Mexico, and Pandemic Influenza Act*, Public Law 109-148 Division C: *Public Readiness and Emergency Preparedness (PREP) Act of 2005* § 2, 109th Congress (December 30, 2005).

[13] For more information on the NRF, see https://www.fema.gov/emergency-managers/national-preparedness/frameworks/response (accessed August 25, 2023).

[14] For more information on the NIMS, see https://www.fema.gov/emergency-managers/nims (accessed August 25, 2023).

Service Act, the various authorizing statutes applicable to specific agencies, and other statutes that might apply to particular types of PHEs (DHS, 2016). The NDRF may be applied to an incident even in the absence of a federal emergency or disaster declaration (DHS, 2016).

The NDRF is a roadmap for promoting successful disaster recovery, especially from large-scale or catastrophic incidents. Although the framework states that its primary role is in the preparedness phase, its end goal is helping local governments, states, and tribes recover quickly from a disaster (DHS, 2016). It provides disaster recovery managers with a flexible structure that lets them work in a unified manner. It also aims to improve the social, health, economic, natural, and environmental aspects of impacted communities and make the United States more resilient (DHS, 2016). The framework seeks to make the best use of existing federal resources and authorities and to use the full power of all sectors to help communities recover (DHS, 2016). Together with the NRF, the NDRF provides guidance for implementing the response and recovery doctrine laid out in 2007's National Homeland Security Strategy (DHS, 2007).

The Recovery Support Functions (RSFs) are six groups of core recovery capabilities that make it easier to solve problems and access resources during disasters and emergencies (DHS, 2016). The RSFs also facilitate collaboration among state and federal agencies, nongovernmental partners, and other stakeholders. Each RSF is directed by a set of primary and coordinating federal agencies with supporting organizations that work with SLTT officials, nongovernmental organizations, and private-sector partners (DHS, 2016). RSFs gather pertinent specialists and stakeholders both during steady state planning and when they are activated post disaster to identify and address recovery issues. RSFs help facilitate local stakeholder participation and promote intergovernmental and public–private partnerships (DHS, 2016).

A federal coordinating officer (FCO) works together with a federal disaster recovery coordinator to coordinate and aid in the transition between the ESFs and RSFs (DHS, 2016). Because each disaster is complex and unique, operations and the methods and pace for transitioning from ESFs to RSFs will differ in each case. The FCO works with state, tribal, and local authorities to decide when to start phasing down ESFs and to start phasing in RSFs (DHS, 2016). In some instances, RSFs may be deployed while ESFs are still active, and the two tend to occur in parallel while ESFs are demobilized. Note that ESFs and RSFs have distinct mission objectives, approaches, partnerships, and structures, and the stakeholders involved in each may differ.

In an effort to make these intersecting frameworks and functions easier to understand, the Federal Emergency Management Agency (FEMA) introduced Community Lifelines in the fourth edition of the NRF.[15] The eight Community Lifelines are services necessary for government and business operations to continue to function in order to protect human health, safety, and economic security (FEMA, 2023). They are interdependent and mutually vulnerable. The Health and Medical Lifeline includes objectives for restoring Medical Care, Public Health, Patient Movement, the Medical Supply Chain, and Fatality Management. Community Lifelines specifically incorporate local civil society and private-sector partners (FEMA, 2023). While ESFs and RSFs are organizational structures, Community Lifelines outline the key components of a community's service infrastructure that need to be prioritized to address the effects of a disaster (FEMA, 2023).

REFERENCES

ASPR (Administration for Strategic Preparedness and Response). 2023a. *Declarations of a public health emergency.* https://aspr.hhs.gov/legal/PHE/Pages/default.aspx (accessed November 13, 2023).

ASPR. 2023b. *A public health emergency declaration.* https://aspr.hhs.gov/legal/PHE/Pages/Public-Health-Emergency-Declaration.aspx (accessed November 13, 2023).

Elsea, J. 2020. *Emergency authorities under the National Emergencies Act, Stafford Act, and Public Health Service Act.* Edited by J. Sykes. Washington, DC: Congressional Research Service.

FEMA (Federal Emergency Management Agency). 2017. *National incident management system.* https://www.fema.gov/emergency-managers/nims (accessed July 21, 2023).

FEMA. 2023. *Community lifelines implementation toolkit version 2.1.* Washington, DC: US Department of Homeland Security.

Jaeger-Fine, T. 2020. *American legal systems: A resource and reference guide.* 3rd ed. Durham, North Carolina: Carolina Academic Press.

Lee, E. A., and B. R. Lindsay. 2021. Stafford Act assistance for public health. *Congressional Research Service Reports.* https://crsreports.congress.gov/product/pdf/IN/IN11229 (accessed July 21, 2023).

Lister, S. A., K. Sekar, A. Dabrowska, F. Gottron, A. Singer, and A. K. Sarata. 2020. Overview of U.S. domestic response to coronavirus disease 2019. *Congressional Research Service Reports* R46219. https://crsreports.congress.gov/product/pdf/R/R46219 (accessed July 21, 2023).

Roberts, P. S. 2013. *Disasters and the American state: How politicians, bureaucrats, and the public prepare for the unexpected.* Cambridge: Cambridge University Press.

WHO (World Health Organization). 2019. *Emergencies: International health regulations and emergency committees Q & A.* https://www.who.int/news-room/questions-and-answers/item/emergencies-international-health-regulations-and-emergency-committees (accessed November 13, 2023).

Wiley, L. F., R. Yearby, and A. Hammond, A. 2021. United States: Legal response to COVID-19. *The Oxford Compendium of National Legal Responses to COVID-19.* https://doi.org/10.1093/law-occ19/e24.013.24.

---

[15] For more information on Community Lifelines, see https://www.fema.gov/emergency-managers/practitioners/lifelines (accessed July 21, 2023).

Appendix B

Health Effects of IPV on Individuals Experiencing IPV Across the Lifespan

Health Effects of IPV on Individuals Experiencing IPV Across the Lifespan
Lisa Fedina, PhD

INTRODUCTION

Intimate partner violence (IPV) has been linked to numerous acute and long-term health consequences among women of all backgrounds. Reviews of research on physical health outcomes associated with IPV document common health problems including chronic pain (e.g., back pain, neck pain), cardiovascular conditions (e.g., hypertension), gastrointestinal disorders (e.g., digestive problems, stomach ulcers), neurological problems (e.g., fainting, seizures, traumatic brain injury), gynecological and reproductive health issues (e.g., pelvic pain, urinary tract infections, sexually transmitted disease), and respiratory conditions (e.g., asthma) (Campbell, 2002; Dillon et al., 2013; Stockman et al., 2015; Stubbs and Szoeke, 2022; Wang et al., 2022). Additionally, the mental health outcomes of IPV are well documented and include anxiety, depression, suicidal ideation and behavior, post-traumatic stress disorder (PTSD), and sleep disorders as well as behavioral health challenges such as alcohol and substance misuse (Dillon et al., 2013; Lagdon et al., 2014; Mason and O'Rinn, 2014; Oram et al., 2022). The physical, mental, and behavioral health outcomes and subsequent health care needs among individuals experiencing IPV are often interrelated and highly comorbid (Mason et al., 2014; Mehr et al., 2022).

Individuals experiencing IPV at various points across the lifespan may be at greater risk for specific health conditions. Understanding age-specific effects of IPV at various points in development can guide immediate health care responses to support health care needs of survivors in various age groups. Relatedly, understanding age-related differences in health outcomes can help tailor health care responses during public health emergencies. This paper addresses two aims: (1) identifies and describes the long-term health effects of IPV among women, including its additive effects on health throughout the lifespan; and (2) discusses the health effects of acute IPV in different age groups including age-related differences in those health effects. Studies on racial/ethnic minority, sexual minority, and transgender women as well as other populations of women (e.g., women with disabilities, pregnant women) are also highlighted to identify health effects and needs within populations of women, and to elucidate potential health inequities associated with IPV at various points across the life course.

LONG-TERM HEALTH EFFECTS OF IPV

Overview

Systematic review and meta-analysis studies on chronic health conditions and health behaviors (e.g., substance use) associated with IPV among adult women identify several key considerations when assessing the knowledge base on long-term health effects of IPV (Banjar et al., 2022; Dillon et al., 2013; Pate and Simonic, 2022; Stubbs and Szoeke, 2022; Stockman et al., 2015; Wang et al., 2022). First, many studies on IPV and health outcomes primarily assess only physical forms of IPV, with fewer studies including measures of sexual violence and psychological abuse (Stubbs and Szoeke, 2022). Psychological forms of IPV are often overlooked in screening and intervention, yet studies that include assessments of psychological IPV link psychological IPV to many of the same chronic health problems associated with physical IPV, including hypertension, diabetes, gynecological symptoms, and HIV (Al-Modallal, 2016; Campbell et al., 2018; Jewkes et al., 2015). Second, studies consistently show a dose–response relationship between IPV and health outcomes. More frequent or severe exposure to IPV as well as exposure to multiple types of IPV (e.g., physical, sexual, psychological, coercive control, stalking) result in compounded and more serious health problems over time (Dillon et al., 2013; Pate and Simonic, 2022; Stubbs and Szoeke, 2022). Finally, early studies on health outcomes associated with IPV have primarily used cross-sectional study designs, which has presented challenges in disentangling health effects of IPV and establishing temporality between victimization and subsequent health outcomes. However, a considerable number of longitudinal studies now exist that are consistent with findings in cross-sectional studies and establish temporal pathways between IPV and health outcomes, particularly for the health outcomes of somatic symptoms, sleep disorders, HIV, and aspects of mental health including depression, anxiety, PTSD, and substance use disorders (Dillon et al., 2013; Mehr et al., 2022).

Cardiovascular Risk/Disease

Several cardiovascular risk factors have been associated with IPV victimization, including obesity, low high-density lipoprotein levels and high triglyceride levels, and hyperlipidemia (Al-Modallal et al., 2016; Bosch et al., 2017; Mason et al., 2021, 2017; Stene et al., 2013). Halpern and colleagues (2017) assessed inflammatory cardiovascular disease biomarkers in a small sample (N = 37) of African American (n = 19) women and non-African American women (n = 18) and found significant correlations between IPV and multiple risk markers. In this same study, researchers found significant disparities by race/ethnicity in women exposed to IPV, including increased expression of inflammatory mediators CRP, IL-1β, IL-6, and MMP9 among African American women (Halpern et al., 2017). One study examined differences in health outcomes among sexual minority women (Anderson et al., 2014). In this study, researchers examined differences in cardiovascular health risks among heterosexual (n = 484) and lesbian women (n = 394) experiencing IPV and found that although lesbian women reported higher rates of adult physical and sexual assault than heterosexual women, no significant differences were found in physical health (i.e., a combined report of hypertension, thyroid conditions, heart disease, and/or diabetes) between lesbian and heterosexual women (Anderson et al., 2014).

In one large data mining study of electronic health records, researchers found significant associations between IPV and cardiovascular disease (Karakurt et al., 2017). Another study by Wright and colleagues (2018, 2019) found that IPV increased 30-year cardiovascular disease by 1 percent; however, these effects were mitigated after controlling for race/ethnicity, health insurance status, and other social and economic factors. Using data from the Nurses' Health Study II (N = 51,431), Mason et al. (2012) found that women reporting severe emotional abuse had a 24 percent increased rate of hypertension compared to women without emotional abuse; however, no significant relationship was found between physical and sexual IPV and hypertension after controlling for confounding variables. Stubbs and Szoeke (2022) note that the relationship between IPV and cardiovascular health is likely a pathophysiological connection, and that psychological IPV, in particular, can affect blood pressure and lead to subsequent health risks.

Endocrine System

Endocrine-related health outcomes assessed in studies of IPV include diabetes, stress and cortisol, and menopause symptoms (Al-Modallal et al., 2016; Basu et al., 2013; Dillon et al., 2013; Gibson et al., 2019; Kim et al., 2015; Mason et al., 2012). In a sample of 238 Palestinian refugee women, Al-Modallal et al. (2016) found that women exposed to psychological IPV were significantly more likely to be diagnosed with diabetes than women without IPV exposure (21 percent vs. 13 percent, respectively). Similar patterns were found in Mason et al.'s (2012) study of 51,431 women from the Nurses' Health Study II, such that women exposed to IPV had significantly higher rates of diabetes even after controlling for other variables and that severe psychological abuse was most strongly associated with diabetes.

Research with smaller samples of women suggest that cortisol-related indicators including lowered cortisol awakening response, dissociative symptoms, flattened diurnal cortisol patterns, and higher midday cortisol have all been positively correlated with IPV (Basu et al., 2013; Kim et al., 2015). In a cross-sectional analysis of women 2,016 women ranging from 40 to 80 years old, Gibson et al. (2019) found that physical and emotional IPV were each associated with increased risk for night sweats and dyspareunia and that sexual IPV was associated with other vaginal symptoms (e.g., dryness, irritation). More research is needed on the effects of IPV on cortisol and mechanisms between IPV and endocrine health, including mediating roles of hormonal changes particularly during menopause (Stubbs and Szoeke, 2022).

Sexual and Reproductive Health

Gynecological symptoms (e.g., pain or burning during urination, pain during intercourse), sexually transmitted disease and infections (STDs/STIs), and HIV/AIDS are all well-established health outcomes of IPV in samples of women from developed and developing countries (Dillon et al., 2013; Stubbs and Szoeke, 2022). An early systematic review of studies (N = 51) published from 1996 to 2006 assessing physical IPV and sexual health found that across numerous studies, IPV was consistently associated with sexual risk behaviors (e.g., inconsistent condom use), risk of STIs, unplanned pregnancy or induced abortion, and gynecological symptoms primarily in the form of chronic pelvic pain (Coker et al., 2007).

Stockman et al.'s (2015) systematic review of studies (N = 36) on racial/ethnic minority women found that IPV was associated with multiple symptoms, including discolored vaginal discharge, burning during urination, unwanted pregnancy, irregularity in menstruation, sexual risk-taking behaviors (e.g., having multiple sex partners, inconsistent condom use), and increased risks for HIV among African American, Latina, and South Asian immigrant women. Further, the research on IPV and HIV status among women suggests that women experiencing IPV are not only at greater risk for contracting HIV, but also for suffering worse outcomes and reduced immune states (e.g., lower CD4+, CD8+, T cells among HIV positive samples of women) (Jewkes et al., 2015; Stubbs and Szoeke, 2022). Researchers have attributed HIV as well as STIs/STDs to reduced sexual decision making and free choice victims have in violent and coercive relationships (Decker et al., 2014; Josephs and Abel, 2009; Stockman et al., 2015).

Neurological Symptoms

Compared with other health outcomes, fewer studies have assessed neurological health outcomes associated with IPV, and among extant studies the findings are mixed. In Dillon et al.'s (2013) review of qualitative and quantitative studies (*N* = 75), headaches, migraines, and dizziness were commonly reported in studies and documented as long-term chronic problems in some samples. Karakurt and colleagues' (2017) study of electronic health records found that commonly reported symptoms among patients with histories of IPV included loss of consciousness, dizziness, disorientation, and memory problems. Headache symptoms have also been documented in samples of women exposed to both physical and psychological IPV, suggesting that psychological abuse may have similar effects on neurological health as physical violence resulting in injury (Stubbs and Szoeke, 2022).

Although research is limited, neurological symptoms associated with IPV may be associated with traumatic brain injury (TBI). In a study of 901 women of African descent, Campbell et al. (2018) found that abused women with a probable TBI were more likely to report increased central nervous system symptoms than abused women without TBI, even after controlling for mental health symptoms (e.g., depression, PTSD). Additional symptoms associated with IPV in Campbell et al. (2018) included blackouts, vision and hearing problems, memory loss, and difficulty concentrating.

Other studies have found similar patterns in smaller samples of service-seeking women and general population convenience samples of women (Maldonado-Rodriguez et al., 2021; Raskin et al., 2023; Valera and Kucyi, 2017). Maldonado-Rodriguez et al. (2021) found that in a sample of 40 women with histories of IPV, brain injury load significantly affected some cognitive functions (i.e., number of targets hit, average hand speed); however, mental health symptoms including PTSD, anxiety, and depression also contributed to these and other cognitive functioning measures. Similarly, Valera and Kucyi (2017) conducted clinical interviews, functional magnetic resonance imagings, and neuropsychological measures with 20 women experiencing TBI resulting from IPV and found that greater TBI severity was associated with resting-state functional connectivity and poor performance on memory and learning-related cognitive tasks. In another recent study, Raskin et al. (2023) recruited survivors of IPV (*n* = 50) and sexual assault (*n* = 35) seeking formal services and a comparison group of women without victimization histories recruited from online advertisements (*n* = 50). In this study, researchers found survivors of IPV with potential TBI scored lower on memory and executive functioning than survivors of sexual assault and women without victimization histories and that cognitive changes were greatest for women experiencing non-fatal strangulation (Raskin et al., 2023).

Some research has explored the long-term effects of non-fatal strangulation on neurological symptoms and cognitive functioning. Monahan et al. (2022) conducted a review of 55 studies addressing short- and long-term effects of IPV-related non-fatal strangulation and found that survivors of non-fatal strangulation report post-concussive symptoms including fatigue, headaches, vision problems, mood disturbances, and sleep problems. In this same review, one study found that survivors of chronic non-fatal strangulation reported more severe symptoms (e.g., lightheadedness, memory loss) than survivors who did not experience chronic non-fatal strangulation. Overall, Monahan and colleagues (2022) note significant challenges in characterizing cognitive consequences resulting from IPV non-fatal strangulation and that few studies on IPV include non-fatal strangulation when discussing IPV-related TBIs, and among existing studies most do not separately report impacts for both strangulation and TBIs.

Chronic Disease

Chronic diseases associated with IPV include gastrointestinal disorders, respiratory diseases, chronic pain, fibromyalgia, and liver and urinary health problems (Al-Modallal, 2016; Banjar et al., 2022; Dillon et al., 2013; Stubbs and Szoeke, 2022; Wang et al., 2022). Banjar et al. (2022) conducted a systematic review of studies (N = 15) on IPV and functional gastrointestinal (FGID) symptoms and found increased risks for FGID symptoms for physical, sexual, and psychological IPV when assessed as singular and combined exposures. In Wang and colleagues' (2022) review of studies (N = 37) on IPV and asthma, findings suggest evidence for increased rates of asthma among women exposed to IPV, including increased asthma exacerbations and worsened asthma control. In smaller studies, some evidence suggests that women exposed to IPV report increased risks for temporomandibular joint disorder and premature telomere shortening indicative of cellular aging and neoplasms (Chandan et al., 2019; Karakurt et al., 2017; Whiting et al., 2017). A review by Cook et al. (2011) on IPV among older adults found evidence for long-term impacts of trauma exposure in older adult women samples including pre-mature aging, premature mortality, cognitive functioning, and dementia. In a sample of women (average age 76) with probable Alzheimer's disease, researchers found that 17.5 percent of women had reported spousal abuse with head trauma (i.e., being struck in the head five or more times and losing consciousness on two or more occasions), with the majority of women experiencing abuse nearly 30 years earlier (Leung et al., 2006).

Mental and Behavioral Health

While there is variation in prevalence of IPV across demographic and cultural contexts, IPV is consistently associated with a range of mental health issues. Dillon et al.'s (2013) review of studies (N = 75) on mental health outcomes associated with IPV found consistent associations between victimization and increased depression, PTSD, anxiety, self-harm, and sleep disorders. A more recent review of studies (N = 29) demonstrates worsened mental health symptoms associated with lifetime IPV, with depression, anxiety, PTSD, and substance misuse most frequently assessed in the research (Pate and Simonic, 2022). Physical, sexual, and psychological IPV have all been independently associated with worsened mental health symptoms (Nur, 2012). However, some research shows that women experiencing stalking (accompanied with fear and threat) is specifically associated with worsened post-traumatic stress severity even after accounting for other forms of IPV and that women with stalking histories experience twice the rate of hyperarousal symptoms (Fleming et al., 2012).

Additionally, certain populations of women may experience compounded mental and behavioral health problems associated with IPV victimization. A review of studies (N = 13) on mental health outcomes associated with IPV among women in the military suggests stronger evidence for an association between IPV and depression and alcohol problems than between IPV and PTSD in this population of women (Sparrow et al., 2017). This same study found differences between active-duty service members and veterans, such that IPV and alcohol misuse were more consistently found among active-duty samples whereas IPV and mental health problems were found more frequently among veterans. Additionally, psychological IPV was more commonly associated with depression and alcohol problems than physical/sexual IPV among active-duty personnel (Sparrow et al., 2017). In another study, Coston (2019) analyzed data from the National Intimate Partner and Sexual Violence Survey and found that women survivors of IPV who had a disability were more likely to report their mental health as poor, difficulty sleeping, difficulty attending school or work, and PTSD than victimized women without disabilities.

AGE-SPECIFIC ACUTE HEALTH EFFECTS

Adolescents and Young/Emerging Adults (18–29)

Research on the acute health effects of IPV at adolescent and young/ emerging adult developmental stages largely include sexual/reproductive health symptoms and behavioral health/mental health symptoms (Exner-Cortens et al., 2013; Glass et al., 2003; Hanson et al., 2010; Reuter et al., 2017). Sexual and reproductive health outcomes associated with IPV at this developmental stage include increased risk for STIs, self-reported HIV status, pregnancy, and sexual risk-taking behaviors such as inconsistent condom use and having multiple sexual partners (Bonomi et al., 2013; Brennan et al., 2012; Fedina et al., 2016; Glass et al., 2003; Hanson et al., 2010; Hill et al., 2019).

Co-occurring forms of IPV likely contribute to poor sexual and reproductive health outcomes, including sexual risk-taking behaviors. For example, Hill et al.'s (2019) study with a clinical health care sample of 550 girls ages 14 to 19 found that respondents who reported both reproductive coercion and relationship abuse were more likely to have had multiple sexual partners, using fewer birth control methods, and to have a partner at least 5 years older. Notably, Glass's review (2003) of studies on adolescent dating violence revealed that several studies found low birthweight in adolescent pregnancies associated with IPV, which researchers note may be due to abusive partners pressuring girls not to gain weight during their pregnancy.

Although limited, some research has documented physical injuries associated with IPV in studies of adolescents and young adults. Tharp and colleagues' (2017) analyzed data from a randomized control trial with adolescents in 8th through 12th grade enrolled in the Safe Dates prevention program. Researchers found that risks for physical injury associated with IPV were elevated for girls and for victims who experienced all three forms of IPV (physical, sexual, psychological). Researchers also found that girls in 8th grade were at highest risk for injury, and that injury risk declined at higher grade levels (Tharp et al., 2017).

Mental and behavioral health outcomes associated with IPV include substance use, depression, suicidal ideation, suicide attempts, smoking and heavy drinking, and eating disorders (Bonomi et al., 2013; Exner-Cortens et al., 2013; Glass et al., 2003; Hanson et al., 2010). In Hanson's (2010) analysis of the Youth Risk Behavior Survey (YRBS), researchers found that female adolescents exposed to IPV victimization were more likely to engage in risky sexual behavior and substance abuse, to contemplate suicide, and to engage in violent behavior at school than girls without IPV victimization. Similarly, Exner-Cortens et al. (2013) analyzed three waves of data from the National Longitudinal Study of Adolescent to Adult Health (Add Health) and found that female participants who reported emotional and/or physical IPV had increased rates of depression, suicidal ideation, smoking, and heavy drinking at adolescent and young adult time periods. Another study of women ages 18–19 (N = 726) found that past psychological IPV was associated with increased psychological distress, whereas physical IPV was associated with depression, loneliness, and stress (Shen and Kusunoki, 2019). Mental and behavioral health effects of IPV have also been documented in sexual and gender minority populations within this age group. A study by Whitton et al. (2019) found that IPV victimization was associated with increased psychological distress among lesbian, gay, bisexual, transgender, queer, and other (+) sexual and/ or gender minority identity (LGBTQ+) youth ages 16–20 across 5 years of data. In this same study, experiencing physical IPV was also associated with marijuana use sustained across several waves of data, with sexual risk behaviors associated with both physical and sexual IPV in the past six months (Whitton et al., 2019).

Midlife (30–64)

Acute health effects of IPV in midlife include physical injuries primarily to the head and neck, anxiety and depression, post-partum depression, substance misuse, somatic symptoms including headaches, and sexual/ reproductive health issues including pregnancy-related diagnoses and STIs (Bachhus et al., 2018; Eaton et al., 2016; Kishton et al., 2022; Wu et al., 2010).

In a study by Eaton et al. (2016), researchers analyzed electronic medical records in two age cohort samples of adult women in midlife (i.e., ages 45–53 vs. ages 54–64). Among both age groups, anxiety symptoms, psychiatric problems other than anxiety and depression, headaches, and injury to the head/neck/jaw were all significantly associated with an IPV ICD-9 diagnosis. Notable differences were found specifically for women of child-bearing age, such that reproductive health concerns were significantly associated with a IPV diagnosis. Mental health symptoms were most strongly associated with an ICD-9 IPV in women ages 45–53 compared with women ages 54–64 (Eaton et al., 2016).

Similar patterns were found by Kishton and colleagues (2022), who analyzed administrative claims from the United Health Clinical Research Database to compare health outcomes among privately insured women with histories of IPV and those without histories. In this study, over twice as many women with histories of IPV had a mental health diagnosis claim, and they also had increased rates of substance use disorder diagnoses, pregnancy-related diagnoses, and STIs (Kishton et al., 2022). Similar to the findings in Eaton et al. (2016), there was a slightly higher percentage of pregnancy-related claims in age-bearing populations (age 30–39). Additionally, women with histories of IPV had comorbidity scores nearly three times greater than women without IPV histories.

As previously discussed, mental and behavioral health symptoms associated with IPV victimization can persist over the life course as long-term health consequences of IPV. However, research also demonstrates acute effects on mental and behavioral health in studies of women in midlife. Bacchus et al.'s (2018) systematic review and meta-analysis of cohort studies (N = 35) examined past-year IPV exposure and mental and behavioral health outcomes among adult women (Bacchus et al., 2018). In this review, eight studies found a positive association between recent IPV and subsequent depressive symptoms, five studies found positive associations between depressive symptoms and subsequent IPV, and five studies found associations between IPV and subsequent postpartum depression. In some studies IPV was found to have a bidirectional relationship between recent IPV and substance use (i.e., hard drug use, marijuana use). However, there was no evidence of an association between recent IPV and alcohol use or STIs. Notably, very few studies measuring recent IPV exposure included measures of substance use, alcohol use, and STIs (Bacchus et al., 2018).

Older Adulthood (65+)

While older adult women experiencing IPV have many of the same mental health outcomes as younger women, they also face additional challenges that compound health outcomes, including decreased physical health and physical mobility, decreased financial stability, loss of independence, and challenges in facing the end of their life (Cook et al., 2011; Roberto et al., 2013). Systematic reviews of research on IPV among older adult women identified strong associations between IPV exposure and mental health symptoms including depression, loneliness, and isolation (Cook et al., 2011; Knight and Hester, 2016). Some evidence also suggests associations between IPV victimization and cognitive challenges, functional impairment, dementia, and greater likelihood of premature death (Cook et al., 2011; Knight and Hester, 2016). Roberto et al. (2013) conducted an integrated review of studies (N = 57) on IPV in late life and found that older women experiencing IPV report increased risks for chronic pain, digestive issues, heart problems, bone and joint concerns, and physical injuries in samples of women 60 and older and increased risk for HIV in samples of women 50 and older (Roberto et al., 2013).

Notably, Knight and Hester (2016) found that much of the research on elder abuse does not differentiate between intimate and non-intimate partner abuse. This presents challenges to distinguishing acute health effects of IPV from other forms of abuse (e.g., non-intimate physical, sexual, psychological, and financial abuse) experienced in late life. Despite these limitations, data suggests that many older adults experience abuse from intimate partners. For example, a nationally representative study of older adults ages 70 and older (N = 2,185) found that among those reporting physical and/or psychological abuse in the past year, 23 percent were abused by intimate partners only, 20.8 percent were abused by both intimate and non-intimate partners, and 56.2 percent were abused by non-intimate partners only. In this study, older adults reporting past-year abuse were more likely to have been currently romantically involved, have current activity limitations, and to experience health care insecurity (i.e., needed to see a doctor in the past year but could not afford it) (Rosay and Mulford, 2017).

Age-Related Differences in Acute Health Effects

Overall, few studies have specifically assessed age-related differences in acute health outcomes associated with IPV. In Bacchus et al.'s (2018) review of studies on past-year IPV and physical health, studies included age primarily as a control variable but did not examine group differences or test interaction effects by age in health outcomes associated with IPV. Some systematic reviews, however, have noted differences in mental health outcomes associated with IPV by age group within studies. Cook et al.'s (2011) review found that psychological symptoms were lower among older adult women reporting IPV than among women in young adulthood and midlife. Similarly, an updated review by Knight and Hester (2016) found that most studies reported lower levels of psychological distress among older adult women experiencing IPV in comparison to younger victims. Knight and Hester (2016) also noted that very little research has compared the impact of IPV on health across age cohorts, but that some evidence suggests that the physical health of older adult victims may be more severely affected than younger victims.

In an older study by Wilke and Vinton (2005), researchers analyzed data from the 1995–1996 National Violence Against Women Survey data examining health outcomes among cohorts of women ages 18–29, 30–44, and 45 and older. In this study, younger women were more likely to report drug use than older women, and women ages 45 and older were more likely to report chronic health conditions and the use of sedatives, antidepressants, and tranquilizers in the past month than women in younger cohorts. Although the health consequences were similar overall for all age groups, the authors found that older women faced more prolonged abuse, and many reported injuries resulting from recent violence.

Using data mining methods, Yilmaz et al. (2023) analyzed data from a private electronic health record database of ambulatory visits to compare health outcomes among women ages 18–65 and older adult women ages 65 and older. Researchers found that poisoning and substance abuse were significantly comorbid with IPV in older women, in addition to numerous mental health diagnoses (i.e., major depression, mood disorder, anxiety, chronic PTSD), alcohol intoxication, and continuous opioid dependence. In particular, older victims of IPV suffered from major depression at four times the rate of younger IPV victims. Additionally, limb deformity and other musculoskeletal conditions were more common among older adult women—an outcome that may be due to IPV injuries, including IPV-related fall injuries. Neoplasm of the stomach was also found to be a significant differential comorbidity among older adult women (Yilmaz et al., 2023).

In a retrospective analysis of data from the 2005–2015 National Electronic Injury Surveillance System (NEISS) All Injury Program (AIP), Khurana and Loder (2022) compared the demographics and injuries of older (60 years or older) and younger (under age 60) IPV patients reporting to emergency departments. Older adults were significantly more likely to sustain trunk fractures, trunk strain/sprains, lacerations, and upper extremity injuries compared with younger patients, and they also had greater hospital admission rates. The younger age cohort of adults were more likely to experience contusion/abrasions, upper extremity strains/sprains, and fractures of both the upper and lower extremities. Overall, the authors suggest that younger victims may be more likely to sustain upper extremity fractures due to being able to physically fight back or resist abusers instead of protecting their trunk or face and may be less likely to have lower extremity fractures due to their physical ability to flee from abusers (Khurana and Loder, 2022).

SUMMARY AND CONCLUSIONS

Systematic review and meta-analysis studies have established multiple long-term health outcomes associated with physical, sexual, and psychological IPV among adult women. These include cardiovascular risks, endocrine disorders, gastrointestinal disorders, gynecological and reproductive health issues, and a range of mental and behavioral health-related consequences (e.g., anxiety, depression, PTSD, substance misuse). Additionally, some evidence has linked IPV to long-term neurological health symptoms, which may be connected to TBIs and non-fatal strangulation. However, research in this area has relied primarily on small convenience samples and does not differentiate between neurological effects of TBIs versus non-fatal strangulation.

The acute health effects of IPV among adolescents and young adults primarily include behavioral health symptoms (e.g., substance misuse), sexual risk-tasking behaviors (e.g., inconsistent condom use), and sexual/reproductive outcomes including increased risks for STIs and unintended pregnancy. Among studies of women in midlife, the documented acute effects of IPV include physical injuries, sexual and reproductive health impacts (e.g., STIs, pregnancy-related diagnoses), somatic symptoms (e.g., headaches), and mental and behavioral health symptoms (e.g., substance misuse, anxiety, postpartum depression). Research on health outcomes among women in older adulthood finds poor mental and emotional health (e.g., loneliness, isolation, depression), cognitive challenges, functional impairment, dementia, chronic pain, digestive problems, and physical injuries.

Studies testing the age-specific effects of IPV are limited. However, existing research suggests some differences in acute health effects based on age primarily related to physical injuries, mental/behavioral health outcomes, and chronic health conditions. Physical injuries more commonly sustained among older adult women may include upper extremity and trunk-related injuries, whereas younger women may experience more upper extremity strains/sprains and fractures of both upper and lower extremities (Khurana and Loder, 2022). Significant age group differences and more severe impacts have been found in mental health diagnoses, alcohol use, substance dependence, and musculoskeletal conditions among older adult women victims ages 65 and older when compared with younger women victims under the age of 65 (Yilmaz et al., 2023). Although dated, one survey study using nationally representative data found significant differences in chronic health conditions and substance use among women aged 45 and older compared with women in younger age cohorts (Wilke and Vinton, 2005).

Notably, there is very little data on potential racial/ethnic differences in acute and long-term health outcomes associated with IPV among women. Stockman's review (2015) on IPV among ethnic minority women noted that most studies did not have sufficient power or conduct data analyses to test group differences. Studies included in multiple systematic reviews (e.g., Bacchus et al., 2018; Pate and Simonic, 2022; Stubbs and Szoeke, 2022) primarily include race/ethnicity as a control variable, in addition to age (as previously noted), without exploring potential differences in health outcomes among women. Relatedly, few studies have examined the health effects of IPV among sexual minority women or have tested for potential differences in health outcomes based on sexual orientation in addition to other pertinent sociodemographic factors (e.g., disability status, socioeconomic indicators) that act as social determinants of health (Davis et al., 2020; Javed et al., 2022; Logie, 2012).

Communities of color, sexual and gender minority populations, and lower-income communities experience increased stressors and discrimination that ultimately lead to health inequities and that also likely exacerbate acute and long-term health effects of IPV among survivors from minoritized backgrounds (Adams and Campbell, 2012; Davis et al., 2020; Stockman et al., 2015; Waltermaurer et al., 2006). Indeed, the social and economic factors contributing to both poor health outcomes and IPV victimization represent a complex and interrelated set of relationships. Structural inequities related to access and discrimination in the areas of education, employment, and housing in particular have been well-researched in the general population and linked to many of the same poor health outcomes associated with IPV (Davis et al., 2020; HealthyPeople 2030, n.d.). Many women experiencing IPV face increased risks for homelessness, housing insecurity, and barriers to accessing health care, which in turn can increase risks for poor health outcomes among survivors (Fedina et al., 2022; Jagasia et al., 2022). Additionally, barriers to accessing affordable and culturally responsive health care affect the acute and long-term effects of IPV. Reviews of research indicate that many survivors report experiences of discrimination and stigma from health care providers (e.g., not being able to privately discuss abuse with health care professionals, being left out of decision-making processes, being dismissed) as well as a lack of availability of inclusive and affirming services, particularly for sexual and gender minorities (Papas et al., 2023; Robinson et al., 2021). Discriminatory experiences not only lead to increased stress, but also influence survivors' decisions to seek needed health care in the future. Researchers highlight the need to attend to stigma and discrimination and broader social, political, cultural, and structural barriers influencing patient–provider communication and survivors' decisions to seek health care in order to prevent adverse health outcomes, particularly for women disproportionately affected by both health inequities and IPV victimization (Pappas et al., 2023; Stockman et al., 2015).

REFERENCES

Adams, M. E., and J. Campbell. 2012. *Being undocumented and intimate partner violence (IPV): Multiple vulnerabilities through the lens of feminist intersectionality.* https://tspace.library.utoronto.ca/bitstream/1807/32411/1/11.1_Adams_%26_Campbell.pdf (accessed June 7, 2023).

Al-Modallal, H. 2016. Effect of intimate partner violence on health of women of Palestinian origin. *International Nursing Review* 63(2):259–266.

Andersen, J. P., T. L. Hughes, C. Zou, and S. C. Wilsnack. 2014. Lifetime victimization and physical health outcomes among lesbian and heterosexual women. *PLoS ONE* 9(7):e101939.

Bacchus, L. J., M. Ranganathan, C. Watts, and K. Devries. 2018. Recent intimate partner violence against women and health: A systematic review and meta-analysis of cohort studies. *BMJ Open* 8(7):e019995.

Banjar, O., M. Ford-Gilboe, C. Wong, D. Befus, and B. Alilyyani. 2022. The association between intimate partner violence and functional gastrointestinal disorders and symptoms among adult women: Systematic review. *Journal of Family Violence* 37:337–353.

Basu, A., A. A. Levendosky, and J. S. Lonstein. 2013. Trauma sequalae and cortisol levels in women exposed to intimate partner violence. *Psychodynamic Psychiatry* 41(2):247–276.

Bonomi, A. E., M. L. Anderson, J. Nemeth, F. P. Rivara, and C. Buettner. 2013. History of dating violence and the association with late adolescent health. *BMC Public Health* 13:821.

Bosch, J., T. L. Weaver, L. D. Arnold, and E. M. Clark. 2017. The impact of intimate partner violence on women's physical health: Findings from the Missouri Behavioral Risk Factor Surveillance System. *Journal of Interpersonal Violence* 32(22):3402–3419.

Brennan, J., L. M. Kuhns, A. K. Johnson, M. Belzer, E. C. Wilson, R. Garofalo, and Adolescent Medicine Trials Network for HIV/AIDS Interventions. 2012. Syndemic theory and HIV-related risk among young transgender women: The role of multiple, co-occurring health problems and social marginalization. *American Journal of Public Health* 102(9):1751–1757.

Campbell, J. C. 2002. Health consequences of intimate partner violence. *Lancet* 359(9314):1331–1336.

Campbell, J. C., J. C. Anderson, A. McFadgion, J. Gill, E. Zink, M. Patch, G. Callwood, and D. Campbell. 2018. The effects of intimate partner violence and probable traumatic brain injury on central nervous system symptoms. *Journal of Women's Health (2002)* 27(6):761–767.

Chandan, J. S., T. Thomas, C. Bradbury-Jones, J. Taylor, S. Bandyopadhyay, and K. Nirantharakumar. 2019. Intimate partner violence and temporomandibular joint disorder. *Journal of Dentistry* 82:98–100.

Coker, A. L. 2007. Does physical intimate partner violence affect sexual health? A systematic review. *Trauma, Violence, and Abuse* 8(2):149–177.

Cook, J. M., S. Dinnen, and C. O'Donnell. 2011. Older women survivors of physical and sexual violence: A systematic review of the quantitative literature. *Journal of Women's Health* 20(7):1075–1081.

Coston, B. M. 2019. Disability, sexual orientation, and the mental health outcomes of intimate partner violence: A comparative study of women in the U.S. *Disability and Health Journal* 12(2):164–170.

Davis, B. 2020. Discrimination: A social determinant of health inequities. *Health Affairs Forefront*. https://www.healthaffairs.org/content/forefront/discrimination-social-determinant-health-inequities (accessed September 3, 2023).

Decker, M. R., E. Miller, H. L. McCauley, D. J. Tancredi, H. Anderson, R. R. Levenson, and J. G. Silverman. 2014. Recent partner violence and sexual and drug-related STI/HIV risk among adolescent and young adult women attending family planning clinics. *Sexually Transmitted Infections* 90(2):145–149.

Dillon, G., R. Hussain, D. Loxton, and S. Rahman. 2013. Mental and physical health and intimate partner violence against women: A review of the literature. *International Journal of Family Medicine* 2013:313909.

Eaton, A., T. L. Temkin, B. H. Fireman, B. R. McCaw, K. J. Kotz, D. Amaral, and R. Bhargava. 2016. A description of midlife women experiencing intimate partner violence using electronic medical record information. *Journal of Women's Health* 25(5):498–504.

Exner-Cortens, D., J. Eckenrode, and E. Rothman. 2013. Longitudinal associations between teen dating violence victimization and adverse health outcomes. *Pediatrics* 131(1):71–78.

Fedina, L., D. E. Howard, M. Q. Wang, and K. Murray. 2016. Teen dating violence victimization, perpetration, and sexual health correlates among urban, low-income, ethnic, and racial minority youth. *International Quarterly of Community Health Education* 37(1):3–12.

Fedina, L., S. M. Peitzmeier, M. R. Ward, L. Ashwell, R. Tolman, and T. I. Herrenkohl. 2022. Associations between intimate partner violence and increased economic insecurity among women and transgender adults during the COVID-19 pandemic. *Psychology of Violence* 13(1):53–63.

Fleming, K. N., T. L. Newton, R. Fernandez-Botran, J. J. Miller, and V. Ellison Burns. 2012. Intimate partner stalking victimization and posttraumatic stress symptoms in post-abuse women. *Violence Against Women* 18(12):1368–1389.

Gibson, C. J., A. J. Huang, B. McCaw, L. L. Subak, D. H. Thom, and S. K. Van Den Eeden. 2019. Associations of intimate partner violence, sexual assault, and posttraumatic stress disorder with menopause symptoms among midlife and older women. *JAMA Internal Medicine* 179(1):80–87.

Glass, N., N. Fredland, J. Campbell, M. Yonas, P. Sharps, and J. Kub. 2003. Adolescent dating violence: Prevalence, risk factors, health outcomes, and implications for clinical practice. *Journal of Obstetric, Gynecologic, and Neonatal Nursing* 32(2):227–238.

Halpern, L. R., M. L. Shealer, R. Cho, E. B. McMichael, J. Rogers, D. Ferguson-Young, C. P. Mouton, M. Tabatabai, J. Southerland, and P. Gangula. 2017. Influence of intimate partner violence (IPV) exposure on cardiovascular and salivary biosensors: Is there a relationship? *Journal of the National Medical Association* 109(4):252–261.

Hanson, M. J. 2010. Health behavior in adolescent women reporting and not reporting intimate partner violence. *Journal of Obstetric, Gynecologic, and Neonatal Nursing* 39(3):263–276.

HealthyPeople 2030. n.d. *Social determinants of health literature summaries.* U.S. Department of Health and Human Services, Office of Disease Prevention and Health Promotion. https://health.gov/healthypeople/priority-areas/social-determinants-health/literature-summaries (accessed June 7, 2023).

Hill, A. L., K. A. Jones, H. L. McCauley, D. J. Tancredi, J. G. Silverman, and E. Miller. 2019. Reproductive coercion and relationship abuse among adolescents and young women seeking care at school health centers. *Obstetrics and Gynecology* 134(2):351–359.

Jagasia, E., J. J. Lee, and P. R. Wilson. 2022. Promoting community institutional partnerships to improve the health of intimate partner violence survivors experiencing homelessness. *Journal of Advanced Nursing* 79(4):1303–1313.

Javed, Z., M. Haisum Maqsood, T. Yahya, Z. Amin, I. Acquah, J. Valero-Elizondo, J. Andrieni, P. Dubey, R. K. Jackson, M. A. Daffin, M. Cainzos-Achirica, A. A. Hyder, and K. Nasir. 2022. Race, racism, and cardiovascular health: Applying a social determinants of health framework to racial/ethnic disparities in cardiovascular disease. *Circulation: Cardiovascular Quality and Outcomes* 15(1):e007917.

Jewkes, R., K. Dunkle, N. Jama-Shai, and G. Gray. 2015. Impact of exposure to intimate partner violence on CD4þ and CD8þ T cell decay in HIV infected women: Longitudinal study. *PLoS ONE* 10(3):e0122001.

Josephs, L. L., and E. M. Abel. 2009. Investigating the relationship between intimate partner violence and HIV risk-propensity in Black/African-American women. *Journal of Family Violence* 24:221–229.

Karakurt, G., V. Patel, K. Whiting, and M. Koyuturk. 2017. Mining electronic health records data: Domestic violence and adverse health effects. *Journal of Family Violence* 32(1):79–87.

Khurana, B., and R. T. Loder. 2022. Injury patterns and associated demographics of intimate partner violence in older adults presenting to U.S. emergency departments. *Journal of Interpersonal Violence* 37(17–18):NP16107–NP16129.

Kim, H. K., S. S. Tiberio, D. M. Capaldi, J. W. Shortt, E. C. Squires, and J. J. Snodgrass. 2015. Intimate partner violence and diurnal cortisol patterns in couples. *Psychoneuroendocrinology* 51:35–46.

Kishton, R., L. Sinko, R. Ortiz, M. N. Islam, A. Frederickson, N. E. Sheils, J. Buresh, P. F. Cronholm, and M. Matone. 2022. Describing the health status of women experiencing violence or abuse: An observational study using claims data. *Journal of Primary Care and Community Health* 13:21501319221074121.

Knight, L., and M. Hester. 2016. Domestic violence and mental health in older adults. *International Review of Psychiatry* 28(5):464–474.

Lagdon, S., C. Armour, and M. Stringer. 2014. Adult experience of mental health outcomes as a result of intimate partner violence victimisation: A systematic review. *European Journal of Psychotraumatology* September 12:5.

Leung F. H., K. Thompson, and D. F. Weaver. 2006. Evaluating spousal abuse as a potential risk factor for Alzheimer's disease: Rationale, needs and challenges. *Neuroepidemiology* 27:3–16.

Logie, C. 2012. The case for the World Health Organization's Commission on the Social Determinants of Health to address sexual orientation. *American Journal of Public Health* 102(7):1243–1246.

Maldonado-Rodriguez, N., C. V. Crocker, E. Taylor, K. E. Jones, K. Rothlander, J. Smirl, C. Wallace, and P. van Donkelaar. 2021. Characterization of cognitive-motor function in women who have experienced intimate partner violence-related brain injury. *Journal of Neurotrauma* 38(19):2723–2730.

Mason, R., and S. E. O'Rinn. 2014. Co-occurring intimate partner violence, mental health, and substance use problems: A scoping review. *Global Health Action* 7:24815.

Mason, S. M., R. J. Wright, E. N. Hibert, D. Spiegelman, J. P. Forman, and J. W. Rich-Edwards. 2012. Intimate partner violence and incidence of hypertension in women. *Annals of Epidemiology* 22(8):562–567.

Mason, S. M., N. Ayour, S. Canney, M. E. Eisenberg, and D. Neumark-Sztainer. 2017. Intimate partner violence and 5-year weight change in young women: A longitudinal study. *Journal of Women's Health* 26(6):677–682.

Mehr, J. B., E. R. Bennett, J. L. Price, N. L. de Souza, J. F. Buckman, E. A. Wilde, D. F. Tate, A. D. Marshall, K. Dams-O'Connor, and C. Esopenko. 2023. Intimate partner violence, substance use, and health comorbidities among women: A narrative review. *Frontiers in Psychology* 13:1028375.

Monahan, K., S. Bannon, and K. Dams-O'Connor. 2022. Nonfatal strangulation (NFS) and intimate partner violence: A brief overview. *Journal of Family Violence* 37:75–86.

Nur, N. 2012. The effect of intimate partner violence on mental health status among women of reproductive ages: A population-based study in a middle Anatolian city. *Journal of Interpersonal Violence* 27(16):3236–3251.

Oram, S., H. L. Fisher, H. Minnis, S. Seedat, S. Walby, K. Hegarty, K. Rouf, C. Angénieux, F. Callard, P. S. Chandra, S. Fazel, C. Garcia-Moreno, M. Henderson, E. Howarth, H. L. MacMillan, L. K. Murray, S. Othman, D. Robotham, M. B. Rondon, A. Sweeney, D. Taggart, and L. M. Howard. 2022. The Lancet Psychiatry Commission on intimate partner violence and mental health: Advancing mental health services, research, and policy. *The Lancet Psychiatry* 9(6):487–524.

Papas, L., O. Hollingdrake, and J. Currie. 2023. Social determinant factors and access to health care for women experiencing domestic and family violence: Qualitative synthesis. *Journal of Advanced Nursing* 79(5):1633–1649.

Pate, T., and B. Simonic. 2021. Intimate partner violence and physical health problems in women: A review of the literature. *Slovenian Medical Journal* 90(7–8):390–398.

Pathak, N., R. Dhairyawan, and S. Tariq. 2019. The experience of intimate partner violence among older women: A narrative review. *Maturitas* 121:63–75.

Raskin, S. A., O. DeJoie, C. Edwards, C. Ouchida, J. Moran, O. White, M. Mordasiewicz, D. Anika, and B. Njoku. 2023. Traumatic brain injury screening and neuropsychological functioning in women who experience intimate partner violence. *Clinical Neuropsychologist* May 24:1–23. 38(2):354-376. https://doi.org/10.1080/13854046.2023.2215489.

Reuter, T. R., M. E. Newcomb, S. W. Whitton, and B. Mustanski. 2017. Intimate partner violence victimization in LGBT young adults: Demographic differences and associations with health behaviors. *Psychology of Violence* 7(1):101–109.

Roberto, K. A., M. C. McPherson, and N. Brossoie. 2013. Intimate partner violence in late life: A review of the empirical literature. *Violence Against Women* 19(12):1538–1558.

Robinson, S. R., K. Ravi, and R. J. Voth Schrag. 2021. A systematic review of barriers to formal help seeking for adult survivors of IPV in the United States, 2005–2019. *Trauma, Violence, & Abuse* 22(5):1279–1295.

Rosay, A. B., and C. F. Mulford. 2017. Prevalence estimates and correlates of elder abuse in the United States: The National Intimate Partner and Sexual Violence Survey. *Journal of Elder Abuse & Neglect* 29(1):1–14.

Shen, S., and Y. Kusunoki. 2019. Intimate partner violence and psychological distress among emerging adult women: A bidirectional relationship. *Journal of Women's Health* 28(8):1060–1067.

Sparrow, K., J. Kwan, L. Howard, N. Fear, and D. MacManus. 2017. Systematic review of mental health disorders and intimate partner violence victimisation among military populations. *Social Psychiatry and Psychiatric Epidemiology* 52(9):1059–1080.

Stene, L. E., G. W. Jacobsen, G. Dyb, A. Tverdal, and B. Schei. 2013. Intimate partner violence and cardiovascular risk in women: A population-based cohort study. *Journal of Women's Health (2002)* 22(3):250–258.

Stockman, J. K., H. Hayashi, and J. C. Campbell. 2015. Intimate partner violence and its health impact on ethnic minority women [corrected]. *Journal of Women's Health (2002)* 24(1):62–79.

Stubbs, A., and C. Szoeke. 2022. The effect of intimate partner violence on the physical health and health-related behaviors of women: A systematic review of the literature. *Trauma, Violence, & Abuse* 23(4):1157–1172.

Tharp, A. T., H. L. M. Reyes, V. Foshee, M. H. Swahn, J. E. Hall, and J. Logan. 2017. Examining the prevalence and predictors of injury from adolescent dating violence. *Journal of Aggression, Maltreatment & Trauma* 26(5):445–461.

Valera, E., and A. Kucyi. 2017. Brain injury in women experiencing intimate partner violence: Neural mechanistic evidence of an "invisible" trauma. *Brain Imaging and Behavior* 11(6):1664–1677.

Waltermaurer, E., C. A. Watson, and L. A. McNutt. 2006. Black women's health: The effect of perceived racism and intimate partner violence. *Violence Against Women* 12(12):1214–1222.

Wang, E., S. Zahid, A. N. Moudgal, S. Demaestri, and F. S. Wamboldt. 2022. Intimate partner violence and asthma in pediatric and adult populations: A systematic review. *Annals of Allergy, Asthma & Immunology* 128(4):361–378.

Whiting, K., L. Y. Liu, M. Koyutürk, and G. Karakurt. 2017. Network map of adverse health effects among victims of intimate partner violence. *Pacific Symposium on Biocomputing* 22:324–335.

Whitton, S. W., M. E. Newcomb, A. M. Messinger, G. Byck, and B. Mustanski. 2019. A longitudinal study of IPV victimization among sexual minority youth. *Journal of Interpersonal Violence* 34(5):912–945.

Wilke, D. J., and L. Vinton. 2005. The nature and impact of domestic violence across age cohorts. *Affilia*, 20(3), 316–328.

Wright, E. N., A. Hanlon, A. Lozano, and A. M. Teitelman. 2018. The association between intimate partner violence and 30-year cardiovascular disease risk among young adult women. *Journal of Interpersonal Violence* 36(11-12):NP6643–NP6660.

Wright, E. N., A. Hanlon, A. Lozano, and A. M. Teitelman. 2019. The impact of intimate partner violence, depressive symptoms, alcohol dependence, and perceived stress on 30-year cardiovascular disease risk among young adult women: A multiple mediation analysis. *Preventive Medicine* 121:47–54.

Wu, V., H. Huff, and M. Bhandari. 2010. Pattern of physical injury associated with intimate partner violence in women presenting to the emergency department: A systematic review and meta-analysis. *Trauma, Violence & Abuse* 11(2):71–82.

Yilmaz, S., E. Gunay, D. H. Lee, K. Whiting, K. Silver, M. Koyuturk, and G. Karakurt. 2023. Adverse health correlates of intimate partner violence against older women: Mining electronic health records. *PLoS ONE* 18(3):e0281863.

Appendix C

Public Session Agendas

January 10, 2023

Keck Center of the National Academies of Sciences, Engineering, and
Medicine and by Webcast
Agenda
1:25–2:55 p.m. Eastern Time

1:25 p.m.   **Welcome and Introductions**
Susan J. Curry, Committee Chair
Crystal J. Bell, Study Director

1:30 p.m.   **Perspective of the Study Sponsor and Q&A**
*Nancy Mautone-Smith and Ellen Hendrix, Health
Resources and Services Administration*

2:15 p.m.   **Presentations from Invited Speaker and Q&A Session**
Dr. Melissa Simon, Northwestern University

2:45 p.m.   **Public Comment Session**

2:55 p.m.   **End Open Session**

MEETING 2: PUBLIC SESSION

February 23, 2023

Beckman Center of the National Academies of Sciences, Engineering, and Medicine and by Webcast
Agenda
12:45–3:20 p.m. Eastern Time

12:45 p.m. **Chair's Open Session Statement**
Susan J. Curry, Committee Chair

12:50 p.m. **Panel 1: IPV in the LGBTQ+ Community Including Unique Care Needs and Novel Care Models**
Athena Sherman, Emory School of Nursing
Rob Stephenson, University of Michigan School of Nursing
Sarah Peitzmeier, University of Michigan School of Nursing

1:35 p.m. **Committee Questions**

2:05 p.m. **Panel 2: IPV Care in Various Care Settings**
Maria Balata, Swedish Covenant Hospital
Ivon Mesa, Community Action and Human Services
  Department of Miami- Dade County
Marianne Gausche-Hill, Los Angeles County Emergency
  Medical Services Agency

2:50 p.m. **Committee Questions**

3:20 p.m. **Break and Open Session Ends**

MEETING 3A: PUBLIC SESSION

March 29, 2023

Virtual
Agenda
12:00–1:05 p.m. Eastern Time

12:00 p.m. **Welcome and Opening Comments**
Sue Curry, Committee Chair
Crystal J. Bell, Study Director

12:05 p.m.	**Panel on IPV Care in Native American Communities**
	Lisa D. Martin, MPH, Senior Research Associate, Center for Indigenous Health, Johns Hopkins University
	Lorena Halwood, Executive Director, ADABI Healing Shelter
12:35 p.m.	**Committee Questions**
1:05 p.m.	**Break and Open Session Ends**

MEETING 3B: PUBLIC SESSION

April 4, 2023

Virtual
Agenda
12:00–1:20 p.m. Eastern Time

12:00 p.m.	**Welcome and Chair's Open Session Statement**
	Sue Curry, Committee Chair
	Crystal J. Bell, Study Director
12:05 p.m.	**Panel on IPV Care in Other Health Care Settings**
	Gregory J. Della Roca, MD, Orthapaedic Surgeon and Inpatient Medical Director, University of Missouri Health Care
	Charisma De Los Reyes, MSW, Coordinator, San Diego County Office of Education's (SDCOE) Foster Youth Services Coordinating Program (FYSCP)
	Hirsch Handmaker, MD, CEO and Chairman, CACTIS Foundation
	Anita Ravi, MD, MPH, MSHP, FAAFP, President, CEO, and Co-Founder, PurpLE Health Foundation
12:50 p.m.	**Committee Questions**
1:20 p.m.	**Break and Open Session Ends**

Appendix D

Biographical Sketches of Committee Members

Sue Curry, Ph.D. (Chair) is emeritus dean and distinguished professor in the Department of Health Management and Policy of the University of Iowa College of Public Health. Previously, Dr. Curry served as director of the Center for Health Studies at Group Health Cooperative where she conducted an extensive portfolio of health system research in chronic disease prevention and management. Dr. Curry is a member of the National Academy of Medicine (NAM). She is an elected member of the NAM Governing Council and serves on the Council's Executive Committee. She is also a member of the Governing Board of the National Research Council. She received her graduate training at the University of New Hampshire and completed post-doctoral work at the University of Washington and Fred Hutchinson Cancer Research Center. Dr. Curry served on the U.S. Preventive Services Task Force from 2009 to 2019 and served as chair of the task force from 2018 to 2019. She was chair of the task force when it released its 2018 recommendations for intimate partner violence screening. Other completed professional activities include service as vice chair of the Board of Directors of the Truth Initiative (formerly the American Legacy Foundation), member of the Board of Scientific Advisors for the National Cancer Institute, and member of the National Academies of Sciences, Engineering, and Medicine Board on Population Health and Public Health Practice. She is a fellow of both the Society of Behavioral Medicine and the American Psychological Association.

Sue Anne Bell, Ph.D., FNP-BC, FAAN, is an assistant professor at the University of Michigan School of Nursing, with expertise in disaster preparedness and response, women's health, and emergency care. Trained as a health services researcher, her work focuses on the health and well-being of vulnerable and at-risk populations in the context of disasters and public health emergencies. She has been active in numerous activities at the National Academies of Sciences, Engineering, and Medicine; as a member of the Committee on Best Practices in Assessing Mortality and Significant Morbidity Following Large-Scale Disasters, as an invited panelist at the Climate Change and Human Health Meeting of Experts, as an invited speaker at the Emerging Leaders Forum, and as a co-author on *Rapid Expert Consultation on Understanding Causes of Healthcare Deaths Due to the COVID-19 Pandemic (December 10, 2020)*. She is currently serving a second 3-year term on the Federal Emergency Management Agency's National Advisory Council. She also serves on the National Advisory Committee for Seniors and Disasters at the U.S. Department of Health and Human Services (HHS) and is a member of the Expert Panel on Environmental and Public Health at the American Academy of Nursing. Her original training is as a family nurse practitioner, and she is clinically active in disaster response through the HHS National Disaster Medical System with over a dozen deployments, including for the COVID-19 pandemic, Hurricane Maria in Puerto Rico, and the 2018 Paradise, California wildfire.

Jacquelyn C. Campbell, Ph.D., is a professor in the Johns Hopkins University School of Nursing. She has published more than 300 articles and 7 books and has been principal investigator of more than 15 major National Institutes of Health (NIH), Centers for Disease Control and Prevention (CDC), and National Institute of Justice grants in her decades of advocacy policy work collaborating with domestic violence survivors, advocates, health care professionals, and marginalized communities. She is particularly known for her research on domestic violence homicide and the development and validation of the Danger Assessment that helps intimate partner violence survivors more accurately assess their risk of being killed or almost killed by their abusive partner that is used widely in the United States and globally. She is an elected member of the National Academy of Medicine, the American Academy of Nursing, is on the Board of Futures Without Violence and was on the boards of four domestic violence shelters. She has consulted for the Department of Health and Human Services, CDC, NIH, World Health Organization, the Office on Violence Against Women, the Department of Defense, the Department of Veterans Affairs, and multiple advocacy organizations on the intersection of gender-based violence and physical and mental health outcomes. Dr. Campbell is a member of the American Academy of Nursing Violence Expert Panel. Dr. Campbell has received numerous awards for her research and has served on three National Academies of Sciences, Engineering, and Medicine committees as well as been the co-chair of the Institute of Medicine (IOM)/NAM Forum for Global Violence Prevention.

Regardt Jacobus Ferreira, Ph.D., is the director of Tulane University's Disaster Resilience Leadership Academy and an associate professor at the Tulane School of Social Work. His main research interest is at the intersection of disaster, climate change, resilience and behavioral health with an emphasis on interpersonal violence; with work conducted in Europe, Africa, North America, the Caribbean and South Asia. His interdisciplinary work includes more than 100 published journal articles, chapters, and scientific abstracts on a variety of trauma, climate change and resilience topics. Dr. Ferreira's work has been recognized with several top teaching awards for his innovative and engaging approaches to teaching and community engagement. He was previously chair for the Disaster and Traumatic Stress Track with the Council for Social Work Education and currently serves as the founding convener of the Climate and Disaster Research Special Interest Group with the Society for Social Work Research. He received his undergraduate degree (BSW) in social work and master's degree in disaster risk management (cum laude) at the University of the Free State in Bloemfontein, South Africa, and his Ph.D. in social work (Dean citation) from the University of Louisville, Louisville, Kentucky.

Francisco Garcia, M.D., M.P.H., is the director and chief medical officer of the Pima County Department of Health in Tucson, Arizona. Dr Garcia is an experienced administrator, highly regarded physician executive, and internationally recognized expert in public health emergency preparedness, border health, and women's reproductive health. Before entering government, Dr. Garcia achieved the rank of tenured Distinguished Outreach Professor of Public Health, Obstetrics and Gynecology at the University of Arizona. There, he served in a variety of leadership roles including as director of the Hispanic Center of Excellence, the Center of Excellence in Women's Health, and the Cancer Disparities Institute of the Arizona Cancer Center. Dr. Garcia's previous National Academies service includes membership on the Committee on Evidence-Based Practices for Public Health Emergency Preparedness and Response, the Roundtable on Health Equity, and the Committee on Preventive Services for Women. He also previously served as a member of the Women's Preventive Services Taskforce.

Rosa M. Gonzalez-Guarda, Ph.D., M.P.H., RN, FAAN, is an associate professor at Duke University School of Nursing and assistant dean of the Ph.D. Program in Nursing. Her research describes the intersection of intimate partner violence, substance abuse, HIV, and mental health among Latinos in the United States and the development of multi-level interventions to address these. She uses a syndemic orientation, mixed methods, and community engaged strategies to influence practice and policy changes to promote health equity for Latinos, survivors of intimate partner violence, and other historically marginalized populations. Dr. Gonzalez-Guarda serves on local and national organizations influencing services and policies addressing violence, abuse, mental health, and health equity for Latinos, including serving as the chair of the Board of Directors of El Futuro, a community-based mental service organization serving Spanish-speaking and uninsured immigrants in North Carolina. She is a member of the Scientific Advisory Board of Esperanza United, a National Technical Assistance provider for community-based organizations addressing Latino and immigrant families affected by violence, and a member of the executive team of LATIN-19 (Latinx Advocacy and Interdisciplinary Network for COVID-19), a local multisector coalition influencing systems change for Latinx inclusion. She also served as a previous chair of the Violence Expert Panel of the American Academy of Nursing. Dr. Gonzalez-Guarda was a member of the IOM committee that produced the landmark *Future of Nursing: Leading Change, Advancing Health* (2010) report and has led various local and national initiatives to promote health equity research careers for populations systemically excluded from health professions. Dr. Gonzalez-Guarda has interdisciplinary training in nursing, public health, and psychology and is a fellow of the Substance Abuse Mental Health Service Administration (SAMHSA) Minority Fellowship Program and the Robert Wood Johnson Foundation Nurse Faculty Scholars program.

Elizabeth Miller, M.D., Ph.D., FSAHM, is Distinguished Professor of pediatrics, public health, and clinical and translational science and medical director of community and population health at the University of Pittsburgh Medical Center Children's Hospital of Pittsburgh. Trained in internal medicine and pediatrics and medical anthropology, she has more than 20 years of practice and research experience in addressing intimate partner and sexual violence prevention and health equity in clinical and community settings, with funding from National Institutes of Health, Centers for Disease Control and Prevention (CDC), Substance Abuse and Mental Health Services Administration, National Institute of Justice, Office on Women's Health, and other foundations. Dr. Miller is recognized for her expertise in partner and sexual violence research as well as clinical care; she contributes to content on sexual and partner violence for a medical resource for health professionals called UpToDate. She has conducted numerous randomized controlled trials to evaluate clinical and community partnered interventions. She has more than 330 peer reviewed research publications, and has authored numerous book chapters, commentaries, and clinical guidelines. She serves as faculty for Health Partners on IPV and Exploitation, a Health

Resources and Services Administration–supported National Training and Technical Assistance Center program led by Futures Without Violence. She has served as a lead investigator on a collaborative project with the American Academy of Pediatrics, CDC, Futures Without Violence, and researchers at University of Pittsburgh on the impact of the COVID-19 pandemic on survivors of partner violence and their children.

Mona Mittal, Ph.D., is an associate professor in the Department of Family Science, School of Public Health, at the University of Maryland (UMD), College Park. She is core faculty for the UMD Center for Healthy Families, and provides mental health services to individuals, couples, and families. She is an affiliate faculty member for the UMD Prevention Research Center, where she focuses on LGBTQ+ mental health. Lastly, she is also an affiliate faculty member at the Maryland Population Research Center, wherein she produces and promotes population-related research. Dr. Mittal is engaged in prevention and intervention research focused on mental health and traumatic stress, particularly intimate partner violence, and sexual and reproductive health outcomes among populations that experience health inequities. Dr. Mittal has received National Institutes of Health funding to develop and test integrated interventions to reduce interpersonal violence and HIV risk among women of color and heterosexual African American couples. In addition, Dr. Mittal is collaborating with U.S. and international researchers to further her program of research and promote capacity building in traumatic stress, particularly intimate partner violence. Dr. Mittal serves on the editorial board for the *Journal of Marital and Family Therapy*. She is also a board member of the Network for Victim Recovery of DC. She earned her Ph.D. in marriage and family therapy from Texas Tech University and a master's degree in clinical investigation from the University of Rochester.

Heidi Nelson, M.D., M.P.H., MACP, FRCP, is a professor of health systems science at the Kaiser Permanente Bernard J. Tyson School of Medicine in Pasadena, California. Previous positions include professor of medical informatics and clinical epidemiology and medicine at the Oregon Health & Science University (OHSU), investigator at the Pacific Northwest Evidence-based Practice Center, and medical director for women and children's programs at Providence Health and Services in Portland, Oregon. Dr. Nelson's research focuses on clinical epidemiology, women's health, and health care guidelines and delivery. She has led nearly 100 evidence reviews for the U.S. Preventive Services Task Force, NIH, the Agency for Healthcare Research and Quality, Veterans Administration, and the Health Resources and Services Administration–sponsored Women's Preventive Services Initiative. Her work has been used to determine national clinical practice guidelines and coverage, including screening for intimate partner violence, affecting millions of Americans, particularly women. Dr. Nelson is board certified in internal medicine. She completed her degrees at the University of Minnesota, residency at OHSU, and fellowship at the University of California, San Francisco. Dr. Nelson was a member of the Institute of Medicine Committee on Preventative Services for Women that identified services to be covered under the prevention care mandate of the Affordable Care Act in 2011.

Usha Ranji, M.S., is the associate director for women's health policy at KFF. Her work addresses the impact of major health policy issues on women and girls, with an emphasis on insurance coverage, access to care, and low-income populations. Ranji has led several analyses and written a number of major reports, including findings from national surveys of women on health care utilization and spending, state-level policies on Medicaid coverage of family planning and perinatal services, and the impact of the Affordable Care Act (ACA) on access to reproductive health services. Ms. Ranji has helped develop several interactive tools available through KFF, including a tracker that summarizes the preventive services recommendations covered by insurance plans as a result of the ACA, such as screening for interpersonal violence. In addition to her work at KFF, Ms. Ranji has published in the peer reviewed literature and speaks extensively on women's coverage, maternity care, and the impact of the ACA to national and local groups. She is a member of advisory committees for the California Maternal Quality Care Collaborative and the California Breast Cancer Research Program.

Merritt D. Schreiber, Ph.D., is a professor of clinical pediatrics in the Department of Pediatrics at Harbor-UCLA (University of California, Los Angeles) Medical Center Lundquist Institute, and a senior advisor for the Terrorism and Disaster Program, National Center for Child Traumatic Stress at the David Geffen School of Medicine at UCLA. He serves as lead for the Mental Health Workgroup for the Western Regional Alliance for Pediatric Emergency Management and is the chair of disaster response for the California Psychological Association (CPA). Dr. Schreiber's work focuses on developing population-level models of a "stepped continuum of mental health care" (e.g., mental health "first aid") in mass-casualty disasters and other traumatic incidents. He also works on enhancing resilience and response of emergency disaster medical workers, pre-hospital first responders, and others, using an evidence-based model. As a result of this work, Dr. Schreiber has developed varied tools and a pediatric disaster mental health concept of operations designed to provide population-level response tactics to all-hazard events impacting children, youth, and families. This includes the PsySTART Mental Health Incident Management System and a stepped "triage to care" of at-risk pediatric patients and emergency medical responders. He is also the developer of "Anticipate, Plan and Deter," a disaster medical provider resilience system and "Listen, protect, and connect," family-to-family Psychological First Aid. Dr. Schreiber received the Joint Meritorious Service Medal serving as Commissioned Corps of the U.S. Public Health Service Reserve Officer on detached service to North American Aerospace Defense Command-U.S. Northern Command, the APA Presidential Citation for 9/11 response, and the CPA Distinguished Humanitarian Award. He previously served on the Department of Health and Human Services (HHS) Secretary's Advisory Board on Emergency Public Information and Communications. He deployed for HHS to Miramar for the COVID-19 response effort. He recently received the HHS Civilian Coronavirus Response Medal for his deployments in support of National Disaster Medical System (NDMS) response to COVID-19 at Marine Air Corps Station Miramar and two other deployments in support of returning NDMS teams in COVID-19 and Hurricane Ian.

Jamila K. Stockman, Ph.D., is professor and vice chief in the Division of Infectious Diseases and Global Public Health at the University of California, San Diego School of Medicine. Dr. Stockman is also co-director of the Health Equity Sociobehavioral Science Core within the San Diego Center for AIDS Research. Dr. Stockman is an infectious disease epidemiologist also trained in qualitative, mixed methods, and intervention research. For the past 15 years, Dr. Stockman has conducted observational intervention research studies addressing the co-occurrence of HIV, gender-based violence, substance use, mental health, and underlying social and structural factors (e.g., discrimination, medical mistrust) affecting socially marginalized populations. Her research is conducted in the U.S., U.S.-Mexico border region, Latin America, and Caribbean. Dr. Stockman's research has been funded by the National Institutes of Health and the California HIV/AIDS Research Program, garnering more than 90 peer-reviewed papers. In addition to her research, Dr. Stockman actively collaborates with local public health departments and community-based organizations to ensure ethical and cultural appropriateness of her research among members of the community. In 2015, Dr. Stockman received the Linda E. Saltzman Award for her accomplishments in the field of domestic violence research.

Mitch Stripling, M.P.A., is the founding director of the New York City Pandemic Response Institute, a resource supporting New York City agencies, organizations, and communities to prepare and respond to critical public health crises. Formerly, he was the national director of preparedness and response for the Planned Parenthood Federation of America, where he directed that organization's COVID-19 response and supporting sexual and reproductive health access initiatives. He has also served as an assistant commissioner at the New York City Department of Health and Mental Hygiene, where he focused on preparedness and response issues. Stripling has responded to more than a dozen federally declared disasters and public health emergencies around the county.

Lindsay F. Wiley, J.D., M.P.H., is a professor of law and founding faculty director of the Health Law and Policy Program at University of California, Los Angles School of Law. She is an internationally recognized expert in health care access and public health law, policy, and ethics. She has published extensively and served as consultant on matters relating to policy-making during public health emergencies, particularly with respect to the use of population-wide non-pharmaceutical interventions. She is the author of *Public Health Law and Ethics: Power, Duty, Restraint* and *Public Health Law and Ethics: A Reader* (with Lawrence O. Gostin, UC Press). Professor Wiley is a former president of the American Society of Law, Medicine, and Ethics and a former member of the National Conference of Lawyers and Scientists. She is currently the United States Rapporteur for the Lex Atlas COVID-19 Project. She is a current member of the Board of Directors of ChangeLab Solutions, LLC and of the Law Professor Panel that advises Local Solutions Support Center. She earned her J.D. magna cum laude from Harvard Law School, her M.P.H. from Johns Hopkins Bloomberg School of Public Health, and her A.B. magna cum laude from Harvard College.